Clinical Manual of Fever in Children

A. Sahib El-Radhi · James Carroll · Nigel Klein (Eds.)

Clinical Manual
of Fever in Children

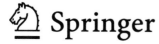
Springer

**A. Sahib El-Radhi, FRCPCH, MRCP,
Ph.D, DCH**
Consultant Paediatrician & Honorary
Senior Lecturer, Medical School
Denver Close
Petts Wood, Orpington
Kent BR6 OSB
United Kingdom

James Carroll, MD
Professor of Neurology, Pediatrics,
and Biochemistry, and Molecular Biology
Vice-Chairman, Department of Neurology
Chief, Section of Pediatric Neurology
The Medical College of Georgia
1120 15th Street
Augusta, Georgia 30912
USA

**Nigel Klein, MBBS, BSc, PhD, MRCP,
FRCPCH**
Professor
Senior Lecturer and Honorary Consultant
in Infection and Immunology
Division of Cell and Molecular Biology
Institute of Child Health
30 Guilford Street
London, WC1N 1EH
United Kingdom

ISBN: 978-3-540-78597-2   e-ISBN: 978-3-540-78598-9

DOI: 10.1007/978-3-540-78598-9

Library of Congress Control Number: 2008926503

Cover design: Frido Steinen-Broo, e-Studio Calamar, Spain

Printed on acid-free paper

9 8 7 6 5 4 3 2 1

springer.com

Preface

Febrile illnesses have their highest incidence in early childhood, and fever is the leading symptom bringing children to see the pediatricians and primary care physicians. Despite the high prevalence of fever and the increased scientific knowledge about fever mechanisms, there is a lack of information about fever pathogenesis and management in pediatric textbooks. Primary care physicians have little time to study the subject. Medical students receive insufficient teaching about fever. Lectures addressing fever are few or nonexistent. Books on the subject of fever are hardly available. One important reason for all these is that there is no specialty or subspecialty to foster and promote the subject.

In the past few decades, remarkable advances have been made in understanding the mechanism of fever and its management. The current knowledge on fever is the result of evidence-based research. The remarkable scientific progress on fever on the one hand and the incomplete dissemination of information of it on the other gave us an impetus to write the book. The results of the research needed conversion into a practical, concise, and reader-friendly text. We are hoping that we have achieved this goal.

Although the book is written primarily for the senior and junior pediatricians, we hope that all medical professionals (primary care physicians and nurses) will find the book useful when dealing with a febrile child. Medical students are usually required to perform scientific projects, including those related to fever, and it is hoped that this book can provide the information they may need to do that.

This Manual provides scientific evidence in the understanding of children with fever. It offers clearly defined, practical, and proven approaches to the major problems affecting these children. This should result in an improved care for the febrile child. In this book, we have attempted to cover the entire spectrum related to fever, emphasizing also facts observed by others and presenting our own concepts of the problems of fever and its management in clinical practice. Chapter 1 introduces fever, its definition, causes and management in various age groups and fever of unknown origin. The chapter also discusses drug fever and whether or not fever can cause malformation. This chapter is followed by hyperthermia (Chap. 2). Many physicians often equate the term fever with hyperthermia. This chapter differentiates the two causes of elevated body temperature, enumerating the causes and features of hyperthermia and their management. Because hyperthermia (or fever) therapy over a century ago had a definite role in the treatment of various infectious diseases, such as syphilis, the subject is included in this chapter.

The remarkable progress made over the past few decades on the pathogenesis of fever is summarized in Chap. 3. The readers will not only confirm the complexity of fever induction but also how effective the temperature regulation is in healthy state and at the height of fever so that body temperature does not climb up relentlessly. Measurement of body temperature (Chap. 4) is a subject that is often neglected in medical teaching. It is also often inaccurately done. The pros and cons of each thermometer and each site to measure body temperature are discussed. Pediatric nurses in particular will find the measurement of body temperature evidence-based and practical when they measure body temperature.

Chapters 5 and 6 are related to fever in infectious and noninfectious diseases, focusing on the incidence and pattern of fever in each disease, a brief management and, whenever possible, on the question whether or not the presence of fever is beneficial for that disease. We did not intend to write an account on infectious diseases as there are excellent books on the market dealing with this subject. It was, however, unavoidable that a short description of each disease was added. Chapter 7 covers the whole aspects of febrile seizures. This subject is included for two reasons. First, fever is an essential precursor of the event and second the degree of fever has an important influence on the recurrence rate of seizures. Chapter 8 reviews the latest advance in hypothermia, its causes in neonates and older children, as well as therapeutic application of hypothermia. As hypothermia in neonates is associated with high mortality in developing countries, preventative measures in delivery room and at home are discussed.

We felt that the book would be incomplete without discussing the important subject "Is fever beneficial" (Chap. 9). Few issues in medicine have been more controversial than this subject. The views of those who consider fever as beneficial and those who consider it as harmful are presented and a conclusion is drawn. Special attention is given to the management of fever (Chap. 10). Despite the intensive research on fever during the past few decades, fever management is often inadequate and not evidence-based. This chapter provides health professionals with almost all clinical information needed to understand how a febrile child should be treated. Antipyretics, their mechanism, doses, and possible side effects are discussed in a concise way. The chapter also includes management of fever in hospital and at home, guidelines for parents, and for the practicing physicians. The chapter ends with a section on "Fever Phobia" and its management.

Alternative medicine (Chap. 11) has become increasingly popular in recent years and many of its methods are used to treat fever. Clinicians need to know whether these methods are effective for fever treatment and whether they can compete with conventional physical and drug antipyretics. Fever may present as the only sign of a disease (e.g. PUO) or in association with other symptoms and signs. Diagnosis in both presentations can be difficult. Chapter 12 ("Differential Diagnosis") provides clinicians with a guide to clinical and laboratory means to reach a diagnosis of the most common febrile diseases. Chapter 13 covers the history of fever from BC to present. In this chapter, the concepts of the ancients, including scholars and lay people, are presented, along with views and practice of Middle Age and European scholars. Finally, we provided the readers with a glossary of the terms related to fever (Chap. 14). The readers will be surprised to see the multiplicity of medical disorders related to the term fever.

Acknowledgements

The authors are grateful to their families for their encouragement and understanding while the book was being prepared. We particularly wish to thank our wives Leena (ASER) and Shirley (JEC) for their patience. A very special thanks is extended to my son Sami (ASER) who has helped in the preparation of this book. The book could not be completed without the facility available at the library of Queen Mary's Hospital, Sidcup, Kent. We wish to thank the librarians Valerie and Sylvia for that. We express appreciation and special thanks to our colleagues, listed later, who contributed a subject, section, or chapter. On this occasion, I cannot forget the encouragement of my brothers and sisters, and for my late parents who taught me important lessons in life. They would have been proud had they been alive to see their son writing this book (ASER).

A. Sahib El-Radhi, James Carroll, and Nigel Klein

Introduction

Man is a homeotherm, that is, he maintains his body temperature within a limited range of ±2°C despite wide variations in ambient temperature. Temperature regulation in health and during fever is maintained by both behavioural and physiological processes. Along with pulse and respiration, body temperature remains the third vital sign.

Of the many symptoms and signs of diseases, fever has received the most attention throughout medical history. For thousands of years, simple palpation has been performed to assess the status of well-being of people by confirming the presence or absence of fever. Many decisions concerning the investigation and treatment of children are based on the results of temperature measurement alone. Without detecting fever a serious underlying illness could be missed, which could result in death.

The views on fever, particularly on its role in disease, have evolved gradually over many centuries. Fever was initially regarded not as a symptom but rather as the disease itself. For most of the history, it was feared by ordinary people as a manifestation of punishment, induced by evil spirits or a marker of death. However, medical scholars of ancient civilizations, particularly the Greeks, believed in the beneficial effects of fever, a concept that prevailed until it underwent a radical transformation in the nineteenth century. Scholars began to regard fever as harmful. The later introduced antipyretics were regarded as beneficial.

During the nineteenth century, fever was still regarded as both part of a symptom complex (as it is today) and a disease in its own right. Examples of fever being regarded as a disease were *autumnal fever, jail fever and hospital fever*. Fever could also be described in terms of the severity of the disease, for example, *malignant fever* or *pestilential fever*, or even in terms of the supposed pathology of the fever, *bilious fever* or *nervous fever*. The multiplicity of names for fever reflects the lack of a breakthrough into an understanding of the causes of febrile illnesses. The breakthrough came with the science of bacteriology, which was able to reveal the aetiology of many infectious diseases, such as the identification of the typhoid bacillus in 1880, and the discovery of the tubercle bacillus in 1882. These discoveries relegated fever to a sign of disease.

With the introduction of fever therapy in the twentieth century, renewed interest in the role of fever began. The best results of fever therapy were observed in gonorrhoea and syphilis, including their complications, such as arthritis, keratitis and orchitis. Approximately 70–80% of the cases treated were arrested using artificial hyperthermia or malarial fever in the range of 40.5–41.0°C. Despite this therapeutic success, the prevailing concepts over two centuries remained negative on the role of fever. Only in the past four decades has there been successful research into the role of fever in disease. The effects of elevated temperatures on body defence have been extensively studied. One of the most important outcomes of this research has been the discovery of a single mononuclear cell product, interleukin-1 (IL-1), whose effects include induction of fever by its action on the hypothalamic centre and activation of T lymphocytes. The fever induction, which occurs simultaneously with lymphocyte activation, constitutes the clearest and strongest evidence in favour of the beneficial role of fever. Despite this recent progress, there is currently no consensus as to whether fever is beneficial, neutral or harmful.

Fever, even when it is associated with multiple symptoms, is often considered as the dominant feature of an illness or as the illness itself. This may be due to *fear of fever* and also by us feeling better when the fever is reduced, thus assuming that the severity of the disease is reduced. It is thought that during infections both fever and pain (such as muscle pain and headaches) are caused by cytokine-mediated production of prostaglandins. Antipyretics, such as paracetamol, reduce both the elevated body temperature as well as the pain. This is the most important reason why the antipyretics have maintained their popularity over a century.

As emphasised throughout the book, fever should not be regarded as a passive by-product of infection. Rather, fever is the result of an active rise in regulated body temperature. As such, fever should not be equated with hyperthermia (e.g. heatstroke), which is unregulated. With fever, unlike hyperthermia, body temperature is well regulated by a hypothalamic set point that balances heat production and heat loss so effectively that the temperature will not climb up relentlessly and does not exceed an upper limit of 42°C. Within this upper range of 40–42°C, there is no evidence that fever is injurious to tissue. If there is morbidity or mortality, it is due to the underlying disease. The associated fever may well be protective.

Contents

5 Fever in Common Infectious Diseases 81
A. Sahib El-Radhi, James Carroll, Nigel Klein, Meaad Kadhum Hassan,
Mahjoob N. Al-Naddawi, Sushil Kumar Kabra, Ovar E.E.G. Olofsson

A. Sahib El-Radhi, James Carroll, Nigel Klein

Contributors

Anthony Abbas
Queen Mary's Hospital, Sidcup
Kent BR6 0SB
UK

Mahjoob N Al-Naddawi
Welfare Children Hospital
Medical City, Baghdad
Iraq

Charles Buchanan
Variety Club Children's Hospital
King's College Hospital
Bessemer Road, Denmark Hill
London SE5 9RS
UK

James Carroll
The Medical College of Georgia
Augusta, GA 30912
USA

Christopher Edwards
Southampton University Hospital
Tremona Road, Southampton SO16 6YD
UK

A. Sahib El-Radhi
Denver Close, PcHs Wood,
Orpington Kent BR6 OSB
UK

Colin Ferrie
Clarendon Wing, Leeds General Infirmary
Belmont Grove
Leeds West Yorkshire LS2 9NF
UK

Meead Kadhum Hassan
Department of Paediatrics
College of Medicine, University of Basrah
Iraq

Graham RV Hughes
The London Lupus Centre
1st Floor, St Olaf House, London Bridge
Hospital, 27–29 Tooley Street
London SE1 2PR
UK

Sushil Kumar Kabra
Pediatric Pulmonology Division
Department of Pediatrics
All India Institute of Medical Sciences
New Delhi 110 029
India

Nigel Klein
Division of Cell & Molecular Biology
Institute of Child Health
30 Guilford Street
London WC1N 1EH
UK

Matthew Kluger
George Mason University
Virginia 22030
USA

Colin Morley
Royal Women's and Royal Children's
Hospitals, Melbourne, VIC 3070
Australia

Orvar EEG Olofsson
University of Children's Hospital
75185 Uppsala
Sweden

Kavita Singh
Darent Valley Hospital
Children's Resource Centre
Darent Wood Road
Dartford, Kent DA2 8DA
UK

Jennie CI Tsao
UCLA Pediatric Pain Program
Department of Pediatrics
David Geffen School of Medicine at UCLA
10940 Wilshire Blvd, Str. 1450
Los Angeles, CA 90037
USA

Anne Walsh
PO Box 1253, Indooroopilly
Queensland, 4068
Australia

Michael Waterhouse
UCLA Pediatric Pain Program
Department of Pediatrics
David Geffen School of Medicine at
UCLA 10940 Wilshire Blvd, Str. 1450
Los Angeles, CA 90037
USA

Fever

Core Messages

> Fever is a very common complaint in children accounting for as many as 20% of paediatric visits to doctors.

> How sick the child looks is more important than the level of fever.

> Normal body temperature does not preclude serious infection.

> Most children aged 0–36 months who have fever have a focus of infection, which can be identified by careful history and examination. A viral upper respiratory tract infection is the most common focus.

> Most children aged 0–36 months without an obvious focus of infection have viral infections, but they may harbor two important serious bacterial infections (SBI): urinary tract infection or bacteremia.

> Febrile neonates and ill-looking children, regardless of age, are at high risk for SBI and need antibiotic coverage, hospital admission, and comprehensive septic work-up. This entails blood and urine cultures, full blood cell count (FBC), C-reactive protein (CRP), and, when indicated, chest X-ray, LP and stool studies.

> Children aged 1–36 months without a focus may be treated more selectively: if the temperature is >39°C, WBC count is >15,000 mm^{-3} and CRP is >40 mg L^{-1}; urine and blood cultures should be ordered; and a third-generation cephalosporin (ceftriaxone or cefotaxime) considered.

> The distribution of the diseases causing pyrexia of unknown origin (PUO) differs according to the geographic area and the socioeconomic status of the country.

> In PUO, atypical presentation of a common disease is more common than a rare and exotic disease.

A.S. El-Radhi et al. (Eds.) *Clinical Manual of Fever in Children.*
Doi: 10.1007/978-3-540-78598-9, © Springer-Verlag Berlin Heidelberg 2009

1.1
Definitions

Fever (pyrexia) may be defined in both pathophysiological and clinical terms:

Pathophysiologically, fever is an interleukin-1 (IL-1) mediated elevation of the thermoregulatory set point of the hypothalamic center. In response to an upward displacement of the set point, an active process occurs in order to reach the new set point. This is accomplished physiologically by minimizing heat loss with vasoconstriction and by producing heat with shivering. Behavioral means of raising body temperature include seeking a warmer environment, adding more clothing, curling up in bed, and drinking warm liquids.

Clinically, fever is a body temperature of 1°C (1.8°F) or greater above the mean at the site of temperature recording. For example, the range of body temperature at the axilla is 34.7–37.4°C, with a mean of 36.5°C; 1°C above the mean is 37.5°C. The following degrees of temperature are accepted as fever (see also Chap. 5):

Rectal temperature	≥38.0°C
Oral temperature	≥37.6°C
Axillary temperature	≥37.4°C
Tympanic membrane	≥37.6°C

The importance of at least 1°C higher than the mean temperature lies in the diurnal variation of normal body temperature, which reaches its highest level in early evening (5–7 p.m.). Diurnal temperature fluctuations are greater in children than in adults and are more pronounced during febrile episodes.

In young children, a relatively high rectal temperature predominates, with a gradual decrease towards adult levels beginning at 2 years of age. This trend stabilizes soon after puberty.

1.2
Patterns of Fever

The importance of febrile patterns has diminished in medical practice because only a few diseases are known to show a specific pattern of fever, and occasionally the same disease may present in different patterns of fever. In addition, the diagnosis can often be established nowadays by means of laboratory investigations, even before a specific pattern emerges. Several patterns may occur in clinical practice, which sometimes have clinical value, such as malaria with its characteristic fever pattern (Table 1.1).

Patterns of fever include the type of onset (insidious or abrupt), variation in temperature degree during a 24-h period and during the entire episode of illness, cycle of fever, and response to therapy. Further patterns are as follows:

* **Continuous or sustained fever** is characterized by a persistent elevation of body temperature with a maximal fluctuation of 0.4°C during a 24-h period. Normal diurnal fluctuation temperature is usually absent or insignificant.

Table 1.1 Fever patterns found in pediatric diseases

Fever pattern	Diseases
Continuous	Typhoid fever, malignant falciparum malaria
Remittent	Most viral or bacterial diseases
Intermittent	Malaria, lymphoma, endocarditis
Hectic or septic	Kawasaki disease, pyogenic infection
Quotidian	Malaria caused by *P. vivax*
Double quotidian	Kala azar, gonococcal arthritis, juvenile rheumatoid arthritis, some drug fevers (e.g., carbamazepine)
Relapsing or periodic	Tertian or quartan malaria, brucellosis
Recurrent fever	Familial Mediterranean fever

* **Remittent fever** is characterized by a fall in temperature each day but not to a normal level. This is the most common type of fever in pediatric practice and is not specific to any disease. Diurnal variation is usually present, particularly if the fever is infectious in origin.
* In **intermittent fever** the temperature returns to normal each day, usually in the morning, and peaks in the afternoon. This is the second most common type of fever encountered in clinical practice.
* **Hectic or septic fever** occurs when remittent or intermittent fever shows a very large difference between the peak and the nadir.
* **Quotidian** fever, caused by *P. vivax*, denotes febrile paroxysms which occur daily.
* **Double quotidian** fever has two spikes within 12 h (12-h cycles).
* **Undulant fever** describes a gradual increase in temperature that remains high for a few days, and then gradually decreases to normal level.
* **Prolonged** fever describes a single illness in which duration of fever exceeds that expected for this illness, for example, >10 days for a viral upper respiratory tract infection.
* **Recurrent fever** is an illness involving the same organ (e.g., urinary tract) or multiple organ systems in which fever recurs at irregular intervals.
* **Periodic and relapsing fevers** are discussed next.

1.2.1
Periodic and Relapsing Fever

* **Periodic fever** (PF) is characterized by episodes of fever recurring at regular or irregular intervals. Each episode is followed by one to several days, weeks or months of normal temperature. Examples are seen in malaria (termed *tertian* when the febrile spike occurs every third day, and *quartan* when the spike occurs every fourth day) and brucellosis.
* **Relapsing fever** (RF) is the term usually applied to recurrent fevers caused by numerous species of *Borrelia* and transmitted by lice (louse-borne RF) or ticks (tick-borne RF). Lice transmit *Borrelia* (*B. recurrentis*) from infected humans to other humans. Ticks

1

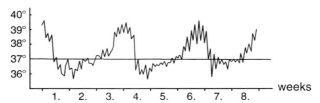

Fig. 1.1 Fever pattern in Pel–Ebstein fever

acquire the *Borrelia* (e.g. *B. duttonii*) from rodents (rats, mice, squirrels). The disease is characterized by rapid onset of high fever, which recurs in paroxysms lasting 3–6 days, followed by an afebrile period of similar duration. The maximum temperature is 40.6°C in tick-borne RF and up to 39.5°C in louse-borne. Associated complaints include myalgia, headache, abdominal pain, and alteration of sensorium. The resolution of each febrile episode may be accompanied within a few hours (6–8 h) by the **Jarish–Herxheimer reaction** (JHR), which usually follows antibiotic treatment. The reaction is caused by the release of endotoxin when the organisms are destroyed by antibiotics. JHR is very common after treating patients suffering from syphilis. It is less commonly seen with cases of leptospirosis, Lyme disease, and brucellosis. Symptoms range from mild fever and fatigue to a full-blown anaphylactic reaction.

- **Rat-bite fever** is another example, caused by *Spirillum minus* and *Streptobacillus moniliformis*. A history of rat bites 1–10 weeks prior to the onset of symptoms suggests the diagnosis.

- **Pel–Ebstein fever** (Fig. 1.1), described by Pel and Ebstein in 1887, was originally thought to be characteristic of Hodgkin's lymphoma (HL). Only a few patients with Hodgkin's disease develop this pattern, but when present, it is suggestive of HL. The pattern consists of recurrent episodes of fever lasting 3–10 days, followed by an afebrile period of similar duration. The cause of this type of fever may be related to tissue destruction or associated hemolytic anemia.

1.2.2
Genetic PF Syndromes (Autoinflammatory Diseases)

Genetic causes of PF syndromes that have been identified in the past few years are shown in Table 1.2. The term autoinflammatory disease has been proposed to describe a group of disorders characterized by attacks of unprovoked systemic inflammation without significant levels of autoimmune or infective causes [1]. Episodes of fever, aphthous stomatitis, pharyngitis, and cervical adenopathy (PFAPA) are the most common clinical features. Each episode is followed by a symptom-free interval ranging from weeks to months. Some of the disorders have regular periodicity, whereas others do not. Most patients have mutations in either the protein pyrin or the TNF-receptor superfamily of molecules. Both play an important role in the inflammatory pathways of the immune system. Pyrin is present in neutrophils and their precursors. It is believed that pyrin decreases inflammation, particularly in neutrophils.

Table 1.2 Hereditary periodic fever syndromes

Disorder	Inheritance	Fever duration	Periodicity	Clinical features	Lab tests/etiology	Amyloidosis	Treatment
FMF	AR	1–3 days	3–6 weeks	Polyserositis (abdominal, chest pain), synovitis, myalgia	Inflammatory markers, gene mutations MEFV on chromosome 16, leading to protein defect	+	Colchicine
Cyclic neutropenia	AD	5–7 days	21 days	Pharyngitis, gingivitis, mouth ulcers, lymph-adenopathy, cellulites	Neutrophils <200, mutations of the gene neutrophils elastase: (ELA2): chromosome 19	No	GCSF
TRAPS	AD	Weeks	Irregular	Muscle cramps, migratory arthralgia, migratory erythematous rash	Inflammatory markers, mutation in TNFRSF1A gene: chromosome 12	Rare	NSAIDs, steroids
HIDS	AR	4–6 days	4–8 weeks	Abdominal pain, headache arthralgia, lymph-adenopathy, diarrhoea	IgD, IgA, TNF-low activity of mevalonate kinase, MVK: chromosome 12	No	Simvastatin?
PFAPA	Sporadic	3–5 days	3–6	Aphthous stomatitis, pharyngitis, Lymphadenitis	Inflammatory marker	No	Steroids, cimetidine
MWS/FCUS/ NOMID/ CINCA	AD	Irregular	Irregular	Urticaria, progressive deafness, arthritis, chronic meningitis, cutaneous rash, arthropathy, abdominal pain	Mutations in CIASI gene on chromosome 1q44	+	Anakinra, NSAIDs, steroids

FMF familial mediterranean fever; *TRAPS* tumor necrosis factor receptor-associated periodic syndrome; *HIDS* hyperimmunoglobuliaemia d and periodic fever syndrome; *NOMID* neonatal-onset multisystem inflammatory disease; *CINCA* chronic infantile neurologic cutaneous and articular syndrome; *PFAPA* periodic fever, aphthous stomatitis, pharyngitis, and adenitis; *MWS* muckle–wells syndrome; *FCUS* familial cold urticaria; *AR* autosomal recessive; *AD* autosomal dominant; *GCSF* granulocyte colony stimulating factor; *NSAIDs* nonsteroidal antiinflammatory drugs

1

1.3
Phases of Fever

Fever is characterized by three phases:

* **The phase of temperature rise** is often characterized by discomfort and is the result of decreased heat loss through vasoconstriction and increased heat production through shivering. The patient feels cold and the skin also feels cold to the touch.
* **The phase of temperature stabilization (fastigium)** then occurs at the new level of the thermoregulatory set point. Heat production and heat loss are balanced as in normal health, but at the higher hypothalamic set point. A flushed or pink appearance signifies that the fever has peaked. Once this phase is reached, the child usually feels comfortable without shivering.
* **The phase of falling temperature or defervescence** occurs either by lysis (falling gradually within 2–3 days to a normal level) or by crisis (falling within a few hours to a normal level).

Table 1.3 shows mechanisms leading to normal and abnormal body temperatures.

1.4
Manifestations during Fever

The subjective perception of fever is generally absent in children, and fever is usually detected by the parents. Manifestations associated with fever vary considerably and depend on the child's age, how acute and how high the fever is, and the nature of the disease that has caused the fever. Common manifestations are summarized in Table 1.4.

* **Symptoms** directly related to fever include chills or rigor, which characteristically herald the onset of high fever. Young children do not often report chills, and the chills may be so subtle that they pass unnoticed. Chills are more characteristic of some

Table 1.3 Peripheral mechanisms responsible for normal and abnormal body temperature

Mechanism	Example	Relation of body temperature to the hypothalamic set point
Heat production = loss	Health, second phase of fever	Body temperature = set point
Heat production > loss	First phase of fever, MH	Body temperature > set point
Heat loss < production	Heat stroke	Body temperature > set point
Heat production < loss	Hypothermia	Body temperature < set point

MH malignant hyperthermia

Table 1.4 Summary of the clinical changes noted during fever

Manifestation	Clinical findings
Symptoms	Chills (rigor), myalgia, headaches, anorexia, excessive sleep, fatigue, thirst, delirium, scanty urine (oliguria)
Signs	Drowsiness, irritability, tachycardia, tachypnoea, increased BP, flushed face, grunting, decrease in GFR, proteinuria. Accentuation (or appearance) of an innocent (functional) murmur and third heart sound
ECG changes	Shortening QT-intervals, increase in supraventricular ectopic beats

BP blood pressure; *GFR* glomerular filtration rate

diseases such as bacteremia and lobar pneumonia. They may also occur in viral diseases and in noninfectious diseases, such as lymphoma. Other symptoms of fever include tachycardia, myalgia, anorexia, and fatigue.

* **Signs** of fever include tachycardia, with the pulse rate rising 10 beats per minute for every 1°C temperature elevation. Tachypnoea during fever is an increase of respiratory rate by approximately 2.5 breaths per minute for each 1°C elevation of body temperature, occasionally associated with grunting (arousing the suspicion of pneumonia). In pneumonia and malaria, the temperature effect on the respiratory rate is even higher at 3.7 breaths per minute per °C [2]. The reason for the difference between 2.5 and 3.7 breaths is related to the comorbid features in these diseases, such as anemia and acidosis and the role of cytokines. While the initial phase of fever is accompanied by a rise in blood pressure and a decrease in glomerular filtration rate (GFR), sustained fever is associated with a fall in blood pressure and a slight increase in the GFR. Proteinuria occurs in 5–10% of children with fever without pre-existing renal diseases.

* An occasionally encountered sign during fever is **relative bradycardia**, which is a pulse rate disproportionately low for the degree of fever. Normally, for every 1°C (1.8°F) rise in fever, the pulse rate increases by 10. For example, a patient with a temperature of 40°C (whose pulse normally is 70 per minute) and a pulse rate lower than 100 per minute has relative bradycardia. Classic causes of relative bradycardia are typhoid fever, drug fever, central nervous system (CNS) lesions, brucellosis, leptospirosis, and factitious fever. **Relative tachycardia** is a pulse rate disproportionately elevated in relation to the degree of fever. Examples include hyperthyroidism and myocarditis.

1.5
Metabolic Effects of Fever

The host metabolic response during fever depends on a number of factors, including the age of the child, the height and duration of the fever, and the severity and duration of the underlying illness. A summary of the metabolic response during fever is shown in Table 1.5. Most of the requirements for cellular energy are supplied by glucose, while free fatty acids

1

Table 1.5 Summary of the metabolic changes [increase (↑) or decrease (↓)] occurring during fever

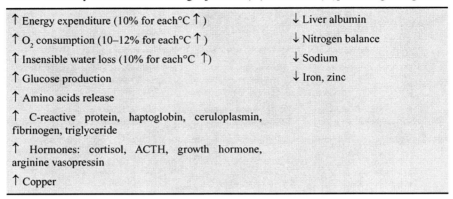

↑ Energy expenditure (10% for each°C ↑)	↓ Liver albumin
↑ O₂ consumption (10–12% for each°C ↑)	↓ Nitrogen balance
↑ Insensible water loss (10% for each°C ↑)	↓ Sodium
↑ Glucose production	↓ Iron, zinc
↑ Amino acids release	
↑ C-reactive protein, haptoglobin, ceruloplasmin, fibrinogen, triglyceride	
↑ Hormones: cortisol, ACTH, growth hormone, arginine vasopressin	
↑ Copper	

are used to a lesser extent. Glucose production is increased in the liver by using amino acids as substrates. These amino acids are released during proteolysis in the muscles and are transported via plasma into the liver. Despite the increase in uptake of amino acids, production of albumin in liver decreases. Nitrogen balance begins to be negative soon after the onset of fever, reaching a loss of about 10 g daily if the fever is high. While plasma iron and zinc concentrations decline rapidly, depriving invading microorganisms of essential nutrients, that of copper increases.

Increase in serum cortisol of up to fivefold may occur in severe bacterial infections. Arginine vasopressin (AVP) is also increased and is responsible for the maintenance of homeostasis of body fluid during fever. Hyponatremia often occurs in association with acute febrile diseases, particularly with pneumonia and meningitis, as a result of inappropriate secretion of AVP. AVP is an endogenous antipyretic, which is secreted in an attempt to control the fever.

Although some of these changes appear harmful, healthy children usually recover rapidly after febrile episodes. Wasting of body fat and muscle may occur if the fever is prolonged.

1.6
Potential Complications (See Box 1.1)

Complications directly related to fever are rare. Morbidity and mortality are closely linked to the severity of the underlying disease but not to the level of fever. Complications are the following:

- **Dehydration** may occur owing to increased body temperature and the therapeutic effects of drugs that promote sweating. Fever and infection increase the metabolic rate to <1.5 times the basal metabolic rate. For every 1°C rise of body temperature, there is a 10% increase of insensible water loss. Dehydrated children are prone to heat stroke,

> **Box 1.1 Practical Tips**
>
> › Fever should not be equated with hyperthermia; the latter is due to imbalance between heat production and loss and is not controlled centrally.
> › Fever is not dangerous. If there is morbidity or mortality, it is due to the underlying disease. The associated fever may be protective.
> › The principal complication of fever is dehydration, which can be easily prevented and treated by providing extra fluid to the child.
> › Fever does not damage the central nervous system. It also does not climb up relentlessly because it is well controlled by a hypothalamic center.

particularly if the child is excessively wrapped. It is essential to prevent this complication by offering oral fluids to the febrile child frequently.

- Three to four percent of genetically susceptible children younger than 5 years experience **fever-induced seizure (febrile seizure)**, which occurs when the temperature of a susceptible child rises rapidly.
- Some young children experience **delirium** in association with a high degree of body temperature. This is a nonspecific sign, occurring in viral as well as with bacterial infections. Delirium often recurs, causing considerable anxiety to the parents.
- **Hyperpyrexia** is a rectal temperature of 41.1°C or higher (for axillary or tympanic temperature, 40°C is taken instead of 41.1°C), as defined by Dubois, who observed this degree of temperature elevation in about 5% of 1,761 patients with severe bacterial infections [3]. In a recent study of 130,828 consecutive pediatric patients seen over a two-year period, only 103 (1 per 1,270 patient visits) had a fever of 41.1°C or higher [4]. Of the 103 subjects, 20 (18.4%) had serious bacterial infection. This report and others [5] emphasized the significant association between such a degree of temperature elevation and serious bacterial infections, such as bacterial meningitis. Apart from infection, hyperpyrexia up to 41.8°C has been reported in newborn infants presenting with intraventricular haemorrhage [6].
- **Herpes labialis** (cold sore) results from activation of a latent herpes simplex infection in association with febrile illnesses. It occurs less often in children than in adults, and is more common with certain bacterial infections, such as pneumococcal or meningococcal infection.

1.7
Classification of Fever (Tables 1.6 and 1.7)

1.7.1
Fever with Localized Signs

Table 1.6 The principal three classes of fever encountered in pediatric practice

Class	Commonest cause	Usual fever duration
Fever with localizing signs	URTI	<1 week
Fever without localizing signs	Viral infection, UTI	<1 week
Fever of unknown origin	Infection, JIA	>1 week

URTI upper respiratory tract infection; *UTI* urinary tract infection; *JIA* juvenile idiopathic arthritis

Table 1.7 Definitions of terms used in Sect. 1.7

Term	Definition
Fever with localization	Acute febrile illness with a focus of infection, which can be diagnosed after a history and physical examination
Fever without localization	Acute febrile illness without apparent cause of the fever after a history and physical examination
Lethargy	Poor or absent eye contact; no interaction with the examiner or parents, no interest in surroundings
Toxic appearance	Clinical signs characterized by lethargy, evidence of poor perfusion, cyanosis, hypo- or hyperventilation
Serious bacterial infections	Suggest serious diseases, which can be life threatening. Examples are meningitis, sepsis, bone and joint infection, enteritis, urinary tract infection, pneumonia
Bacteraemia and septicemia	Bacteremia indicates the presence of bacteria in blood, evident by a positive blood culture; septicemia indicates in addition tissue invasion of the bacteria, causing tissue hypoperfusion and organ dysfunction

Table 1.8 Main causes of fever due to diseases of localized signs

Group	Diseases
Upper airway infections	Viral URTI, otitis media, tonsillitis, laryngitis, herpetic stomatitis
Pulmonary	Bronchiolitis, pneumonia
Gastrointestinal	Gastroenteritis, hepatitis, appendicitis
CNS	Meningitis, encephalitis
Exanthems	Measles, chickenpox
Collagen	Rheumatoid arthritis, Kawasaki disease
Neoplasma	Leukaemia, lymphoma
Tropics	Kala azar, sickle cell anaemia

URTI upper respiratory tract infection

The most common febrile illnesses encountered in pediatric practice belong to this category (Table 1.8). Fever is usually of short duration, either because it settles spontaneously or because a specific treatment, such as an antibiotic, is administered. Diagnosis may be suggested by the history and physical examination and confirmed by simple investigation, such as a chest X-ray. As children <36 months experience the highest rate of febrile illnesses with localizing signs, a brief discussion of this subject in this age group is presented.

Fever in children <3 days of age

Fetal temperature. Fever is unusual in the fetus, rare in neonates, and infrequent in the pregnant mother before parturition. It has been assumed that fever suppression in these groups may be caused by the action of the arginine vasopressin hormone, which acts as an endogenous antipyretic. Fetal temperature at about 38.0°C is 0.5–0.9°C higher than the mean maternal core temperature, allowing a continuous heat transfer along the gradient from the fetus to the mother through the umbilical circulation. At birth, the body temperature of the neonate and mother briefly maintains this difference. Heat is produced via nonshivering thermogenesis, which begins shortly after birth.

Fever in children 1–3 days of age, elevated body temperature (fever or hyperthermia) in the first hours of life may be caused by the following:

- **Maternal fever**. The major cause of such an intrapartum fever is the use of epidural anesthesia, occurring in about 15% of women (7). The longer the labor, the greater the risk of fever development in women who are given an epidural.
- **Maternal infection**. A less frequent cause of intrapartum fever is maternal infection, such as chorioaminionitis. Infants of women who are febrile during labor are more likely to be evaluated for sepsis and to receive antibiotics than infants of afebrile women. These infants may also need resuscitation because of low Apgar score and hypotonia.
- Hyperthermia. Elevated body temperature during the first 1–3 days of life may be caused by placing the neonate under a radiant warmer or dehydration. Infection as a cause of fever at this age is rare.

Fever in children 4 days to <3 months of age

Children at this age have the highest incidence of serious bacterial infection (SBI), estimated to be 12% in neonates and 6% in children aged 1–2 months. Overall, children younger than 3 months of age have a 21-times higher risk of SBI than those older than 3 months [8]. Definite identification of SBI requires a positive culture of the cerebral spinal fluid (CSF), blood, stool, or urine or an identifiable bacterial focus by physical examination or radiograph.

Despite the high incidence of infection, febrile episodes are uncommon in this age group, and some seriously ill infants are hypothermic. In a series of consecutive infants younger than 3 months of age evaluated at an ambulatory clinic, only 1% had a rectal temperature >38.0°C, with a temperature >40.0°C occurring in only 6% of these febrile episodes [9]. The rate of SBI has been shown to be proportional to the height of fever, occurring in 9.5% with a temperature <40°C and in 36% with a temperature of 40°C and greater [10]. A normal temperature did not exclude infection: 30% of infants with SBI were afebrile on admission[11].

Infants usually present with nonspecific and subtle symptoms (Table 1.9). Organisms causing SBI are shown in Table 1.10.

Management of febrile children at this age is summarized in Fig. 1.2.

Table 1.9 Symptoms and signs of a child with serious bacterial infection

General	Reduced activity, weak cry, poor eye contact, absent smile
Body temperature	Instability, fever, hypothermia
Signs of shock	Clammy, mottled skin, reduced CRT
Respiratory	Apnoea, tachypnoea, shallow respiration, grunting
Gastrointestinal	Poor feeding, vomiting, abdominal distension, diarrhea
CNS	Drowsiness, sometimes alternating with irritability (in case of meningitis: bulging fontanelle, other meningeal signs such as neck stiffness are usually absent)

CNS central nervous system; *CRT* capillary refill time

Table 1.10 The most common organisms causing SBI in children younger and older than 3 months of age.

Children <3 months	
Developed countries	
Early-onset	GBS, *E. coli*
Late-onset	*E. coli*, GBS, CONS, *N. meningitidis*, *S. pneumoniae*, *Salmonella*, *Listeria monocytogenes*
Developing countries	
	Klebsiella, *E. coli*, *Pseudomonas*, *Salmonella*, *Staphylococcus aureus*, *H. influenzae*, *S. pneumoniae*, *S. pyogenes*
Children >3 months	*S. pneumoniae*, *N. meningitidis*, *Salmonella*

GBS group B streptococcus; *CONS* coagulase negative staphylococci; *S. Streptococcus*; *N. Neisseria*, *H. Haemophilus*

Fever in children 3 to 36 months of age

Children aged 3–36 months have the highest incidence of fever during childhood, with approximately six febrile episodes per year. An upper respiratory tract infection (URTI) is the most common infection, occurring in 50% of all febrile episodes. The highest degrees of fever are found in this age group. Temperature >40°C is common, occurring in 20% of all febrile episodes. Such a degree of fever may accompany bacterial or viral infection. In contrast to younger children, the vast majority of febrile illnesses are benign and self-limited. SBIs are uncommon (about 2–3%). Table 1.11 summarizes factors that increase the risk of SBI.

Management of a child with fever includes history, physical examination, and laboratory investigation. The most important challenge facing a physician is to determine the etiology of the illness, in particular confirming or excluding a serious disease. Management includes the following:

- **History taking**, focusing on:

  - Onset and duration of fever, the degrees of temperature recorded at home, and the temperature-taking method

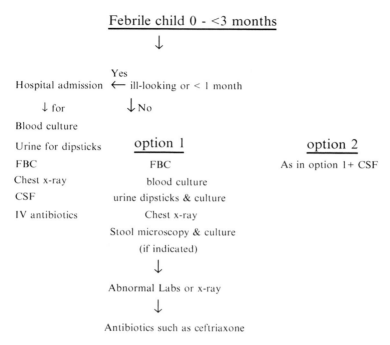

Fig. 1.2 Management of a child aged 0 to <3 months without a focus of infection

- - Presence of similar symptoms in other family members
- - Pattern of feeding, degree of activity, playfulness at home
- - Features suggestive of SBI (Tables 1.9, 1.11, and 1.12)
- - Pre-existing disease
- - Previous administration of antibiotics

- **Physical examination**, performed in two parts, consisting of:

    - - Observation of items to predict SBI (shown in Table 1.12). These items, combined with a history and physical examination, can identify most serious diseases in children. Those children who are unwell require immediate admission to hospital, appropriate investigation, and treatment. Those who appear well are managed according to the algorithm shown in Fig. 1.3
    - - Physical examination, looking particularly for a focus to explain the fever

- **Investigation**, taking into consideration that:

    - - In a child with localized signs of infection, investigation should be minimal and focus on the diagnostic test most likely to provide a diagnosis
    - - Screening tests include full blood cell count (FBC), looking particularly at the white blood cell (WBC) count, C-reactive protein (CRP) and urine dipsticks

1

Table 1.11 Factors that increase the prediction of SBI

Age	Infants <3 months
Temperature	
Neonates	Any degree of fever
Older child	>39.0°C, particularly >40°C
Pre-existing disorder	
Neonates	Prematurity, premature rupture of membrane, maternal infection, GBS
Older child	Sickle cell anaemia, immunosuppression, nephrotic syndrome, splenectomy, HIV-infection
Others	Venous catheter, skin petechiae
History and signs	See symptoms and signs in Table 1.9
Laboratory findings	WBC >15,000, CRP >10 (neonates); >40 (older child)
	CSF: >8 WBC mm^{-3}
	Urine: positive nitrate on dipsticks, urinalysis showing >10 WBC per hpf
	Chest radiograph: infiltrate
	Stool: >5 WBC per hpf stool smear

hpf high power field; *CRP* C-reactive protein; *WBC* white blood cell; *CSF* cerebro spinal fluid

Table 1.12 Summary of observation items to identify a child with SBI

Item	Unwell	Very unwell
Appearance	Ill looking (lethargy, reduced activity)	Absent eye contact, does not recognize parents, no activity
Quality of cry	Whimpering	Weak cry, high-pitched cry
Response to cuddling	Slow response, unwilling	Too weak to respond
Alertness	Drowsiness	Frequently falls asleep, difficulty to arouse
Hydration	Slightly dry mouth	Dry mouth, sunken fontanelle, doughty skin
Color	Peripheral cyanosis or pallor	Mottled, pale face or ashen
Sociability/stimulation	Brief smiling and response	Not smiling, anxious face, expressionless

- In small children, chest auscultation is frequently unreliable and chest X-ray is usually necessary to establish the diagnosis of pneumonia
- Blood culture is an important test in a child thought to have SBI, particularly in a child who has no focus of infection.
- Pulse oximetry is a mandatory test for any ill child.

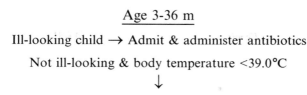

Age 3-36 m

Ill-looking child → Admit & administer antibiotics

Not ill-looking & body temperature <39.0°C
↓
Urine dipsticks, review if condition worsens

Body temperature >39.0°C
↓
Evaluate for SBI

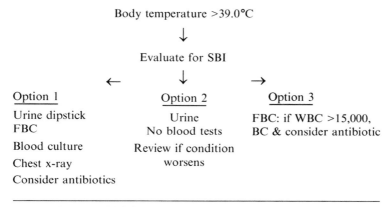

Option 1	Option 2	Option 3
Urine dipstick	Urine	FBC: if WBC >15,000,
FBC	No blood tests	BC & consider antibiotic
Blood culture	Review if condition	
Chest x-ray	worsens	
Consider antibiotics		

SBI Serious bacterial infection; *FBC* Full blood count; *BC* Blood culture

Fig. 1.3 Management of a child 3–36 m of age without a focus of infection

* Antibiotic treatment, depending on the underlying disease, how ill the child is, age of the child, and the height of the fever. It is indicated for:
  - Any ill-appearing child, irrespective of age
  - Neonates
  - Children whose focus of infection is likely to be caused by bacteria
  - Children aged 1–2 months who appear well but the initial laboratory tests (e.g., CRP) are abnormal

For children 3 months of age and older, antibiotics are not indicated in most infections, which tend to be viral as an underlying cause.

1.7.2
Fever without Localized Signs (Bacteremia)

About 20% of all febrile episodes demonstrate no localizing signs on presentation. The most common cause is a viral infection, mostly occurring during the first few years of life. Such an infection should be considered only after exclusion of urinary tract infection

Table 1.13 Usual causes of fever without localized signs

Causes	Examples	Clues for diagnosis
Infection	Bacteremia/sepsis	Ill looking, high CRP, leukocytosis
	Most viruses (HH-6)	Well appearing, normal CRP, WBC
	UTI	Urine dipsticks
	Malaria	In malarial area
PUO	JIA	Pre-articular, rash, splenomegaly, high ANF (antinuclear factor), CRP
Post-vaccination	Triple vaccination, measles	Time of fever onset in relation to the time of the vaccination
Drug fever	Most drugs	History of drug intake, diagnosis of exclusion (see Sect. 1.9)

HH-6 human herpes-6; *UTI* urinary tract infection; *JIA* juvenile idiopathic arthritis; *CRP* C-reactive protein; *WBC* white blood cell

(UTI) and bacteremia. Table 1.13 shows the most common causes of this group. SBIs include UTI, malaria in malaria endemic areas, and bacteremia.

Bacteremia indicates the presence of bacteria in blood, while septicemia suggests the tissue invasion of the bacteria, causing tissue hypoperfusion and organ dysfunction. Neonates and young infants more often have septicemia rather than bacteremia. The overall incidence of bacteremia in febrile children is around 1%, but higher risks exist in:

- Children aged 3–24 months who have the highest incidence, estimated to be 3–4%, with children aged 7–12 months demonstrating twice the incidence of those aged 13–18 months
- Association with high fever. While the risk of bacteraemia is negligible with temperatures of 38–39°C, a strong correlation exists between the incidence of bacteremia and higher temperatures. The incidence is 7% with temperatures of 40–40.5°C, 13% with a temperature of 40.5–41.0°C, and 26% with a temperature higher than 41.0°C

Symptoms and signs of bacteremia are often those noted in children with SBI (Table 1.9). Abnormal findings on physical examination may be absent, with fever above 39.0°C and ill general appearance being the only manifestations of the disease. Occasionally, bacteremic patients may present with alarming symptoms such as hypotension, impairment of consciousness, disseminated intravascular coagulopathy (DIC), and renal failure.

Although bacteremia occurs more frequently as a primary isolated disease, many infectious diseases are known to be associated with septicemia. These include meningitis (in up to 80% depending on organisms and age), pneumonia (in about 10%), and otitis media (1.5%) [12]. Bacteremic pneumococcal pneumonia has been found to have an increased fatality compared to cases of pneumococcal pneumonia without bacteremia [13].

The predominant bacteria isolated from blood culture in the neonatal period are group B streptococcus (GBS), which were responsible for over 50% of early-onset neonatal septicemia in a series of 410 cases from Finnish hospitals, followed by *E. coli* [14]. Prior to the discovery of the H influenzae type b (Hib) vaccine, Hib was the most common causative bacteria of bacteremia and bacterial infection in older children. In recent years *S. pneumoniae* has become the most common causative agent.

The prognosis of bacteremia is generally good, provided the possibility is considered in any febrile child without a focus of infection and appropriate antibiotic is initiated early. Recent reports indicate a spontaneous resolution of bacteremia without antibiotics in 40–60% of cases. The remainder may develop bacterial complications, including bacterial meningitis in about 10% of cases. (See Box 1.2)

1.7.3
Persistent Pyrexia of Unknown Origin (PUO)

This term is usually applied when fever without localizing signs persists for 1 week during which evaluation in the hospital fails to detect the cause. In 1961 PUO was defined as a duration of fever of at least 3 weeks and uncertainty of diagnosis after a 1 week investigation in the hospital [15]. As the progression of disease in children is more rapid and has more profound effects on the child's health than in an adult, using the duration of fever of 3 weeks is impractical in children.

Several comments are of practical importance to the diagnosis of PUO:

• The patient's history should be searched for animal exposure, travel abroad, and prior use of antibiotics.
• Repeated physical examinations are more helpful in establishing a diagnosis than extensive investigations.

Table 1.14 Principal causes of PUO

Cause	Reason for being a case of PUO
Infection (60%–70%)	
Localized	
Sinusitis	Standard sinus radiograph not performed or negative
Endocarditis	Previously unsuspected of having a cardiac defect
Occult abscess (abdomen, dental)	Absence of clinical signs
Systemic	
Viral (e.g. EBV)	Fever as the only sign of the disease
TB	Extrapulmonary, tuberculin test negative
Kawasaki disease	Incomplete presentation, diagnosis not considered
Brucellosis	Diagnostic test for brucella not performed
Collagen (about 20%)	
JIA	Prearthritic manifestation
SLE	Atypical manifestations
Neoplasma (5%)	
Leukaemia	Atypical presentation; blood tests negative
Lymphoma	Unusual localization
Neuroblastoma	Disseminated
Miscellaneous (5–10%)	
Drug fever	Diagnosis not considered, suspected drug not stopped
Factitious fever	Diagnosis not considered, thermometer left to patient

EBV Ebstein–Barr virus; *JIA* Juvenile idiopathic arthritis; *SLE* systemic lupus erythematosus

* A child with the initial diagnosis of PUO on presentation to the hospital may often prove to have either a self-limiting benign disorder, such as viral infection, or a common disease that can be diagnosed easily with simple initial investigations, such as urine culture or a chest X-ray. Therefore, provided that the child's condition is satisfactory, extensive investigations initially are not required. An atypical presentation of a common disease is more common than a rare and exotic disease.
* With the exception of bone marrow aspiration, an invasive technique such as laparotomy, laparoscopy, or biopsy is rarely indicated nowadays to diagnose PUO. Rheumatoid arthritis in a child with established diagnosis of PUO is often the single most common diagnosis.

Table 1.14 shows the main causes of PUO.

* Infections are the most common causes, accounting for 60–70% of all cases. The younger the child, the higher the relative percentage of infection. Although most viral infections rarely cause prolonged fever, about 15% of the infectious cases of PUO are due to viral infection.
* Collagen diseases account for about 20%, of which the most common cause is rheumatoid arthritis as a pre-arthritic presentation.
* Malignancy presenting as fever without other manifestations is unusual in children compared to adults, but may occur in up to 5%.

* Miscellaneous diagnoses account for 5–10% and undiagnosed in the remaining 5%. Previously, a high percentage of PUO (up to 25%) was categorized as undiagnosed, but with recently developed techniques, in particular imaging, the percentage of undiagnosed cases has greatly decreased.

Physical examination of a patient with PUO should include the following:

* A thorough examination on admission, which should be repeated during hospitalization
* Measurement of temperature by a nurse attending to the procedure to eliminate the rare possibility of factitious fever, occurring in <1% of PUO in children
* Checking for tenderness over the sinuses, bones, and muscles, and palpation of lymphnodes
* Eye examination (looking in particular for uveitis as an early clue for rheumatoid arthritis, bulbar conjunctivitis for leptospirosis, choroid tubercles, and toxoplasmosis lesions)
* Noting that an absence of sweat with high fever may suggest heat stroke, dehydration, anhidrotic ectodermal dysplasia, or familial dysautonomia

The tempo of laboratory investigation (Table 1.15) is based on the child's condition, while the extent of investigation is based on clues obtained from history:

* Travel abroad
* Exposure to animals
* Ingestion of raw milk
* Exposure to infection
* Consideration of ethnic group

Initial investigations (chest X-ray, blood and urine culture) may rapidly establish a diagnosis of unexplained fever. If these investigations fail to reach a diagnosis, further investigations and occasionally invasive techniques will be required.

Table 1.15 Suggested investigations for a case with PUO

Initial tests	Further investigations
FBC, CRP, ESR, blood film	Serum albumin: globulin ratio
Blood culture	Serology for brucellosis, toxoplasmosis
Urine (microscopy and culture)	Cytomegalovirus, mononucleosis
Stool (microscopy and culture)	*Salmonella*
Chest X-ray	Viral study
Tuberculin test	Radiology of sinuses, mastoid
Lumbar puncture	Ultrasound of abdomen and heart (for vegetation)
Liver function tests	Bone marrow aspiration
Antinuclear antibody	Isotope bone scan

FBC full blood count; *CRP* c-reactive protein; *ESR* erythrocyte sedimentation rate

The prognosis of PUO is better in children than in adults, mainly because of the higher incidence of infection and lower incidence of malignancy. Fatality may occur in <5% of the patients primarily due to neoplastic cases.

1.8
Fetal Malformation and Fever

A woman early in pregnancy with high body temperature increases her skin blood flow and ventilation at the expense of blood flow to the uterus and placenta. This reduces the heat removal efficiency of the placenta and results in a high fever in the fetus, which, theoretically, may lead to the loss of the fetus.

Fever or hyperthermia has been shown to be teratogenic in experimental animals, and several retrospective studies have suggested a casual relationship between fever (or hyperthermia) during pregnancy and congenital anomalies in human [16,17]. Fever of 38.9°C or higher or the use of a hot sauna for 15 min or longer was used as the marker of excessive heat [18]. As shown in Table 1.16, a wide variety of fetal malformations have been reported, particularly involving the CNS. It has been postulated that during early gestation at the time of neural tube closure (22–28 days), the rapidly proliferating cells may be sensitive to heat, causing a disruption of mitosis. Skeletal malformations, such as arthrogryposis, were found to occur in animal experiments at a higher temperature than those associated with abnormalities in the CNS [19].

Despite these reports, evidence for maternal fever or hyperthermia causing fetal malformations is inconclusive because:

Table 1.16 List of reported congenital defects

Location	Defect
CNS	Neural tube defect Anencephaly Encephalocele Microcephaly Mental deficiency
Face	Micrognathia Microphthalamia Cleft palate
Heart	Congenital defects (atrial septal defect Hypoplastic left heart syndrome)
Limb/skeletal	Clubfoot Arthrogryposis Limb reduction defect
Genitals	Hypospadias Micropenis
Intestine	Hirschsprung's disease

- Most studies were based on birth registries, and history was ascertained as far as 10 years back. The accuracy of such a history is therefore difficult to evaluate.
- A temperature of 38.9°C or higher is not uncommon with infection during pregnancy. If there is, indeed, a relationship between temperature elevation and fetal malformation, it is difficult to explain the rarity of these congenital malformations. A large prospective study involving 55,000 women could not confirm an association between febrile illness during pregnancy and fetal malformation [20]. A more recent study from Denmark involving over 24,000 women found no evidence that fever in the first 16 weeks of pregnancy was associated with the risk of fetal death [21].
- The use of saunas as a possible source of teratogenic hyperthermia has been challenged by Finnish authors on the grounds that their surveys did not show an increase in CNS abnormalities and that the incidence of anencephaly is very low in Finland [22] (only 0.32/1,000 in contrast to an incidence of 1/1,000 in other European countries and the United States). In general, pregnant Finnish women are not advised against the use of saunas. Ten to thirty minutes in an ambient temperature of 70–100°C usually does not raise body temperature higher than 38.5°C. Body temperature rises by 1.6°C during a 10-min sauna in children under 5 years of age and 0.9°C in those over 15 years of age.

1.9
Drug Fever (DF)

DF is a common condition, with fever often appearing as the sole manifestation of an adverse reaction of drugs.

- **Definition**: A disorder characterized by elevation of body temperature with the administration of a drug and the disappearance of the fever after discontinuation of the drug, with no other cause for the fever evident after a careful physical examination and laboratory investigation [23].
- **Diagnostic features include.**

  - DF is a diagnosis of exclusion.
  - Definite tests to confirm the diagnosis are usually absent, and a rechallenge is generally discouraged.
  - A characteristic fever pattern is lacking.
  - Drug fever may develop immediately following initiation of therapy but more commonly is delayed for 7–10 days.
  - Diagnosis is suggested by prompt defervescence (usually within 24 h) after discontinuation of the offending drug.
  - Conditions predisposing to the development of DF include atopic disorders, severe infection (e.g., meningitis) and systemic lupus (SLE).
  - Patients usually do not appear toxic, and the body temperature is usually of moderate degree. However, a high temperature may occur, including hectic patterns and chills. The highest temperatures are caused by cytotoxic drugs and by those drugs inducing hyperthermia.

1

– Cutaneous manifestations are frequently observed, particularly urticaria, along with eosinophilia, and a pulse that is disproportionately low in relation to the degree of temperature (relative bradycardia).

Drugs may induce fever by several mechanisms:

* IL-1 can be produced by an antigen–antibody complex with leukocytes; the drug acts as an antigen. An example of this mechanism is penicillin.
* Antibiotics and some cytotoxic drugs, such as bleomycin and aspraginase, are derived from microorganisms and may occasionally be contaminated by endotoxin, which can provoke fever.
* Cytotoxic drugs often cause immunosuppression with subsequent infections and are responsible for most febrile episodes.
* Drugs can also elevate the body temperature by inducing hyperthermia in several ways: by increased heat production (e.g., drugs inducing malignant hyperthermia, severe salicylate intoxication, and thyroxine), by reduction of sweating (e.g., anticholinergic drugs such as atropine), or by inducing vasoconstriction, as with adrenaline (see Chap. 2).
* Some drugs, for example cocaine, may have a direct pyrogenic effect on the hypothalamic center.
* Almost any drug may provoke a temperature rise as an adverse reaction. However, certain drugs have more predictable pyrogenic effects in causing hyperthermia/fever, which are shown in Table 1.17.

Other drugs that are associated with high incidence of fever include:

A neonate with suspected congenital heart defect, especially a ductus arteriosus-dependent defect (e.g., pulmonary stenosis, tricuspid atresia, hypoplastic left heart syndrome) should receive prostaglandin infusion as soon as possible to maintain the

Antimicrobial	Antihypertensive
Penicillin	Hydralizine
Ampicillin	Methyldopa
Rifampicin	Oxprenolol
Sulphanamide	
Isoniazid	Antiepileptic
Cephalosporins	Carbamazepine
Co-trimoxazole	Diphenylhydantoin
Nitrofurantoin	
Amphotericin B	Phenothiazines
	Promethazine
Cytotoxic drugs	Chlorpromazine
Bleomycin	Haloperidol
Chlorambucil	
6-Mercaptopurine	Others
Daunorubicin	Blood
L-Asparaaginase	Aspirin
	Quinidine
	Procainide

Table 1.17 The main drugs that can cause a rise of body temperature

patency of the ductus. The procedure is particularly important if the child is born outside a tertiary center (with facility of cardiac surgery) so that the baby is transported to an appropriate center for surgery. The most frequent complication of prostaglandin infusion is fever, with an incidence of around 60%. This complication should disappear once the dose is moderately reduced. Other side effects include apnoea and tachycardia (or bradycardia, hypotension, and cardiac arrhythmia).

● **Interferon treatment.**
Interferon are endogenous pyrogens capable of inducing fever (see Chap. 3). Interferon-α has been the most effective treatment for patients suffering from hepatitis B and C, and melanoma. In a study of 100 children (mean age 7 years) treated for hepatitis B, fever was observed in 72%, occurring either periodically or throughout the whole 20-week treatment [24].

References

Periodic Fever

1. Padeh S. Periodic fever syndromes. Pediatr Clin North Am 2005; 52: 577–609

Manifestations of Fever

2. O'Dempsey TJD, Laurance BE, McArdle, et al. The effect of temperature reduction on respiratory rate in febrile illnesses. Arch Dis Child 1993; 68: 492–95

Potential Complications

3. Dubois EF. Why are fever temperatures over 106°F rare? Am J Med Sci 1949; 217: 361–8
4. Tautner BW, Caviners AC, Gerlacher GR, et al. Prospective evaluation of the risk of serious bacterial infection in children who present to the emergency department with hyperpyrexia (temperature of 106°F). Pediatrics 2006; 118: 34–40
5. Press S, Fawwett NP. Association of temperature greater than 41.1°C (106°F) with serious illness. Clin Pediatr 1985; 24: 21–5
6. Pomerance JJ, Richardson J. Hyperpyrexia as a sign of intraventricular haemorrhage in the neonate. Am J Dis Child 1973; 126: 854–5

Fever with Localized Signs

7. Lieberman E, Lang J, Richardson DK, et al. Intrapartum maternal fever and neonatal outcome. Pediatrics 2000; 105: 8–13
8. Pantell RH, Naber M, Lamar R, et al. Fever in the first six months of life. Clin Pediatr 1980; 19: 77–82
9. O'Shea JS. Assessing the significance of fever in young infants. Clin Pediatr 1978; 17: 854–6

10. McCarthy PL, Dolan TF. The serious implication of high fever in infants during their first three months. Clin Pediatr 1876; 15: 794–6
11. Bonadio WA, Hegenbarth M, Zachariason M. Correlating reported fever in young infants with subsequent temperature pattern and rate of serious bacterial infections. Pediatr Infect Dis J 1990; 9: 158–60

Fever without Localizing Signs

12. Teele DW, Pelton SI, Grant MJA, et al. Bacteraemia in febrile children under 2 years of age: results of cultures of blood of 600 consecutive febrile children seen in a "walk in" clinic. J Pediatr 1975; 87: 227–30
13. McCabe WR, Treadwell TL, De Maria A. Pathophysiology of bacteraemia. Am J Med 1983; 75: 7–17
14. Vesikari T, Janas M, Grönroos P, et al. Neonatal septicaemia. Arch Dis Child 1985; 60: 157–60

Persistent Fever of Unknown Origin

15. Pertersdorf RO, Besson PB. Fever of unexplained origin: report of 100 cases. Medicine 1961; 40: 1–30

Fetal Malformation and Fever

16. Ivarsson SA, Henriksson P. Septic shock and hyperthermia as possible teratogenic factors. Acta Paediatr Scand 1984; 73: 73: 855–6
17. Fraser FC, Skelton J. Possible teratogenicity of maternal fever. Lancet 1978; 3: 634
18. Pleet H, Graham JM, Smith D. Central nervous system and facial defects associated with maternal hyperthermia at four to 14 weeks gestation. Pediatrics 1981; 67: 785–9
19. Edwards MJ. Congenital defects in guinea pigs. Acta Pathol 1967; 84: 42–8
20. Clarren SK, Smith DW, Ward HR, et al. Hyperthermia-a prospective evaluation of a possible teratogenic agent in man. J Pediatr 1979; 95: 81–3
21. Andersen AN, Vastrup P, Wohlfahrt J, et al. Fever in pregnancy and risk of fetal death: a cohort study. Lancet 2002; 360: 1552–6
22. Rapola J, Saxon L, Granroth G. Anencephaly and the sauna. Lancet 1978; 2: 1162

Drug Fever

23. Mackowiak PA. Drug fever: mechanisms, maxims and misconception. Am J Med Sci 1987; 294: 275–86
24. Liberek A, Luczak G, Korzan M, et al. Tolerance of interferon-alpha therapy in children with chronic hepatitis B. J Paediatr Child Health 2004; 40: 265–9

Hyperthermia

2

Core Messages

› Hyperthermia is a peripherally (skin and muscle) mediated elevation of body temperature, which greatly differs from fever. Temperature is uncontrolled because the hypothalamic centre is not involved.

› Hyperthermia, in contrast to fever, is uncommon, but it has to be considered in the differential diagnosis of elevated body temperature.

› Although hyperthermia and fever cannot usually be differentiated clinically on the basis of the height of temperature, a temperature above 42°C suggests hyperthermia. A normal temperature excludes fever but not hyperthermia.

› Hyperthermia has different causes, symptoms and signs than fever. Its management is specific and is also different from that of fever, e.g. antipyretics are ineffective while physical methods are effective.

› Drugs play a major role in causing hyperthermia. In contrast to fever hyperthermia can largely be prevented.

› Hyperthermia has many causes of which malignant hyperthermia (prototype of increased heat production) and heat stroke (prototype of decreased heat production) are the most common and serious causes.

2.1
Definition

Hyperthermia is a state of thermoregulatory failure resulting from the inability to dissipate heat at a sufficient rate (e.g. heat stroke) or excessive heat production with a normal rate of heat loss (e.g. malignant hyperthermia). Dehydration, the most common cause of hyperthermia, leads to vasoconstriction and decreased sweating, which impair heat dissipation causing a rise of body temperature. Hyperthermia may coexists with fever: hyperthermia,

A.S. El-Radhi et al. (Eds.) *Clinical Manual of Fever in Children.*
Doi: 10.1007/978-3-540-78598-9, © Springer-Verlag Berlin Heidelberg 2009

Table 2.1 Main differences between fever and hyperthermia

Criteria	Fever	Hyperthermia
Occurrence	Commonest sign	Relatively rare
Clinical findings	Feeling cold, cold skin	Feeling hot, dry flushed skin
Temperature	Usually 38–41°C	May exceed 42°C
Principal therapy	Antipyretics	Physical measures
Central regulation	Yes	No
Central set-point	Elevated	Normal
Mortality	Unusual	High (excluding minor forms such as dehydration)

caused by dehydration, may occur on top of fever due to infection, or a febrile seizure caused by infection may lead to hyperthermia from intense muscular contractions.

In contrast to fever, hyperthermia is not mediated by pyrogen or Interleukin-1 (IL-1), and the body temperature is higher than the hypothalamic set-point, which is usually normal. Because hyperthermia is not regulated centrally, a temperature in excess of 42°C is common, and the presence of such makes hyperthermia a likely diagnosis. This very high degree of temperature rarely occurs, if ever, with fever alone, even with the most severe infections. Despite this difference, a febrile range of temperature of 38–42°C does not exclude hyperthermia. Table 2.1 shows the main differences between fever and hyperthermia.

Characteristically, patients with hyperthermia feel warm and attempt to eliminate the heat by stretching out, drinking cold liquid, seeking a cooler environment and removing clothes.

2.2
Physiology

The body temperature is regulated by mechanisms involving the autonomic nervous system (mainly via skin) and the hypothalamus. These are:

- Heat production by muscle activity (increase in muscle tone or shivering) and cellular metabolisms, mainly within the liver, heart and brain through the catabolism of the intracellular proteins, carbohydrates and fats.
- Heat dissipation from the skin and, to lesser extent, the lungs, through conduction, convection, radiation and evaporation. The loss is dependent on the humidity and the ambient temperature of the body's surroundings.

Heat production and loss are usually so balanced that a constant body temperature is maintained between 36.6°C and 37.9°C measured rectally.

During the neonatal period, the dominant source of heat production is through non-shivering thermogenesis that increases the metabolic rate without shivering. This may begin as early as 15 min after birth. The site of non-shivering thermogenesis is brown adipose tissue, which is found predominately in the interscapular area, axillae, peri-renal area and around the large vessels in the chest.

When the body is exposed to extreme levels of heat, excessive heat production or impaired heat loss, the thermoregulatory system fails, causing heat stress and hyperthermia.

2.3
Effects of Hyperthermia

Not all forms of hyperthermia are dangerous. Hyperthermia is a physiological response to intense exercise, and a moderate temperature of 39–40°C can be found in athletes during hard exercise.

Hyperthermia, particularly when excessive, can induce cellular damage. The brain is especially sensitive to extremes of body temperature. Although it has been difficult to establish a thermal threshold or **critical thermal maximum (CTM)** in man (defined as the temperature above which tissue damage may occur), a temperature of 42°C is likely to induce such damage [1]. Complications and mortality above this temperature are related more to the severity of the underlying disease than to the height of the temperature. The upper thermal limit for the survival of most organisms is about 45.0°C because proteins tend to denature above this temperature. However, it has been difficult to differentiate the clinical effects caused by hyperthermia per se from those caused by related manifestations or complications of hyperthermia, such as hypoxia, hypotension, metabolic acidosis, disseminated intravascular coagulation (DIC), azotaemia, hypoglycaemia, circulatory failure or seizures. These secondary disturbances may play a part in the pathogenesis of organ damage and in the poor prognosis of hyperthermia. Table 2.2 summarizes the effects of hyperthermia.

2.4
Causes of Hyperthermia

There are several causes for hyperthermia (Table 2.3). (See also Chap 12 for the differential diagnosis of the forms of hyperthermia).

Table 2.2 Summary of the effects of hyperthermia

• Cardiac: decreased output by direct damage of the myocardium
• Respiratory: hyperventilation or apnoea, hypoxia
• Renal: failure, acute tubular necrosis, hyperkalaemia
• Gastrointestinal: diarrhoea, liver damage, pancreatitis
• Blood: haemoconcentration, DIC, leukocytosis
• Neurologic: confusion, seizure, cerebral oedema
• Muscular: rhabdomyolysis, increased creatinine kinase, myoglobulinaemia
• Fetal malformation? (discussed in Chap. 1)
• Therapeutic effects (see "Therapeutic Hyperthermia")

Hyperthermia caused by increased heat production	**Table 2.3** Causes of hyperthermia
• Malignant hyperthermia	
• Neuroleptic malignant syndrome	
• Serotonin syndrome	
• Drug-induced	
• Exercise-induced hyperthermia	
• Endocrine hyperthermia	
• Miscellaneous clinical disorders	
Hyperthermia caused by decreased heat loss	
• Neonatal hyperthermia	
• Dehydration	
• Heat stroke	
• Haemorrhagic shock and encephalopathy	
• Sudden infant death syndrome (SIDS)	
• Drug-induced	
Unclassified	
• Factitious fever	
• Induced illness	
• Induced illness by proxy	

2.4.1
Hyperthermia Caused by Increased Heat Production

Malignant Hyperthermia

Malignant hyperthermia (MH), usually induced by anaesthetic agents, is an autosomal dominant myopathy causing a massive heat production. The condition is due to several gene mutations, the commonest being in the skeletal ryanodine receptor gene (*PYR1*) located on chromosome 19q 13.1. Patients with this gene defect are usually asymptomatic. Some patients have no detectable gene defect.

During an acute episode of MH, intracellular calcium increases in skeletal muscle, causing uncontrolled muscle contractions and hyperthermia. The hypothalamic thermo-regulatory center functions normally and therefore antipyretics are ineffective. Most of the commonly used anaesthetic agents and muscle relaxants can induce MH, but the agents most commonly incriminated are halothane, isoflurane, enflurane and succinylcholine. Normothermia does not exclude MH.

MH is a potentially fatal condition with a mortality rate ranging between 50% and 70% if untreated. The reported incidence ranges from about 1/10,000 to 1/50,000 anaesthetic procedures, with children being at higher risk (1/15,000) than adults. Even very young children may be affected. Risk factors for MH include:

* Genetically susceptible patients with an underlying, sub-clinical muscle disease, who appear normal.
* Susceptibility to heat stress, such as exertional heat stroke.
* Parents of babies who died of SIDS related to high body temperature.
* Patients with chronic myopathy, e.g. central core disease, Duchene muscular dystrophy, chondrodystrophic myotonia (Schwartz–Jampel syndrome) and those with Noonan syndrome. Interestingly, MH and central core disease have been found to reside near one another on chromosome 19q13.1.
* Some patients with characteristic clinical features, including spinal deformities, ptosis and cryptorchidism.

The presence of the disease can be identified by:

* Elevated serum CPK screening.
* An in vitro response of the patient's biopsied muscle to halothane (caffeine-halothane contracture test) confirms the diagnosis.
* Deoxyribose nucleic acid (DNA) markers to identify the region on chromosome 19 that carries the gene for MH susceptibility.
* Molecular genetic sampling for MH in the umbilical cord blood [2].

Clinical features resulting from the abnormal muscular contractions are:

* Muscle rigidity, particularly of masseter muscle, causing rhabdomyolysis.
* An increase in end tidal carbon dioxide, which is often an early sign.
* Tachycardia, rising blood pressure, cardiac arrhythmia, tachypnoea and hyperpnoea (as a result of respiratory and metabolic acidosis).
* A rapid rise in body temperature, 0.5–1.0°C every 5–10 min, reaching a temperature as high as 44.0°C.

Investigations depend on the organ affected and are shown in Table 2.2. To identify susceptible patients pre-operatively, the following steps should be taken:

* Obtain history of hyperthermia or death among relatives during anaesthesia.
* Screen with serum CPK (a normal CPK does not exclude MH).
* Local anaesthesia other than lignocaine should be used whenever possible, e.g. procaine. Also spinal, epidural or regional blocks are recommended.
* For general anaesthesia, thiopentone (or diazepam) and nitrous oxide are safe.

Treatment in established cases during surgery includes:

* Local anaesthesia other than lignocaine should be used whenever possible, e.g. procaine. Also spinal, epidural or regional blocks are recommended. For general anaesthesia, thiopentone (or diazepam) and nitrous oxide are safe.
* Termination of anaesthesia and surgery while continuing ventilation.
* Initiating rapid and aggressive total body cooling with ice-packs or ice-water, through a naso-gastric tube, i.v and rectally. Antipyretics are ineffective.

- 100% oxygen.
- Correction of acidosis with sodium bicarbonate (1 mg kg^{-1} and higher).
- Other medications: i.v furosemide (1 mg kg^{-1}) and mannitol (1 g kg^{-1} as 20% solution) to maintain urine output and reduce cerebral oedema; insulin and dextrose to treat hyperkalaemia; hydrocortisone (100 mg every 4 h).
- Dantrolone, the specific antidote, given in a dose of 2.5 mg kg^{-1} and then every 5–10 min. The drug prevents an increase in cytoplasmic calcium. (Mortality rate in MH has been reduced to 10% using dantrolone.)
- Arrhythmia treatment with lignocaine or procainamide hydrochloride.

Neuroleptic Malignant Syndrome (NMS)

This is a rare drug-induced syndrome, which has the following features:

- Increased extrapyramidal disturbance and hyperthermia.
- An incidence, which varies between 0.02% and 3.2% of patients treated with neuroleptics [3]. (Drugs triggering NMS are shown in Table 2.4.)
- Current occurrence of cases mostly after intake of typical or atypical antipsychotic drugs.
- Certain diagnostic criteria [4], which are shown in Table 2.5.
- Symptoms, which usually subside 5–7 days after discontinuation of the triggering drug. (The symptoms may last longer with the use of depot preparations.)

This complication of neuroleptic drugs is to be distinguished from the more common and benign side-effects of these drugs, which may produce fever. Infants with dehydration, fever or co-existing brain damage are at higher risk of developing NMS.

The hyperthermia, often in excess of 41°C, is partly due to sustained muscle contraction and partly due to central disturbance of dopaminergic pathways within the hypothalamic

Table 2.4 Medications that can induce neuroleptic malignant syndrome

Phenothiazine
  Thioridazine
  Chlorpromazine
	Monoamine oxidase inhibitors
	  Phenelzine

Benzodiazepine
  Diazepam
	Antimanics
	  Lithium

Butyrophenones
  Haloperidol
	Tricyclic antidepressants
	  Imipramine
	  Amitriptyline

Anticonvulsants
  Carbamazepine
  Phenytoin
	Serotonin reuptake inhibitors (SSRI)
	  Fluoxetine

Atypical antipsychotic
  Olanzapine
  Risperidone
	Thioxanthenes

Table 2.5 Diagnostic criteria for NMS (modified from [4])

Essential	Recent use of antipsychotics (or recent use of other dopaminergic or recent discontinuation of dopamine agent)
Major	Elevated body temperature >38.0°C No other cause is found for the temperature Muscular rigidity Elevated CPK (>3 times normal)
Minor	Tachycardia, arrhythymia, dystonia, tremor, Tachypnoea, altered consciousness, unstable blood pressure (high or low), myoglobulinuria

thermoregulatory center. NMS is a potentially life-threatening disorder with a reported mortality rate of 11.6% [5].

Laboratory findings are those resulting from affected organs (Table 2.2). Therapy is similar to that of malignant hyperthermia, including stopping medication, rapid cooling measures, close monitoring and the use of dantrolone as a muscle relaxant. Bromocriptine has been used with success. Anticholinergics are of little value.

Serotonin Syndrome (SS)

SS overlaps with NMS. Although clinical features are common to both disorders (elevated body temperature, muscle rigidity, delirium, autonomic instability and high CPK), more typical presentation of SS includes other features:

* Behavioural: confusion and agitation
* Autonomic: tachycardia, hypo- or hypertension, mydriasis
* Neurologic: myoclonus seizures, clonus, tremor, hyperreflexia
* Intestinal: diarrhoea

Hyperthermia of SS is a less consistent finding, compared to MH and NMS, and is present in about 50% of cases [6]. The syndrome is caused by excessive serotonin stimulation. It has been most commonly associated with an intake of monoamine oxidase inhibitors with tricyclic antidepressants, amphetamines, selective serotonin reuptake inhibitors (SSRIs), the use of cocaine, amphetamine and ecstasy.

Drug-Induced Hyperthermia

Sympathomimetics are the most common drugs in causing hyperthermia. They interfere with heat loss and increase heat production through increased muscle activity. Life-threatening hyperthermia caused by these agents is idiosyncratic and not related to duration and mode of administration. The most used drugs are:

* **Ecstasy** (3,4-methylenedioxymethamphetamine) is an amphetamine derivative, which causes sympathomimetic activity by releasing serotonin from neurons in the CNS. It

was used briefly in the 1970s and 1980s as an adjunct to psychotherapy. Since then, this drug has become popular and is abused by teenagers and young adults as an illicit drug, causing a number of adverse events and fatalities. The hyperthermia is mainly attributed to "rave" parties involving high ambient temperatures, excessive dancing and dehydration. In severe cases, particularly with co-use of other illicit drugs, rhabdomyolysis, DIC, seizures, renal and liver failure, and cardiac arrest may occur. There is a correlation between the extent of hyperthermia and survival rates in patients taking ecstasy.

* **Cocaine and amphetamine** can cause similar symptoms and signs. Intoxication with these two drugs can cause mortality, which is directly related to the degree of the hyperthermia.
* **Methylphenidate** is a CNS stimulant which is widely used for the management of ADHD in children. Side-effects with the usual daily dose of 10–60 mg include insomnia, irritability, tachycardia and jitteriness. With overdose, symptoms are similar to those of amphetamine overdose, such as agitation, hallucinations, psychosis, tremors, seizures and hyperthermia.
* **Baclofen.** This drug is used for spasticity and is being increasingly given intrathecally via an implantable pump, where it achieves a high CSF concentration (100 times greater than that achieved by oral route). Its rapid withdrawal (e.g. pump or catheter malfunction) causes a syndrome characterized by altered mental status, tachycardia, hypo- or hypertension, seizures, rebound spasticity (causing muscle rigidity that sometimes progresses to fatal rhabdomyolysis) and hyperthermia, which results from increased muscle activity. Baclofen is known to inhibit sympathetic activity at the spinal cord level, and so its withdrawal may cause rebound sympathetic activity. The syndrome may be fatal unless treated promptly by restoration of the drug intrathecally, supportive care and the use of benzodiazepines.

Exercise-Induced Hyperthermia (Exertional Heat Stroke)

This may occur in older children following intense and prolonged exercise, particularly in a hot climate. Maximal exercise produces a nearly 15-fold increase in cutaneous blood flow. The greater surface area to mass ratio in children compared to adults allows greater transfer of heat. For example, an 8-year-old child has a surface area to mass ratio of 360–380 cm^2 kg^{-1} as compared to 240–260 cm^2 kg^{-1} in a medium sized adult [7]. Although the greater surface area produces more sweat, the resulting dehydration may eventually limit heat loss. Children generate more metabolic heat per mass unit than do adults, as evidenced by the higher oxygen uptake seen in children performing the same work as adults. Children have a limited capacity for sweating: secretion per gland in the adult is nearly 2.5 times as high as that in an 8- to 10-year-old child.

For these reasons, the American Committee on Sport Medicine [8] has recommended the following measures:

* Caution should be used with prolonged (over 30 min) and intense exercise in environmental temperatures exceeding 30°C and relative humidity of more than 90%.
* Periodic drinks should be available, e.g. 150 ml of cold tap-water every 30 min.

* Clothing should be light, limited to one layer of absorbent material to facilitate evaporation, and sweat-saturated garments should be replaced with dry ones.

Endocrine Hyperthermia (EH)

Endocrine hyperthermia is a rare endocrine disorder in children, compared to adults. Table 2.6 summarizes the main endocrine disorders that may increase body temperature.

Hyperthyroidism. About two-thirds of all endocrine hyperthermia is due to thyroid diseases [9]. Thyrotoxic crisis and subacute thyroiditis (de Quervain disease) may cause a raised body temperature by increasing the metabolic rate. In contrast to the extreme hyperthermia in thyrotoxic crisis, hyperthermia due to subacute thyroiditis is usually low-grade, (rarely with high fever with chills), often associated with tenderness and pain in the thyroid area, tachycardia and high ESR. It may present with fever alone as a case of PUO. The thyroiditis, which is caused by a viral infection, can be confirmed by abnormal thyroid function tests (high or low T4/T3 levels) with reduced isotope uptake on thyroid scan.

Diabetes mellitus. Hyperglycaemic, hyperosmolar nonketotic syndrome (HHNS) is usually associated with type 2 diabetes mellitus (DM) and is rare in children. Recently, several cases of malignant hyperthermia-like syndrome have been reported in children in association with HHNS in type 1 DM, resulting in rhabdomyolysis and fatality [10]. The underlying aetiology remains unclear (defect in fatty acid oxidation? genetic predisposition?). A rare endocrine abnormality is insulinoma that may be associated with elevation of body temperature and severe hypoglycaemia [11]. A removal of the tumour normalizes the body temperature.

Phaeochromocytoma with increased catecholamine production may cause excessive heat production as well decreased heat loss subsequent to peripheral vasoconstriction. Exercise may trigger both sudden hyperthermia and hypertension.

In **adrenal insufficiency**, elevated temperature may be due to dehydration related to polyuric hypercalciuria and electrolyte imbalance.

Table 2.6 Summary of the main endocrine disorders causing hyperthermia

Disorder	Underlying mechanisms of hyperthermia
Hyperthyroidism	Combination of increased metabolic rate and Enhanced sensitivity to amines
Diabetes Mellitus	Similar mechanisms to malignant hyperthermia
Phaeochromocytoma	Catecholamines causing excessive heat production, peripheral vasoconstriction, IL-6 may be present in the tumour acting as an endogenous pyrogen
Adrenal insufficiency	Dehydration, possibly due to polyuric hypercalciuria
Etiocholanolone fever	Stimulate formation of leukocyte pyrogens

Hyperparathyroidism.

Etiocholanolone fever, the best recognized steroid causing fever, may produce fever by stimulating the formation of leukocyte pyrogen.

2.4.2
Hyperthermia Caused by Decreased Heat Loss

Neonatal Hyperthermia

A rapid rise in body temperature on the second and third day of life may be due to:

* Dehydration (so called dehydration fever) as a result of fluid loss or exposure to a high environmental temperature. This problem results from the infant's greater surface area per unit weight as compared to adults, causing a higher fluid loss through the skin. This condition was identified in 68 out of 358 (19%) febrile neonates, making it the third most common cause of temperature elevation after infection and birth trauma [12]. Table 2.7 shows the main difference between neonatal hyperthermia and infection. Up to 10% of breast-fed children are said to develop this complication due to insufficient breast secretion and/or infant's reluctance to feed. This incidence can be lowered to about 1% following fluid supplement, which is about the same incidence found in formula-fed babies.
* Overheating from mechanical or electrical failure of a warming device, servocontrolled incubators can cause overheating if the skin sensor becomes detached from the infant. Overwrapped infants left in a warm room or under a powerful radiant warmer are also at risk of hyperthermia. Radiant heat from sunlight may overheat the infant without initially warming the air in the surrounding environment.

Table 2.7 Differentiating neonatal hyperthermia from fever due to infection

Criteria	Hyperthermia	Fever
Incidence	1–10%	1%
Main risk	Dehydration, overheating	Prematurity, PRM[a]
Appearance	Well	Unwell
Symptoms	Usually none if hyperthermia is short, sometimes irritability	Numerous (See Chap. 1)
Response of C to fluid	Rapid normalisation	No change
Leg-rectal temperature[b]	<1.5°C	>3.2°C
Laboratory findings	Hypernatraemia, high urea	High CRP, leukopenia

[a] Premature rupture of membrane
[b] Measurement of the skin temperature of the anterior mid-lower leg simultaneously with rectal temperature or tympanic temperature

* A rise in body temperature occurring on the second and third day of life may result from birth trauma. This phenomenon occurred in 86 out of 358 (24%) infants [12]. Temperature usually subsides within 1–3 days, but occasionally persists in the presence of excessive restlessness or convulsions. A probable cause of this hyperthermia is the inability of the sick infant to maintain normal body temperature owing to inadequately developed thermo-regulatory mechanisms.

The treatment of hyperthermia in the newborn consists of cooling the infant rapidly by undressing and exposing him or her to room temperature. If the skin temperature is higher than 39.0°C, sponging with tepid water at about 35.0°C should be initiated until the skin temperature approaches 37.0°C.

Dehydration

Dehydration is the most common cause of hyperthermia. Loss of body fluid causes cutaneous vasoconstriction and decreased sweating, which leads to decreased heat loss and hyperthermia. The increase of body temperature with dehydration is usually mild.

Heat Stroke

Clinical descriptions of 14 different heat-related disorders are recognized in the medical literature, (e.g. heat cramps, heat exhaustion, sunburn, etc.), of which heat stroke is the most important in children and in adults. It is sometimes called siriasis, based on the biblical reference that occurred coincidentally with the appearance of the Dog Star, Sirius [13]. Heat stroke was described in medicine over 1,000 years ago as "another form of fever" by Rhazes (Chap 13: History of fever). Its recognition in Europe did not occur before the eighteenth century when soldiers were sent to warm countries. Risk factors predisposing to heat-related illness are shown in Table 2.8.

Normally, sweat increases in proportion to body temperature. The mechanism is regulated by cyclic discharge of cholinergic, sympathetic nerve fibers of the sweat glands. Over 2,100 kJ (500 kcal) of heat is lost per liter of sweat evaporated.

Heat stroke is due to failure of the heat-regulating mechanisms of the hypothalamus subsequent to inhibition of sweating. The exact mechanisms responsible for this failure are unknown, but the two principal causes are high ambient temperature and water deprivation. Initially, there may be sweat loss leading to dehydration, which aggravates a subsequent temperature rise due to sweat cessation.

Heat stroke has been reported from a number of geographical areas:

* In the USA, in infants who were left sleeping in a parked automobile under the sun with inadequate ventilation: In 2003, the number of children reported to have died from heat stroke after being left unattended in motor vehicles was 42 [14].
* In the UK and other European countries where excessive wrapping is sometimes practiced in infants (mainly from lower socioeconomic classes) overheating may occur. This swaddling, which is an ancient practice, has become increasingly popular as a sleep-promoting intervention, sometimes resulting in fatalities [15].

Table 2.8 Risk factors predisposing to heat-related illness

Age	Environmental
Very young and old	High ambient temperature
Dehydration	High humidity
Fever	Lack of wind
Inadequate fluid intake	Drugs
Gastroenteritis	Lithium
Diuretic use	beta-blockers
Sport	Antiepileptics
Clothing	Condition
Wrapping	Physical or mental disability

* In Melbourne, Australia, heat stroke occurred during a recent heat wave.
* In the tropics heat stroke may occur in children as a result of combined salt and water deprivation, or severe sunburn.

The cardinal features of heat stroke include:

* Body temperature: >40.5°C (lower temperature has been reported)
* Skin: hot, dry (sweating may or may not be present)
* CNS abnormalities: alteration of consciousness, dizziness, headache, convulsion and coma, uncontrollable muscle twitching
* Cardiac: Tachycardia, arrhythmia and failure as a result of extensive haemorrhage in the myocardium
* Gastrointestinal: nausea, vomiting, cramps

In addition, children are usually in shock (due to maldistribution of blood to the circulation), with metabolic acidosis. Clinical evaluation may confirm the presence of renal failure, DIC, rhabdomyolysis (due to severe muscular contraction), hepatic enlargement with elevation of the enzymes and anaemia due to increased RBC destruction, thrombocytopenia and hyperkaliaemia, with characteristic ECG abnormalities.
A child with heat stroke should:

* Be referred to an intensive-care unit with facilities for continuous monitoring and ventilation. The two most important goals of therapy are cooling and support of circulation.
* Undergo rapid cooling, best achieved by removing the clothes, sponging with ice water (or better immersing into ice-water) until body temperature reaches 38.5°C. Then the patient is moved to a bed and wrapped in a blanket. In severe or resistant cases iced-intravenous solution, iced-saline gastric lavage and cold saline enema may be needed.

Additional measures are:

* Vigorous massage to promote vasodilatation and fanning to increase convection. Continuous oxygen therapy is usually given routinely.

* IV fluid therapy aimed at correction of dehydration and balancing electrolytes. Plasma expanders and mannitol (1 g kg^{-1} of 20% solution, infused over 15–20 min) are required to treat cerebral oedema and renal under-perfusion.
* Treating hyperkalaemia with glucose and insulin. Renal failure may require early dialysis, along with adequate fluid, electrolytes and bicarbonate.

Despite intensive treatment, the prognosis of heat stroke is poor, with a mortality ranging from 17% to 70%, depending on the severity of the heat stroke and age of the patient. Post-mortem examination reveals cerebral oedema and haemorrhage in various organs.

Haemorrhagic Shock and Encephalopathy (HSE)

This form of hyperthermia was described by Levin et al. in 1983 [16]. Despite extensive investigations, including viral and bacteriological studies, no specific cause has been found. Although clinical features are similar to heat stroke, the majority of reported cases had no evidence of wrapping, fluid deprivation or high environmental temperature. It was later suggested that HSE may be a manifestation of a genetic defect in the production or release of serum protease inhibitor alpha-1-trypsin [17].

The median age of affected children is 5 months (range 17 days – 15 years) and nearly 90% have been less than 1 year of age. Usually, the children have been completely well with only mild non-specific symptoms, such as an upper respiratory tract infection or febrile gastroenteritis, 2–5 days prior to the onset of HSE. Then abruptly they develop:

* Severe shock, manifested clinically by collapse, pallor, cyanosis and mottled skin. Hypotension is a late sign of shock.
* Encephalopathy manifested with sudden onset of seizures and coma.
* Hyperthermia a constant finding, with a temperature usually above 41°C.
* Bleeding due to DIC, with diarrhoea, may be striking, resulting in severe anaemia requiring transfusion.

Examination reveals hepatomegaly and acidosis with shallow respirations. During the next few hours renal failure becomes established with increased creatinine, hyperkalaemia and acidosis. Additional laboratory abnormalities include leukocytosis, hypernatraemia, elevated serum levels of creatinine phosphokinase (CPK), liver enzymes and trypsin, hypoglycaemia and hypocalcaemia, thrombocytopenia, reduced factors II, V, hyperfibrinogaemia and alpha-1-antitrypsin

Haemorrhagic shock and encephalopathy must be differentiated from:

* Heat stroke with its history of fluid deprivation and high ambient temperature
* Septicaemia with its less abrupt presentation
* Reye's syndrome with its elevated plasma ammonia and characteristic histological findings of the liver; possible aspirin intake
* Haemolytic uremic syndrome with its haemolysis, pronounced anaemia
* Toxic shock syndrome and Kawasaki disease (both have a less dramatic onset); and accidental intake of toxin

There is no specific treatment for HSE and management is similar to that discussed for malignant hyperthermia and heat stroke. Prognosis is poor with a mortality of 80% and severe neurological squeal in the majority of surviving cases. CT scan and autopsy show focal haemorrhage in many organs and cerebral oedema.

Sudden Infant Death Syndrome (SIDS)

This important subject is included because of its possible link to hyperthermia.
The accepted definition of SIDS is:

* An infant's sudden and unexpected death, which remains unexplained after thorough post-mortem examination.
* A thorough investigation of the death-scene.
* A diagnosis of exclusion. Symptoms such an upper respiratory tract infection with possible fever, which do not have serious effects on the child's condition, do not exclude the diagnosis.

Although SIDS is still the leading cause of death in infants 1–12 months of age, its rate has declined since the start of the "Back to Sleep" campaign in 1991 (UK) and 1992 (USA):

* In the USA, the rate in 1992 was 1.2 death per 1,000 live births, which decreased to 0.56 death per 1,000 live births (a reduction of 53%) over 10 years [18]. During this period, the prevalence of prone positioning has decreased from 70% to 11.3%.
* In the UK, there has been a remarkable fall in incidence to 0.4 death per 1,000 live births in the year 2,000 and a further fall to 0.26 in the year 2003 [19].

Despite extensive research over the past decades, the cause of SIDS is unknown. The predominant hypothesis is that certain infants have mal-development or delayed maturation of the brainstem neural network, which is thought to be involved with arousal, chemosensitivity, respiratory drive, thermoregulation, and blood pressure response. A multi-factorial cause, rather than a single one, appears likely. Risk factors associated with SIDS are shown in the Table 2.9. The risk peaks at 2–4 months of age and is low during the neonatal period (only about 4% of all SIDS cases). The two important factors are prone position and maternal smoking.

   Although the vast majority of infants who sleep prone are not in danger of SIDS, up to 88% of SIDS victims were found in this position. A child in prone position may have limited head movement and thus limited access to fresh air. This factor may also explain the low incidence of SIDS in Asian children, who usually sleep in a supine position.

   SIDS and Hyperthermia. Hyperthermia (e.g. in the form of heat stroke) has been implicated as a cause of SIDS. It may cause apnoea as a result of transient loss of respiratory chemoreceptor sensitivity. The most convincing evidence of the relationship between SIDS and hyperthermia was reported by Stanton [20], who found that 32 of 34 cases (94%) of SIDS victims were excessively clothed in an unusually warm environment or were hot and sweaty when found dead. In these cases, sweat and high rectal temperature suggested the presence of hyperthermia.

   The mechanisms leading to hyperthermia in SIDS include:

Table 2.9 Risk factors that contribute to SIDS

General factors	Hyperthermic factors
Maternal smoking	Prone position
Low birth weight	Bed-sharing with parents
IUGR	Excessive bedding
Twins	
Opiate addiction	
Young maternal age	
Maternal alcohol consumption	
Deprived socio-economic status	
Polystyrene-filled cushions	
Sibling with a history of SIDS	

* Excessive wrapping, thick bedding, high environmental temperature (such as proximity to a heat source) and a prone position, which may further limit heat loss through the face in the presence of over-wrapping. Side-sleeping is not as safe as supine sleeping.
* Mild infection, commonly preceding SIDS, may produce fever, which in combination with excessive wrapping could produce heat stroke and SIDS.
* Bed-sharing infants experience warmer thermal environment than those sleeping in a cot.
* In addition, a period of thermoregulatory imbalance may exist during infancy where heat production in relation to surface area reaches a maximum by about 5 months of age while dissipation of heat by sweating develops more slowly over the first year of life.

Drug-Induced Hyperthermia

* Anticholinergic poisoning. The dominant clinical features are:

Central: confusion, agitation, hallucination and seizures
Peripheral: dry mucous membranes, thirst, flushed face, blurred vision, dilated pupils and hyperthermia

The hyperthermia is mainly caused by decreased sweating.
Drugs with anticholinergic activity include:

Antispasmodic:	e.g.	belladonna, propantheline
Antiemetic	e.g.	hyoscine, cyclizine, promethazine
Atypical antipsychotic	e.g.	Olanzapine
Bronchodilator	e.g.	Ipratroprium
Antihistamine	e.g.	Chlorpheneramine
Antidepressant	e.g.	amitriptyline, imipramine

Hyoscyamine is one of the principal alkaloid components of belladonna. Hyoscyamine sulphate drops are sometimes prescribed for infantile colic. Herbal tea and Chinese herbal medicine have also caused anticholinergic poisoning and hyperthermia.

Treatment includes rapid and aggressive cooling. The specific antidote is physiostigmine. Benzodiazepines are also effective.
Other hyperthermia-induced drugs include:

* Topiramate is an anticonvulsant drug with a beneficial effect on various seizure disorders. Side-effects include hypohidrosis (or anhidrosis) causing hyperthermia, which is manifested as prolonged or intermittent elevated body temperature. The decreased production of sweat can by confirmed by pilocarpine iontophoresis sweat test.

In a study of 277 children on topiramate, 161 (58%) developed adverse events, including nervousness, weight loss and hyperthermia [21]. These side-effects disappeared in most cases after reducing the dose. They are rare on monotherapy. The hyperthermia is probably due to inhibition of carbonic anhydrase in human eccrine sweat glands.

* Salicylate poisoning: see Chap. 10, Management of fever

2.4.3
Unclassified Hyperthermia

Factitious Hyperthermia (FF)

The creation of fever by manipulation (usually thermometer manipulation) is rare in children, particularly below the adolescent age. However factitious hyperthermia is occasionally encountered in the differential diagnosis of PUO, occurring in about 2% of a large study of mainly adult cases [22]. It can be the most difficult diagnosis to establish. For example, an adolescent of 15 years of age from the USA with an 8-month history of fever was described [23]. It is true to say that the question as to whether a patient actually has a fever or not is rarely raised.

Many patients with FF appear to seek attention and feel protected in a hospital environment. Occasionally it is an escape from intolerable conditions at home. Methods commonly used by these patients to induce FF include holding the thermometer next to a hot-water bottle, rubbing it against bedclothes, rinsing the mouth with a hot liquid before inserting a thermometer or switching thermometers.

Diagnostic clues include:

* Discrepancy between the generally well appearance and the recorded "fever"
* The absence of warm skin, sweating, tachycardia and the usual diurnal variation of the fever
* Normal laboratory findings, e.g. inflammatory markers: leukocytes, CRP
* Normal body temperature when a nurse attends the temperature recording

Induced Illness (Factitious Illness, Munchausen's syndrome)

This is the most extreme form of factitious disorder. In 1951, Asher described patients who fabricated illnesses and subjected themselves to medical investigations and treatment, including operation [24]. Although principally an adult disease, the syndrome has also been reported in children [25] and is characterized by features shown in Table 2.10.

In a review of literature over 30 years [26], 42 children (mean age 13.9 years) with falsified illness were identified. The most commonly falsified conditions were fevers (13%). The deception was carried out by warming thermometers with heating pads.

Induced Illness by Proxy (Factitious illness by proxy)

In 1977 Meadow reported two children whose parents by fabrication caused them to undergo innumerable, harmful medical procedures [27]. In a second report in 1982 [28] Meadow presented 19 children under the age of 7 years (above this age children are likely to reveal the deception) of which four had fever as the fabricated sign (incidence of fever generally is around 10%). Meadow considered epilepsy to be the most frequently fabricated illness. Mortality rate among children diagnosed is 9%.

The syndrome involves a parent or caregiver who fabricates an illness in a child. The motivation for the perpetrator's behaviour is a psychological need to have the child assume the sick role. The perpetrator tends to be young and articulate, and often has personality disorders and significant family dysfunction. The syndrome is characterized by:

* Discrepancy between history, clinical findings and the child's healthy appearance
* Mother appears less worried about the child's illness than medical staff
* The child's "illness" is recurrent and cannot be explained medically
* There is a history of multiple medical procedures
* Symptoms and signs disappear in the mother's absence
* Mother usually attentive and present in hospital
* Once confronted, the perpetrator typically denies any knowledge

Clinical presentations generally follow two patterns:

* Apnoea, seizures, and cyanosis (seen commonly during infancy)
* Diarrhoea, vomiting, and fevers (seen commonly in older children)

Table 2.10 Main features of induced illness

Essential features
Pathologic lying
Simulation of a disease
Wondering
Minor features
Unusual or dramatic history
Previous treatment in hospital
Previous diagnostic procedures
Multiple scars
Experience in a medical field
Antisocial personality trait

Although the majority of fabricated illnesses are not life threatening, recurrent episodes of cardio-respiratory arrest induced by a mother have been reported, suggesting that Munchausen syndrome by proxy is a form of child abuse. A report of 56 children supported this view: a substantial proportion of the victims sustained failure to thrive, non-accidental injury, inappropriate medication or neglect [29].

The possibility of fabrication needs to be considered in any child with:

* Unexplained, persistent or recurrent illnesses
* Discrepancy between the fabricated symptom and the general health of the child
* Disappearance of the illness when the mother is away from the child

2.4.4
Therapeutic Effects of Hyperthermia

It has been known for thousands of years that hyperthermia helps the body against some diseases. In the 1970s and 1980s several trials showed that hyperthermia combined with radiation or chemotherapy produced better anticancer treatment over radiation and chemotherapy alone. Therapeutic application of hyperthermia and the means to produce it are shown in the Table 2.11. Its potential use includes:

* **Infectious diseases.** Hyperthermia stimulates the immune system, including production of interferon (INF). Examples of diseases treated by hyperthermia are:

  - Wagner von Jauregg in 1917 treated neurosyphilis with malarial fever, for which he won the Nobel Prize (see Chap. 13). The best results of fever therapy were observed in gonorrhoea and syphilis, including their complications, such as arthritis, keratitis and orchitis. Approximately 70–80% of the cases treated were arrested using artificial hyperthermia or malarial fever in the range of 40.5–41.0°C for about 50 h administered in several sessions.
  - Viral naso-pharyngitis: Nasal insufflations of humidified air at 43°C showed suppression of symptoms in 78% of patients [30].

Table 2.11 Therapeutic application of hyperthermia (or fever) and means of producing it

Application of heat:	Local
	    Deep (<3 cm under the skin)
	    Superficial
	Regional
	    Deep (<3 cm under the skin)
	    Superficial
	Whole body

Externally-produced heat	Microwave, thermal blanket, lasers, heating rods, infrared radiation, high frequency electrotherapy, ultrasound, extracorporeal
Internally-produced heat	Pyrogens (bacterial substance producing fever; Fever Therapy)

- Human immunodeficiency virus (HIV)-Infection: Temperatures of $\geq 42°C$ maintained for ≥ 25 min have been shown to inactivate approximately 25% of the HIV [31]. A daily use of such temperatures lower the population of actively infected cells by 40%. A reduction of the virus by 40% would effectively reverse the depletion of T-cells. HIV-infected cells are more sensitive to heat than healthy lymphocytes. This susceptibility increases when the cells are pre-treated with tumour necrosis factor.

* **Musculoskeletal disorders.** Local and regional hyperthermia has been used since ancient times to treat musculoskeletal disorders. Tissue heated at 44°C increases extensibility of the tissue, decreases joint stiffness and muscle spasms. These effects occur mainly through increased blood flow. Whole body hyperthermia also induces soluble tumour necrosis factor receptors (TNF-R), which is an anti-inflammatory product.
* **Cancer.** Therapeutic hyperthermia as an adjunctive therapy has been used since the 1970s to treat patients with cancer, yielding some positive results with complete or partial remission of the tumours. There is evidence that hyperthermia of 42°C or greater is tumouricidal. Hyperthermia has been shown to synergistically enhance the radiation response and cytotoxicity of chemotherapy. This effect of cell death is mainly caused by protein denaturation at a hyperthermic range of 40–44°C. Hyperthermia also causes acidosis, which decreases cell viability.

Hyperthermia in combination with chemotherapy has been shown to be effective in:

* Some patients with advanced malignancies, e.g. renal cell carcinoma [32]
* Lymphomas regress better than with chemotherapy alone
* In the management of retinoblastoma, which has gradually changed over the past 10–15 years: enucleation is preferable only for a large tumour that fills most of the globe [33]. Over 95% of children with retinoblastoma are cured with modern techniques. These include the use of transpupillary thermotherapy alone or in combination with systemic chemotherapy (chemothermotherapy).

Most normal tissues are undamaged by treatment for one hour at a temperature of up to 44°C. Possible adverse reactions include pain, unpleasant sensation and burn at the site of hyperthermia and rarely, neuropathy.

References

Clinical Effects of Hyperthermia

1. Bynum GD, Pandolf KB, Schuette WH, et al. Induced hyperthermia in sedated humans and the concept of critical thermal maximum. Am J Physiol 1978; 235: R228–36

Malignant hyperthermia (MH)

2. Girard T, Joehr M, Schaefer C, et al. Perinatal diagnosis of malignant hyperthermia susceptibility. Anesthesiology 2006; 104: 1353–6

3. Caroff SN, Mann SC. Neuroleptic malignant syndrome. Med Clin North Am 1993; 77: 185–202
4. Nierenberg D, Disch M, Manheimer E, et al. Facilitating prompt diagnosis and treatment of the neuroleptic malignant syndrome. Clin Pharmacol Ther 1991; 50: 580–6
5. Shalev A, Hermesh H, Munitz H. Mortality from neuroleptic malignant syndrome. J Clin Psychol 1989; 50: 18–25

Serotonin sydrome (SS)

6. Halloran L, Bernard DW. Management of drug-induced hyperthermia. Curr Opin Pediatr 2004; 16: 211–5

Exercise-Induced Hyperthermia

7. Bar-Or O. Climate and the exercising child-review. Int J Sports Med 1980; 1: 53–65
8. Committee on sports medicine. Climatic heat stress and the exercising child. Pediatrics 1982; 69: 808–9

Endocrine Hyperthermia

9. Simon HB, Daniels GH. Hormonal hyperthermia, endocrinological causes of fever. Am J Med 1979; 66: 257–63
10. Kilbane BJ, Mehta S, Backeljauw PF, et al. Approach to management of malignant hyperthermia-like syndrome in pediatric diabetes mellitus. Pediatr Crit Care Med 2006; 7: 169–73
11. Goodman EL, Knochel JP. Endocrine hyperthermia. Heat stroke and other forms of hyperthermia. In: Mackowiak P (ed.). Fever: Basic Mechanisms and Management. Raven, New York, 1991; 281

Neonatal Hyperthermia

12. Craig Ws. The early detection of pyrexia in the newborn. Arch Dis Child 1963; 38: 29–39

Heat Stroke

13. Knochel JP. Environmental heat loss. Arch Intern Med 1974; 133: 841–65
14. McLaren C, Null J, Quinn J. Heat stroke from enclosed vehicles: moderate ambient temperatures cause significant temperature rise in enclosed vehicles. Pediatrics 2005; 116: e109–12
15. Van Gestel JPJ, L'Hoir MP, ten-Berge M, et al. Risk of ancient parties in modern times. Pediatrics 2002; 110: e78

Hemorrhagic shock and encephalopathy (HSE)

16. Levin M, Kay JDS, Gould JD, et al. Hemorrhagic shock and encephalopathy. A new syndrome with high mortality in young children. Lancet 1983; 2: 64–7
17. Levin M, Pincott JR, Hjelm M, et al. Haemorrhagic shock and encephalopathy: clinical, pathologic, and biochemical features. J Pediatr 1989; 114: 194–203

Sudden death infant syndrome (SIDS)

18. American Academy of Pediatrics. The changing concept of SIDS: diagnosis, coding shifts, controversies regarding the sleeping environment. New variables to consider in reducing risk. Pediatrics 2005; 116: 1245–55.
19. Blair PS, Sidebotham P, Berry PJ, et al. Major epidemiological changes in SIDS: a 20-year population-based study in the UK. Lancet 2006; 367: 314–9
20. Stanton AN. Overheating and cot death. Lancet 1984; 3: 1199–201

Drug-Induced Hyperthermia

21. Grosso S, Franzoni E, Iannetti P, et al. Efficacy and safety of topiramate in refractory epilepsy. J Child Neurol 2005; 20: 893–7

Unclassified Hyperthermia

Factitious hyperthermia

22. Rumans LW, Vosti KL. Factitious and fraudulent fever. Am J Med 1978; 65: 745–55
23. Edwards MS, Butler KM. Hyperthermia of trickery in an adolescent. Pediatr Infect Dis J 1987; 6: 411–4

Induced Illness

24. Asher R. Munchausen's syndrome. Lancet 1951; 1: 339–41
25. Sneed RC, Bell RF. The dauphin of Munchausen: factitious passage of renal stones in a child. Pediatrics 1976; 58: 127–30
26. Libow JA. Child and adolescent illness falsification. Pediatrics 2000; 105: 336–42

Induced Illness by Proxy

27. Meadow R. Munchausen syndrome by proxy: the hinterland of child abuse. Lancet 1977; 2: 343–5
28. Meadow R. Munchausen syndrome by proxy. Arch Dis Child 1982; 57: 92–8

29. Bools CN, Neale BA, Meadow SR. Co-morbidity associated with fabricated illness (Munchausen syndrome by proxy). Arch Dis Child 1992; 67: 77–9

Therapeutic Effects of Hyperthermia

30. Yerurshalmi A, Lwoff A. Traitement du coryza infectieux et des rhinitis persistantes allergiques par la thermotherapy. C R Seances Acad Sci D 1980; 291: 957–9
31. Pennypacker C, Perelson AS, Nys N. Localized or systemic in vivo heat inactivation of HIV: a mathematical analysis. J Acquir Immune Defic Syndr Hum Retrovirol 1995; 8: 321–9
32. Ismail ZRS, Zhavrid EA, Potapnev MP. Whole body hyperthermia in adjuvant therapy of children with renal cell carcinoma. Pediatr Blood Cancer 2005; 44: 679–81
33. Shields CL, Meadows AT, Leahey AM, et al. Continuing challenges in the management of retinoblastoma with chemotherapy. Retina 2004; 24: 849–62

Pathogenesis of Fever

3

Core Messages

> Although infection is the most common cause of fever, fever is also a common finding in hypersensitivity reaction, autoimmune diseases, and malignancy.

> Febrile response is mediated by endogenous pyrogens (cytokines) in response to invading exogenous pyrogens, primarily microorganisms or their direct products (toxins).

> These endogenous pyrogens act on thermosensitive neurons in the hypothalamus, which ultimately upgrade the set point via prostaglandins.

> The body reacts by increasing the heat production and decreasing the heat loss until the body temperature reaches this elevated set point.

> Fever, in contrast to hyperthermia, will not climb up relentlessly because of an effective central control of the hypothalamic center.

> Cytokines play a pivotal role in the immune response by activation of the B cells and T lymphocytes. The production of fever simultaneously with lymphocyte activation constitutes the clearest and strongest evidence in favor of the protective role of fever.

> The protective processes of the immune response are optimal at high temperature (around 39.5°C).

> Not all effects resulting from fever generation benefit the host; some are harmful and even lethal. This occurs mainly by overproduction of the cytokines or imbalance between cytokines and their inhibitors, such as severe and fulminate infections and septic shock.

A.S. El-Radhi et al. (Eds.) *Clinical Manual of Fever in Children.*
Doi: 10.1007/978-3-540-78598-9, © Springer-Verlag Berlin Heidelberg 2009

3

3.1
History of Research

Research in fever has been centered on the hypothesis that fever results from physiological processes that are set in motion by an external stimulus. Egyptian scholars recognized that local inflammation was responsible for fever. In 1868, Billroth (1829–1894) attempted to confirm this ancient observation by injecting pus into animals, thereby producing a febrile response. In 1943, Menkin carried out similar experiments and isolated a product termed "pyrexin" [1]. Beeson in 1948 isolated a fever-inducing substance from a leukocyte, leukocyte pyrogens, which later became known as endogenous pyrogen (EP). Interleukin-1 (IL-1) was first identified as a cytokine by Gery and Waksman and proved to be identical with EP [2].

3.2
Definitions

* **Fever (pyrexia)** is a regulated body temperature above the normal range occurring as a result of IL-1-mediated elevation of the hypothalamic set point. Once fever is established, body temperature is regulated, as in health, by a net balance between heat production and loss.
* **Hyperthermia** is unregulated elevated body temperature above the normal range due to imbalance between heat production and loss. Interleukins are not involved and therefore the hypothalamic set point is normal.
* A **pyrogen** is a substance (infectious organisms or their product toxins, or cytokines) that provokes fever.
* **Exogenous pyrogens** are substances that originate outside the body and that are capable of inducing interleukins.
* **Endogenous pyrogens** are substances that originate inside the body and that are capable of inducing fever by acting on the hypothalamic thermoregulatory center. IL-1, tumour necrosis factor (TNF) and interferon (INF) are endogenous pyrogens.
* **Cytokines** are proteins produced throughout the body, mainly by monocytes, macrophages, and T cells to regulate the immune responses within the body and control inflammatory and haematopoietic processes and may induce fever. As they enter the circulation and act on distant organs, they are considered as hormones. Cytokines are pro-inflammatory cytokines, anti-inflammatory cytokines, interleukins, or lymphokines.
* **Pro-inflammatory cytokines** (IL-1, IL-6, TNF-α, INF-γ, granulocyte-macrophage colony-stimulating factor, GM-CSF) are responsible for initiating an effective defense against exogenous organisms. Their overproduction may be harmful by causing shock, multiple organ failure, and death.
* **Anti-inflammatory cytokines** (IL-1 receptor antagonist, IL-4, IL-10) antagonize pro-inflammatory cytokines. Their overproduction may also be harmful by suppressing the immune function.
* **Interleukins** are cytokines acting specifically as mediators between leukocytes, and hence their name. If their amino acid sequence is known, they are assigned an

interleukin number. If their sequence is not known, then they are named according to the biological property. IL-1 and IL-6 play a major part in the pathogenesis of fever.

* **Lymphokines** are cytokines that are secreted by lymphocytes (IL-2, IL-3, IL-4, IL-5, IL-6, IL-9, IL-10, IL-13, IL-14, TNF-β).
* **Acute-phase response** is the term used for haematological, endocrinological, and metabolic changes that follow (within hours or days) the onset of fever in response to local damage to a tissue. These changes are induced by several cytokines and are beneficial to the host. During the response, various acute-phase proteins, notably C-reactive protein (CRP) and serum amyloid A, are synthesized by liver and released into circulation in large amounts. CRP plays a role in complement activation, opsonization (engulfing and destroying microbes by phagocytes), and increasing platelet aggregation.

3.3
Exogenous Pyrogens (Fig. 3.1)

Exogenous Pyrogens (ExPs) initiate fever, usually within 2 h of exposure, by interacting with macrophages or monocytes, leading to IL-1 induction. Other mechanisms to initiate fever include the following:

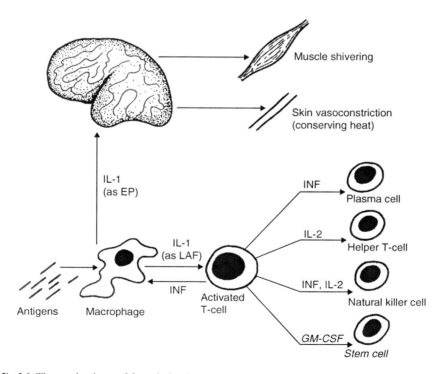

Fig. 3.1 The mechanisms of fever induction

3

- Some endotoxins, produced by bacteria, act directly on the hypothalamus to alter the set point. IL-1 is not involved. Radiation of the hypothalamus, DDT (dichloro-diphenyl trichloroethane) poisoning, and scorpion venom may also induce fever by a direct effect on hypothalamus.
- ExPs may activate lymphocytes to secrete lymphokines, particularly INF-y, which in turn stimulate macrophages and monocytes to produce IL-1.
- Some bacteria produce exotoxins that stimulate macrophages and monocytes to release IL-1. This mechanism operates in scarlet fever and toxic shock syndrome. In toxic shock syndrome, the shock is due to the toxin. Diseases involving exotoxins produced by Gram-positive bacilli are less fever inducing than those produced by pyrogenic Gram-positive cocci.
- *Borrelia spirochetes* (the cause of relapsing fever) do not contain endotoxin, and the attachment of these bacteria to the mononuclear cells induces the production of IL-1.
- Other bacteria, such as pneumococci, have no endotoxin or other pyrogens, and the mechanisms responsible for fever are presumably immunological.

3.3.1
Microbial Pyrogens

- **Gram-negative bacteria.** The pyrogenicity of Gram-negative bacteria (e.g., *Escherichia coli*, Salmonella) is due to a heat-stable factor, endotoxin. The active components are lipid and carbohydrate (lipopolysaccharide, LPS) elements of the outer membrane of these bacteria. Endotoxin causes a dose-related progressive increase in temperature. In severe cases, it causes vasodilatation, capillary leakage, and hypotension. Infection with Gram-negative endotoxin (e.g., septicemia) does not elicit fever in many situations:
  - **Neonates**, young infants, children with fulminating infection with septic shock (complicates septicemia in 20% of cases) and with malnutrition may present with normal temperature or hypothermia.
  - **Septicemia** presenting with hypothermia is a well-known clinical entity possibly due to inhibition of IL-6 and IL-1 by IL-10 [3].
- **Gram-positive bacteria.** The main pyrogen of staphylococci is peptidglycan of the cell wall. Endotoxin is more active per unit weight than peptidoglycan, which may explain the comparatively worse prognosis associated with Gram-negative infection.
- **Viruses.** It is well known in clinical practice that viruses cause fever. Mechanisms by which viruses may produce fever include direct invasion of macrophages, immunological reaction to viral components involving antibody formation, induction by INF, and necrosis of cells by viruses.
- **Fungi.** Live or killed fungal products are exogenous pyrogens that induce fever. The induction of fever mainly occurs when the fungi are in the bloodstream. Children with neoplastic diseases who develop fever associated with neutropenia are at high risk for developing invasive fungal infection.

3.3.2
Non-Microbial Pyrogens

* **Phagocytosis** is largely responsible for fever in blood transfusion reactions (once an infection is excluded) and immune hemolytic anaemia.
* **Antigen–antibody complexes.** An exogenous antigen may react with circulating, sensitized antibodies to form a complex that induces IL-1 production (immune fever). Examples of immunologically mediated fever include systemic lupus erythematosis and adverse drug reactions. Fever associated with penicillin hypersensitivity results from interaction of antigen–antibody complexes with leukocytes, which release IL-1.
* **Other non-microbial pyrogens** include some hormones, drugs, and intracranial lesions such as bleeding and thrombosis.
* **Steroids.** These are endogenous antipyretics, which suppress fever development through its inhibitory effects on IL-1 and TNF-α production. Certain steroids, however, are pyrogenic in humans. The most known steroid is etiocholanolone, an androgenic metabolite that may induce the release of IL-1. This steroid produces fever only when injected intramuscularly (not intravenously), hence fever may result from IL-1 released by subcutaneous tissue at the injection site. This steroid is thought to be responsible for fever in a few patients with adrenogenital syndrome and fevers of unknown origin.

3.4
Monocyte–Macrophage System (Fig. 3.2)

Mononuclear cells are leukocytes (3–8% of the leukocytes) and are largely responsible for the production of IL-1 and fever induction. Polymorphonuclear granulocytes are no longer thought to be responsible for IL-1 production because fever may occur in their absence, for example agranulocytosis. The mononuclear cells are either circulating monocytes in the peripheral blood or tissue macrophages (histocytes) scattered in organs such as lung (alveolar macrophages), lymphnodes, placenta, peritoneal cavity, and the subcutaneous tissue. The origin of both monocytes and macrophages is the granulocytes–monocyte colony-forming unit (GM–CFU) in the bone marrow. Monocytes enter the circulation either to remain there for a few days as circulating monocytes or to migrate to the tissue where they undergo functional and morphological transformation into macrophages, when their life span is several months. These cells play an important role in:

* Host defense, including engulfing and destroying the microbe (phagocytosis), recognition of antigen, and presenting it to attached lymphocytes and
* Activation of T lymphocytes and tumor cell destruction.

Situations associated with reduced function of the monocyte–macrophage system (MMS) include newborn infants, corticosteroid and other immunosuppressive therapy, systemic lupus erythematous, Wiskot–Aldrich syndrome (immune deficiency involving B and T cells, eczema, and thrombocytopenia), and chronic granulomatous disease. The two major monocyte–macrophage products (cytokines) are IL-1 and TNF.

3

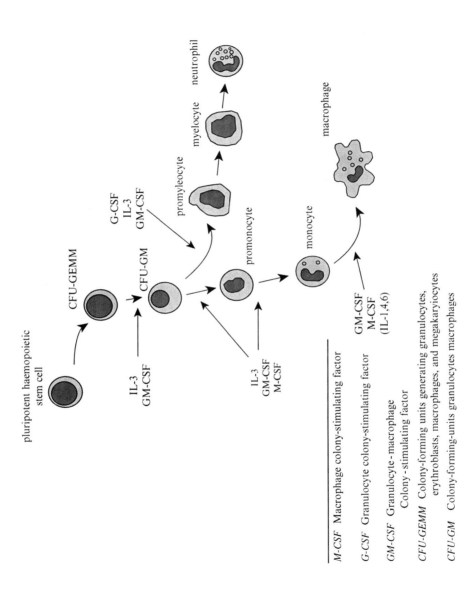

Fig. 3.2 Monocytes and Macrophages

3.5
Endogenous Pyrogens

3.5.1
Interleukin-1 (IL-1)

IL-1 is stored in an inactive form in the cytoplasm of secreting cells and is enzymatically converted to an active form before it is released across the cell membrane into the circulation. It affects distant organs and therefore acts as a hormone. The kidney is the principal site for its removal.

IL-1 consists of three structurally related polypeptides, two agonists (IL-1 α and IL-1β), and an antagonist (IL-1 receptor antagonist = IL-1ra) that inhibits the activities of the two agonists. The relative amount of IL-1 and IL-1ra in a disease influences whether the inflammation remains active or suppressed. IL-1 is produced by:

- Macrophages as the main source of IL-1 production.
- Hepatic Kupffer cells, keratinocytes, pancreatic Langerhans's cells.
- Astrocytes in the brain tissue, which may contribute to the immunological responses within the CNS and the fever secondary to CNS bleeding.
- Cells from certain malignant tumors (e.g., Hodgkin's disease, acute leukemia and renal carcinoma). This explains the frequent association of fever in these conditions in the absence of infection. and
- Monocytes in the circulation and reticuloendothelial system.

Interleukin-1 has multiple functions (Fig. 3.3):

- Induction of fever by acting on the hypothalamus to raise its set point.
- Playing a primary role in the induction of inflammatory responses, such as neutrophil accumulation and adherence, and vascular changes. IL-1 also mediates to neuro-inflammation and cell death in head injury.
- Playing an essential role in T-cell and B-cell proliferation and activation.

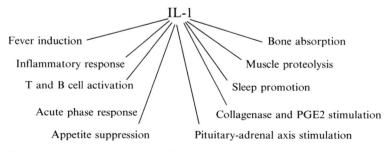

Fig. 3.3 Summary of the main functions of IL-1

- Stimulating the liver to synthesize certain acute-phase proteins, such as fibrinogen, haptoglobin, ceruloplasmin, and CRP. At the same time, the synthesis of albumin and transferrin decreases. Characteristically, there is a decreased concentration of iron and zinc and an increased concentration of copper. The low iron is the result of reduced intestinal assimilation of iron and increased liver storage of iron. These changes contribute to host defense by depriving invading microorganisms of essential nutrients, such as iron and zinc (The process is referred to as nutritional immunity).
- Appetite suppression, which results in a significant reduction of food intake, seen commonly in febrile illness [4]. This process occurs within the brain. IL-1 receptor antagonist attenuates the appetite-reducing effects by IL-1.
- Stimulating osteoclast differentiation and activation, resulting in bone loss.
- Production of Factor S, a peptide identical to IL-1 with sleep promotion effect leading to slow-wave sleep. It is produced in astrocytes of the brain. The factor may explain the observation of increased sleep in febrile illnesses.
- Stimulating the production of collagenase and prostaglandin E2 (PGE2), which play a major role in the pathogenic progression of various arthritides, particularly rheumatoid arthritis.
- Stimulating the pituitary–adrenal axis, causing increasing production of glucocorticoid hormones.
- Increasing protein breakdown, leading to myalgia, which commonly accompanies fever. This proteolysis, mediated by PGE2, is blocked by the PGE2 inhibitor indomethacin. Amino acids released during proteolysis can be metabolized within the muscle as a direct source of energy and are reused for the synthesis of new proteins. Other amino acids may become substrates for gluconeogensis.

In all these circumstances the activity of IL-1 is enhanced at elevated temperatures. Antagonism of IL-1 (IL-1ra) has therapeutic effects in many diseases, including:

- Various forms of hereditary periodic syndromes and neonatal-onset multisystem inflammatory disease (Chap. 1).
- HIV replication. IL-1ra has suppressive effects on the virus.
- Bone erosions and loss, occurring, for example, in rheumatoid arthritis.

There is little or no IL-1 in healthy humans at rest. A long list of diseases, including meningitis, septicemia, Crohn's disease, rheumatoid arthritis, neonatal hypoxic–ischaemic encephalopathy, and acute organ rejection are associated with increased levels of IL-1 and poor outcome for the patients. Malnutrition (kwashiorkor and marasmus), on the other hand, is associated with a significant impairment of macrophage function and IL-1 production.

3.5.2
Tumour Necrosis Factor (TNF)

TNF, discovered in 1968, is a cytokine produced by monocytes and microphages (TNF-α), lymphocytes (TNF-β), natural killer cells, Kupffer cells, and astrocytes of the brain in response to invasive or injurious stimuli. Like IL-1, TNF is regarded as an endogenous pyrogen because its acts on the hypothalamus to induce fever. Unlike IL-1, TNF has no direct effect on stem-cell and lymphocyte activation. TNF in small quantities has diverse beneficial biological effects, including:

* Sharing many biological properties with IL-1, for example, enhancing host defense against infection, promoting normal tissue remolding, including wound healing, and enhancing chemotaxis of macrophages and neutrophils as well as increasing their phagocytic and cytotoxic activity.
* Being the earliest and most important mediator of inflammation.
* Stimulating IL-1 production.
* Having a direct effect against certain tumor cells (e.g., by damaging the nuclear DNA and producing free radicals). Its use against human cancers, however, has been associated with poor outcome, mainly due to its systemic side effects.

When large amounts are released in tissue, however, TNF may lead to.

* Lethal tissue injury and shock (septic or toxic shock).
* Wasting (TNF is identical to cachectin), by inhibiting the activity of lipoprotein lipase, and producing negative nitrogen balance and glucose release, often associated with chronic infection and some tumors.

High serum levels of TNF correlate with the activity and prognosis of many infectious diseases, including bacterial meningitis, leishmaniasis, human immunodeficiency virus (HIV) infection, malaria, and intestinal inflammatory diseases. Increased TNF production in Kawasaki disease may play a role in the immune activation and damage to vascular endothelial cells occurring in the disease.

3.5.3
Interleukin-6

IL-6 is the third most studied cytokines. It is:

* A pro-inflammatory cytokine that is secreted by macrophages and T lymphocytes to stimulate immune response
* Synergistic with IL-1 and TNF-α, including induction of fever (Il-6 responds earlier than IL-1) and acute phase response. It parallels the duration of fever. Il-6 is an early marker (within 3–4 h of endotoxin stimulation)
* A stimulator on both B and T cell function
* Increased in many diseases, for example, sepsis, autoimmune diseases and juvenile idiopathic arthritis, Kawasaki disease, and epidural fever [5]

Anti-IL-6 receptor is available to treat IL-6-related immune-inflammatory diseases.
Other cytokines with their main effects are shown in Table 3.1.

Table 3.1 Common lymphokines produced by T cells and their main effect/use

Interleukin	Effects
IL-3	Stimulatory effect on haematopoietic cells (important after myelotoxic treatment with chemotherapy)
IL-4 (and IL-13, 14)	B-cell differentiation, induces IgE
IL-5	B-cell differentiation, eosinophil and IgA production
IL-7 (and IL-27)	Regulates B and T cells, natural killer (NK) cells
IL-8	Proinflammatory cytokine, potent neutrophil chemo-attractant and activator
IL-9	Stimulation the growth of mast cells and erythroid progenitor cells
IL-10 (& IL-20)	Inhibition of Th1 cell production, including Th1-dependent IL-2, and proinflammatory cytokines, implicated in inflammatory process of JIA and development of haematopoietic cells
Il-11 (and IL-22)	Production of acute phase proteins. IL-11 is effective for chemotherapy-induced thrombocytopenia
IL-12	Inhibition of IL-1 synthesis; plays a role in defence against mycobacteria and salmonella
IL-13 (and IL-14, 17)	Stimulating activated B cells to proliferate and produce IgM, IgG, and IgE
IL-16	Chemo-attracts immune cells
IL-17 (and IL-23)	Mediating the inflammatory differentiation of T cells
IL-18	Induces IFN-γ from T lymphocyte and natural killer cells but does not induce fever
Il-28 (and IL-29)	Playing a role in host defense against microorganisms
Il-31 (and IL-32, 33)	Induction of cytokines (TNF, Il-8) and helper T cells

3.6
Activated Lymphocytes

The antigen-specific cells of the immune system are lymphocytes, of which there are two main types:

- B cells are responsible for antibody production, whereas;
- T cells regulate antibody synthesis and mediate cytotoxic function as well as inflammatory response of delayed-type hypersensitivity. T-cells are either:
  - Th1 cells, which produce INF-γ, IL-2, and TNF-β and promote cell-mediated immunity and phagocytic activity, or
  - Th2 cells that produce Il-4, IL-5, IL-6, IL-9, and IL-10. These promote antibody production and play a crucial role in allergic responses (immediate-type hypersensitivity).

IL-1 has an essential role in the activation of lymphocytes. The T lymphocyte recognizes antigen only after the antigens are processed and presented to them by macrophages; only then do T lymphocytes become active.

3.6.1
Interferon (INF)

Interferon is known for its ability to 'interfere' (hence the name) with viral replication in infected cells. There are three molecules, TNF-α, β, and γ, differing in biological activity and amino-acid sequences. INF-α and INF-β are produced by a variety of cells (such as leukocytes, fibroblasts, and macrophages) in response to viral infection, whereas synthesis of INF-γ is restricted to T lymphocytes. Although the T cells from normal neonates function as effectively as those in adults, INF (particularly INF-γ) is considerably reduced, which may contribute to the increased severity of viral infections in newborn infants. The functions of the INF-γ include:

- Macrophage and fever inducing, either by acting indirectly on macrophages to release IL-1 (a macrophage-activating factor) or directly on the hypothalamic thermoregulatory
- Stimulating B cells to increase antibody production
- Potentiating the antiviral and cytolytic activity of TNF
- Increasing the efficiency of natural killer cells
- Exhibiting antitumor activity either directly by inhibiting cell division through increasing the length of the cell multiplication cycle or indirectly by altering the immune response

The antiviral and antitumor activities of INF are enhanced at elevated temperatures. IL-4, which induces the synthesis of immunoglobulins IgE and IgG4, is blocked by INF-γ and α, indicating that these cytokines act as antagonists of IL-4.
INF is used as a treatment for a variety of illnesses, including

- Various viral infections, such as hepatitis B, C by INF-α
- Upper respiratory tract infection. INF-α in a nasal spray is capable of significantly reducing symptoms due to rhinoviruses, but not those due to influenza viruses, parainfluenza viruses, or coronaviruses
- Thrombocytosis associated with myeloproliferative disorders
- Hairy-cell leukaemia, which remains one of the most important indications for INF-α therapy, showing a response rate of more than 90%
- Childhood angiomatous disease results from INF-antiproliferative effect and
- Non-Hodgkin's lymphoma, malignant melanoma, basal cell carcinoma and chronic myelogenous leukaemia

Toxic effects of INF preparations are numerous, which include fever, chills, arthralgia, myalgia, severe headaches, somnolence, and vomiting. Fever may occur in over 50% of the patients who receive INF and may reach 40.0°C. These side effects are responsive to paracetamol and prednisolone. Severe side effects include hepatic and cardiac failure, neuropathy and pancytopenia. INF therapy is contraindicated in pregnancy owing to its antiproliferative effect.

3.6.2
Interleukin-2 (IL-2)

IL-2 is probably the second most important lymphokine (after INF) that is released by activated T lymphocytes in response to IL-1 stimulation. It has an essential effect on the growth and function of T cells, natural killer cells, and B cells. Cases of severe congenital combined immunodeficiency due to a specific defect in the production of IL-2 have been reported. Its effects are:

* Antitumor cytotoxicity (e.g., against neuroblastoma, melanoma) as a result of proliferation and activation of activated cytotoxic T lymphocytes and
* Stimulating the release of other cytokines, including IL-1, TNF, and INF-γ

IL-2 immunotherapy often causes side effects such as

* A reversible defect of neutrophils chemotaxis, leading to increased susceptibility to infection and
* Those that include malaise, fever, anorexia, and myalgia

3.6.3
Granulocyte-Macrophage Colony-Stimulating Factor (GM-CSF)

Of the four hematopoietic-colony stimulating factors (erythropoietin, granulocyte-colony stimulating factor (G-CSF), macrophage-colony stimulating factor (M-CSF), and granulocyte-macrophage-colony stimulating factor (GM-CSF)), the latter (GM-CSF) appears to have the most potential clinical benefits .[6] It is a proinflammatory cytokine, which is produced mainly by lymphocytes, although monocytes, macrophages, and mast cells are also capable of producing it. GM-CSF's principal function and potential therapeutic uses are the following:

* As a treatment and prophylaxis of neonatal sepsis, possibly due to improved INF-γ secretion. Neonatal neutrophils lack INF-γ
* To stimulate hematopoietic progenitor cells to proliferate and differentiate into granulocytes and macrophages and regulate some of their functions at maturity
* To treat chemotherapy-induced neutropenia, myelodysplasia, aplastic anemia, and bone marrow transplant regimens

The administration of GM-CSF may be associated with the development of fever, which is blocked by nonsteroidal anti-inflammatory drugs such as ibuprofen.

3.7
Thermoregulation

Thermoregulation requires intact peripheral mechanisms that balance heat production and loss, and a functioning hypothalamic thermoregulatory center regulating these mechanisms.

3.7.1
Heat Production

Heat production occurs by various mechanisms:

* At rest, as many organs such as brain, muscles, viscera, liver, heart, thyroid, pancreas, and adrenal glands contribute to heat production at the cellular level involving adenosine triphosphate (ATP).
* In the newborn infant, brown fat localized mainly in the neck and scapular area produces heat through nonshivering thermogenesis. This tissue is highly vascularized and contains a large quantity of mitochondria. Fatty acid oxidation in these mitochondria can increase heat production to twofold in response to cold.
* Older children and adults conserve heat by vasoconstriction and generate heat by shivering in response to cold. Blood flow, regulated by the CNS, plays a vital role in distributing heat throughout the body. In a warm environment or when core temperature is elevated, the hypothalamic thermoregulatory center activates efferent fibers of the automatic nervous system to produce vasodilatation. The increased blood flow to the skin causes heat loss from the core through the skin surface to the surroundings in the form of sweating. In colder environments or with decreased core temperature, reduced skin blood flow promotes retention of body heat.

Pathological uncontrollable increase of heat production occurs in malignant hyperthermia (Chap. 2)

3.7.2
Heat Loss

In response to a rise in body temperature, heat is lost from the body via the four physical modalities of radiation, evaporation, convection, and conduction. Failure of heat loss has been incriminated as the cause of infantile heat stroke, which carries a high mortality rate. Heat loss occurs through the following mechanisms:

* In general, 60% of the total heat is lost by radiation, which is the transfer of heat from the skin surface to the external surroundings by mean of electromagnetic waves.
* About one-quarter is lost by evaporation from the skin and lungs, which occurs as water is converted from liquid to gas: 243 kJ (58 kcal) is lost for every 100 ml of water.
* Convection (12% of the heat loss) is the transfer of heat through the movement of air or fluid surrounding the skin surface.
* Conduction (3% of the heat loss) is the heat transfer between two objects in direct contact and at different temperatures. This is the primary mode of heat loss from the core to the surface. A child in the lying position with a large contact surface has a higher heat loss through conduction than in the standing position.

Simultaneously, the hypothalamus stimulates vasodilatation to increase insensible loss (for every 1°C elevation of body temperature, there is a 10% insensible loss) and activates the sweat glands to increase perspiration production.

Physical factors obviously affect the ability to respond to temperature changes. The greater heat loss in the newborn infant is mainly due to a greater surface area compared to that of an older child. Failure of heat loss occurs in anhidrotic ectodermal dysplasia and during anticholinergic drug overdose.

3.7.3
Temperature Regulation at the CNS Level

Fever generation includes the following stages:

* The specific area of the IL-1 action is the pre-optic and anterior hypothalamus, which contains clusters of thermosensitive neurons localized within the rostral wall of the third ventricle. The site is called organum vasculosum laminae terminalis (OVLT), which has emerged as an interface between circulation and brain. The firing rate of these thermosensitive neurons changes according to the temperature of the area's blood supply and the input from the skin and muscular thermoreceptors. Warm-sensitive neurons have firing rates that increase with warming and decrease with cooling, whereas the firing rates of cold-sensitive neurons increase with cooling or decrease with warming.
* IL-1 enters the perivascular space of the OVLT through the fenestrated capillary wall to stimulate cells to produce PGE2, which diffuses into the adjacent pre-optic/hypothalamic region to cause fever.

    The view that the OVLT is the major port of entry for pyrogenic cytokines has recently been challenged [7]. In the endothelial and perivascular cells of the blood–brain barrier (BBB), pyrogenic cytokines are switched to PGE2. These cells probably represent a structure termed *circumventricular organ system* (CVOS), which consists of small clusters of neurons and is adjacent to the BBB. This structure serves as a communication channel between blood and neurons of the hypothalamus. When circulating pyrogenic cytokines are detected by the CVOS, PGE2 is induced [8].
* The ultimate result of these complex mechanisms is an upward shift of the thermostatic set point to a febrile level that signals efferent nerves, especially sympathetic fibers innervating peripheral blood vessels, to initiate heat conservation (vasoconstriction) and heat production (shivering). This is aided by behavioral means aimed also to increase body temperature, such as seeking a warmer environment or covering up with a blanket. The resulting temperature increase continues until body temperature approximates to the temperature of the elevated set point. The cations Na^+ and Ca^{2+} as well as cyclic adenosine monophosphate (camp) may also contribute to the alteration of body temperature, although their exact role is not yet clear. The raised set point is reset back to normal if the concentration of IL-1 falls or if antipyretics are administered, which blocks prostaglandin synthesis. Recently, the peptide angiotensin 11 has been shown to lower body temperature at the final step of fever [9].

Prostaglandin E2 has been found to exert a negative feedback on the release of IL-1, thereby tending to terminate the mechanisms that initially induced the fever. In addition, arginine vasopressin (AVP) acts within the CNS to reduce pyrogen-induced fevers. The normalization of temperature is initiated by vasodilatation and sweating through increased skin blood flow controlled by sympathetic fibers.

3.8
Summary of Fever Induction

The generation of fever involves the following steps:

* Numerous substances from outside the body, exogenous pyrogens, initiate the fever cycle. Endotoxin of Gram-negative bacteria, with their pyrogenic component lipopolysaccaride, is the most potent ExP. Fever is also a common finding in children without obvious evidence of infection, for example, hypersensitivity reaction, autoimmune diseases, and malignancy.
* The ExPs stimulate monocytes, fixed-tissue macrophages, and reticuloendothelial cells to produce and release identical substances, now collectively termed IL-1, which has multiple biological functions essential for the immune response.
* IL-1 acts on the hypothalamic thermoregulatory center through mediators, of which PGE2 is the most important, to raise the thermostatic set point. IL-1 thereby acts as an endogenous pyrogen. The hypothalamic thermoregulatory center accomplishes heat production by inducing shivering and heat conservation through vasoconstriction. At an established degree, fever is regulated (even at a temperature of over $41.0^\circ C$) and heat production approximates loss, as in health, though at a higher level of the set point. Therefore fever does not climb up relentlessly.
* In addition to the function as an endogenous pyrogen, IL-1 activates T lymphocytes to produce various factors, such as INF and IL-2, which are vital for immune response. The production of fever simultaneously with lymphocyte activation constitutes the clearest and strongest evidence in favor of the role of fever.

References

1. Menkin V. Chemical basis of fever. Science 1944; 100: 337–8.
2. Gery I, Waksman BH. Potentiation of the lymphocyte response to mitogens: Cellular source pf potentiating mediators. J Exp Med 1972; 136: 143–54
3. Conti B, Tabarean I, Andrei C, et al. Cytokines and fever. Front Biosci 2004; 9: 1433–49
4. Reyes TM, Sawchenko PE. Involvement of the accurate nucleus of the hypothalamus in interleukin-1 induced anorexia. J Neurosci 2002; 22: 5091–99
5. Goetzl L, Evans T, Rivers J, et al. Elevated maternal and serum interleukin-6 levels are associated with epidural fever. Am J Obstet Gynecol 2002; 187: 834–8.
6. Modi N, Carr R. Promising stratagems for reducing the burden of neonatal SEPSIS. Arch Dis Child Fetal Neonatal Ed 2000; 83: 150–3
7. Romanovsky AA, Almeida MC, Aronoff DM, et al. Fever and hypothermia in systemic inflammation: Recent discoveries and revisions. Front Biosci 2005; 10: 2193–216
8. Biddle C. The neurobiology of the human febrile responses. AANA J 2006; 74: 145–51
9. Watanabe T, Miyoshi M, Imoto T. Angiotensin II: Its effects on fever and hypothermia in systemic inflammation. Front Biosci 2004; 9: 438–47

Measurement of Body Temperature

4

Core Messages

> Body temperature measurement is mainly indicated to confirm the presence or absence of fever.

> There remains considerable controversy among professionals regarding the most appropriate thermometer and the best anatomical site for temperature measurement.

> Medical staff should be aware of those clinical conditions that require accurate temperature measurement (e.g., febrile neutropenia) and those in which screening for fever may be adequate (maternal intrapartum).

> Core temperature is generally defined as the temperature measured within the pulmonary area.

> In an environment where ambient temperatures are stable (e.g., neonatal units), temperature recorded from the axilla is nearly as accurate that recorded from the rectal site.

> Although rectal temperature is a satisfactory reference standard for core temperature, it is reliable only if the body is in thermal balance and reacts slowly to changes in temperature.

> There is evidence to suggest that tympanic temperature accurately reflects pulmonary artery temperature even when body temperature is changing rapidly.

A.S. El-Radhi et al. (Eds.) *Clinical Manual of Fever in Children.*
Doi: 10.1007/978-3-540-78598-9, © Springer-Verlag Berlin Heidelberg 2009

4

4.1
Introduction

Body temperature measurement is most commonly performed to confirm the presence or absence of fever. Many decisions concerning the investigation and treatment of children are based on the results of temperature measurement alone. An incorrect temperature measurement could result in the delayed detection of a serious illness or alternatively an unnecessary septic workout.

Despite the plethora of instruments that have become available in the last 30 years, there remains considerable controversy as to the most appropriate thermometer and the best anatomical site (Fig. 4.1).

This chapter discusses different sites for temperature measurement, includes advantages and disadvantages of currently available techniques, and describes how the instruments work together with comments on their accuracy. It also makes recommendations based on available evidence and personal experience.

4.2
History of the Thermometer

The history of the thermometer began with the invention of the thermoscope by Heron of Alexandria who lived in the 1st century B.C [1]. This instrument was a glass vessel with a water column that was displaced in proportion to the amount of heat applied. The instrument was reinvented by Galileo Galilei (1564–1642) at the end of the sixteenth century. Temperature was recorded by transmission of air through a tube from the mouth to a container of water (Fig. 4.2, 4.3).

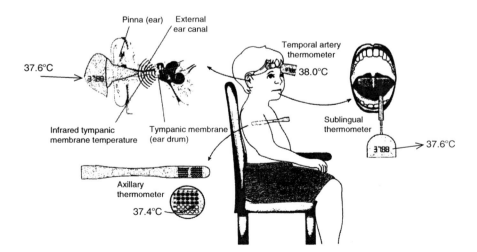

Fig. 4.1 Anatomical site of temperature readings showing febrile recordings from different sites

In the eighteenth century, thermometry made significant advances (Fig. 4.4). Gabriel Fahrenheit, a Polish physicist, invented the mercury thermometer in 1714, using salt, water, and ice. The freezing point of the system was 32°F and the boiling point 212°F. Anders Celsius of Sweden established the centigrade scale in 1742. A comparison of Celsius and Fahrenheit scales is shown in Fig. 4.5.

Carl Wunderlich, a professor of medicine in Leipzig, began in 1851 to collect data on one million measurements of body temperature. He used a foot-long thermometer, which had to be read *in situ* (under the axilla) and required 15–20 min to equilibrate. He noted that children react with higher temperature in response to infection as compared to adults. His work greatly influenced medical practice, ushering in the routine use of the thermometer.

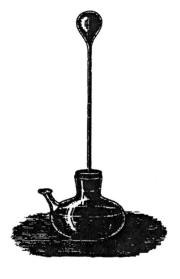

Fig. 4.2 The thermoscope, as invented by Galileo Galilei in 1592, was the first instrument to measure temperature. When the air in the bulb was warmed, the water column fell accordingly. (From Goerke H. *Medizin und Technik.* Verlag Callway, Munich, 1988)

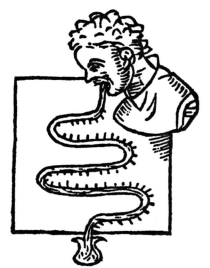

Fig. 4.3 The thermoscope, as invented by Santorio Sanctorius. The bulb was placed into the mouth of a patient. The rate of fluid displacement (measured by the equal graduations shown) indicated whether the patient had a fever. (From Goerke H. *Medizin und Technik.* Verlag Callway, Munich, 1988)

Measurement of Temperature

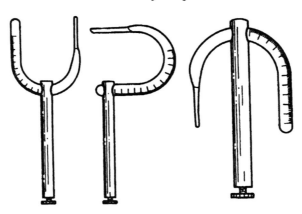

Fig. 4.4 The first thermometer was designed for insertion under the patient's tongue. (From *Br Med J* 1912; 1:1137)

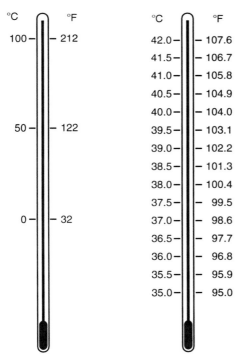

Fig. 4.5 A comparison of Celsius and Fahrenheit scales. NB: °C = (°F − 32) × 5/9; °F = (°C × 9/5) + 32

In 1867 Allbutt of Leeds made a 6 in. glass thermometer that recorded temperature in 5 min. Two physicians in the United States, William Draper and Edward Sequin, designed the first bedside chart in the 1880s. Since then, temperature measurement belongs to the three vital signs, along with pulse and respiration [2].

4.3
The Value of Temperature Measurement

The presence of fever or hypothermia and its severity can be vital indicators of conditions that need careful investigation and prompt treatment. The accuracy of body temperature measurement may be particularly important in the following situations:

* **Fever in neutropenic children with cancer** is frequently caused by bacterial infection, which is among the leading causes of death in these patients. Admission to hospital and administration of intravenous antibiotics are often based on the presence of fever alone. Children with sickle cell anemia are particularly susceptible to overwhelming bacterial infections, and detection of fever commonly has similar implications as with neutropenic febrile children.
* **Drowning and near-drowning** can cause hypothermia. Cardiac arrhythmia and death may occur when the body temperature is <30°C.
* As epilepsy is defined by recurrent nonfebrile seizures, the only outward difference between a **febrile and an epileptic seizure** at the onset of the seizure is the presence of fever in febrile seizure. Since the investigation, treatment, and the prognosis of children with febrile seizure and epilepsy are different, measurement of body temperature at the onset of a convulsion is of paramount importance.
* **Critically ill children** such as those in a pediatric intensive care unit (ICU) who need to be monitored.
* **Hypothermia** (body temperature <35°C) has been recognized as a significant contributor to neonatal mortality in developing and developed countries [3]. There is an association between low body temperature of neonates on admission to neonatal ICU and increased mortality. Induced hypothermia has been used in recent years as a neuroprotectant in encephalopathic newborn infants after acute perinatal asphyxia, either as whole body hypothermia or selective head cooling.
* Accurate temperature measurement is critical in **infants younger than 3 months of age.** In this age group a temperature over 38°C has been associated with serious bacterial infection in 3–15% of patients [4].
* **Maternal intrapartum fever** is a risk factor for neonatal sepsis, and therefore it is essential to monitor maternal temperature during labor.
* **During anesthesia** continuous body temperature monitoring is essential because of the common risk of perioperative hypothermia caused by inhibition of thermoregulation by anesthesia and the patient's exposure to a cool environment. Monitoring is also required to detect the rare complication of malignant hyperthermia.
* A body temperature of >42°C suggests **hyperthermia**. Whereas fever (interleukin-1 mediated elevation of the thermoregulatory set point of the hypothalamic center) does

4

not climb relentlessly beyond 42°C, hyperthermia may exceed this level as a result of malfunction in the mechanisms modulating peripheral heat production and loss.

● The finding of a **difference between core (central) and peripheral (skin) temperature** is valuable in the diagnosis, management, and prognosis of shock and correlates with clinical criteria of brain death in children (>4.0°C) [5].

Often, trends in body temperature are more important than actual values. The pattern of fever may have diagnostic value such as periodic paroxysms of fever in malaria, continuous fever in typhoid fever, hectic fever in Kawasaki disease, and double quotidian in kala azar. While the severity of hypothermia has been found to correlate closely with the rate of survival [6], the higher the fever the greater the likelihood the infection has a bacterial etiology, and the infection is more severe [7].

In outpatient practice, accurate temperature measurement is often not possible or considered necessary, as physicians are usually interested only in the presence or absence of fever. Also small differences between different sites and instruments may not be of clinical importance.

4.4
Core Temperature

There is no uniform core temperature throughout the body. The hypothalamus is the site where body temperature is set and where the highest body temperature is recorded. Since the hypothalamus is inaccessible, core temperature is generally defined as the temperature measured within the pulmonary artery [8]. Other standard core temperature monitoring sites (distal esophagus, bladder and nasopharynx) are accurate to within 0.1 to 0.2°C of core temperature [9] and are useful surrogates for deep body temperature. During anesthesia, bladder temperatures correlated well with mesophageal and pulmonary artery temperature. This correlation was maintained during rapid body re-warming, with an insignificant bias of 0.04°C [10].

Since these deep-tissue measurement sites are clinically inaccessible, physicians have utilized the rectum as a practical site to monitor body temperature in the belief that this site most accurately reflects core temperature.

Any temperature measurement should take into consideration the normal diurnal temperature fluctuation of up to 1°C (1.8°F), with a peak at 5–7 p.m. and a minimum between 2 a.m. and 6 a.m. This diurnal variation, which begins to develop at the age of 4 months, can be so wide that a "normal" temperature in an individual is impossible to identify, but rather a range and a mean of body temperatures.

4.5
Measurement of Body Temperature

Body temperature measurements vary depending on the temperature site. Table 4.1 shows the ranges and means of these temperatures [11,12].

Table 4.1 Normal temperatures at different sites [11,12]

Body site	Type of thermometer	Range (Normal Mean) (°C)	Fever °C
Axilla	Hg-in-glass, electronic	34.7–37.3 (36.4)	37.4
Sublingual	Hg-in glass, electronic	35.5–37.5 (36.6)	37.6
Rectal	Hg-in-glass, electronic	36.6–37.9 (37.0)	38.0
Ear	Infrared emission	35.7–37.5 (36.6)	37.6

Table 4.2 Presence and type of home thermometer in nonmedical households, compared to those households where a parent was a doctor or nurse

	Mercury-in glass: no. (%)	Electronic (axillary): no. (%)	Fever scan: no. (%)	Ear thermometer: no. (%)	No Thermometer: no. (%)
Mothers (*n* = 126)	9 (7)	26 (21)	37 (29)	17 (13)	37 (26)
Nurses (*n* = 62)	25 (40)	11 (18)	4 (6)	0 (0)	22 (35)
Doctors (*n* = 77)	25 (32)	9 (12)	4 (5)	2 (2.5)	37 (48)
Total (*n* = 265)	59 (22)	46 (17)	45 (17)	19 (7)	96 (36)

Where relevant, the medical history should include questions as to how the temperature was taken at home and with which particular device. The recordings of temperature by the parents should be noted.

In a survey [13], mothers, nurses, and doctors were asked whether they had a thermometer at home and if so what type (Table 4.2). Most parents had thermometers: approximately 3 in 4 mothers, 2 in 3 nurses and 1 in 2 doctors have a thermometer.

4.5.1
Tactile Assessment

Simple palpation has been used for thousands of years to assess body temperature. Even nowadays with the availability of electronic and infrared thermometers, tactile assessment is still the most widely used method of evaluating body temperature. Some physicians advocate its use on the grounds that the thermometer holds no advantage over tactile methods when evaluating children with fever [14].

This method of palpation is far from accurate mainly because of lowering of skin temperature during the early phase of fever due to vasoconstriction. When medical staff carried out palpation as a screening method, the presence of fever was accurately predicted in only 42% of cases [15]. Mothers, on the other hand, made the correct prediction in over 80% of cases [16]. Thus palpation by mothers was more sensitive than by medical personnel. An African study[17] investigated the ability of medical students and mothers to use touch to determine whether 1090 children had fever. It was concluded touch overestimated the incidence of fever and that a child who feels hot needs to have a temperature taken before fever is confirmed.

4.5.2
Instrumentation

An ideal thermometer should:

* Accurately reflect core body temperature in all age groups
* Be convenient, easy, and comfortable to use by patient and practitioner, without causing embarrassment
* Give rapid results
* Not result in cross infection
* Not be influenced by ambient temperature
* Be safe
* Be cost effective

In practice, the ideal thermometer involves a combination of the best instrument and the most appropriate site. A tympanic thermometer appears to offer such a combination (see later).

4.6
Site of Temperature Measurement

Body temperature measurements vary depending on the site at which the temperature is taken (Table 4.1).

4.6.1
Axilla

When measuring axillary temperature (AT):

* ensure the mercury level is at minimum when a mercury thermometer is used
* place the bulb high in the apex of a dry axilla halfway between the anterior and posterior margins of the axilla, with the arm extended. The arm is then placed against the chest wall to hold the thermometer for 5 min. While using an electronic thermometer, the duration is reduced to 3 min
* use the same axilla for consecutive recording for accuracy

This site has several **advantages**:

* It is safe, easily accessible, and reasonably comfortable.
* In neonatal units, where ambient temperatures are stable, axillary temperature measurements were found to be as accurate as rectal measurements [18]. However, these studies involved afebrile neonates in a nursery where environmental temperatures and humidity were maintained at optimal levels.

There are several **disadvantages**:

● It requires supervision; otherwise displacement may occur. AT measurement takes longer than rectal or sublingual measurement (takes 5 min with mercury-in-glass and 40–80 s with an electronic thermometer), which is not cost effective with regard to nursing time.

● Temperature measurement at this site is notoriously inaccurate. At the onset of fever when peripheral vasoconstriction is intense, the skin temperature may fall as the core temperature rises. In addition, the effects of sweating and evaporation cause the axillary temperature to be lower than the core body temperature. Therefore, correlation between axillary temperature and core temperature is poor. The sensitivity of axillary temperature to detect fever has been reported to be only 27.8–33% [19,20]. In this study, rectal and axillary temperatures differed by up to 3°C and axillary temperature was occasionally very low.

In summary, the evidence suggests that AT with its low sensitivity should not be relied upon to detect fever in children and should be avoided if possible. AT is not a recommended method to screen for fever and certainly not where accurate temperature measurement is required (except on a neonatal unit) since the aim of temperature measurement is usually to detect or exclude the presence of fever and measurement at this site has a poor detection rate of fever.

4.6.2
Skin

Several companies have introduced reusable, or single-use disposable, plastic-encased **thermophototropic liquid crystals** for forehead application. The substance changes color as the temperature rises. They are most suitable for home use. Their advantages over conventional thermometers are obvious: convenient instruction, ease of use, safety, comfort, and rapid results.

A **temporal artery thermometer** has been introduced for use in hospitals and office settings. It is a noninvasive device that scans the surface infrared temperature from the forehead to behind the ear, with the highest temperature being over the temporal artery. Although this device was found to be easy to use (a gentle stroke across the forehead and then placement behind the earlobe), its accuracy remains a problem.

Estimation of body temperature is limited at the onset of fever because skin temperature is not elevated (and may even be decreased) due to vasoconstriction. Several studies have shown that measurement of skin temperature by these devices is inaccurate and frequently records a normal temperature despite elevated body temperature [21]. Similar inaccuracies were found with the recently used liquid crystal skin-surface thermometers, which were introduced for intraoperative temperature monitoring. The correlation between skin and core temperatures was reported to be poor [22]. High false-positive rates were also associated with continuous temperature measurement in the emergency department [23].

4.6.3
Sublingual (Oral Temperature)

When measuring oral temperature (OT):

- ensure the mercury level is at minimum when a mercury thermometer is used
- place the bulb of the thermometer under the tongue at the mouth floor. As there is variation of temperature recorded from this site (Fig. 4.6), the bulb should be at the area of maximal temperature
- instruct the child to keep the mouth closed and breathe through the nose and
- allow a minimum of 3 min before reading the recorded measurement

This site is often used in children over 5 years of age. Its **advantages** are:

- It is less affected by ambient temperature and is more accurate than the axillary site.
- It is also easily accessible. The mean oral temperature measured by an electronic thermometer or a chemical indicator is about 0.4°C below the simultaneously measured mean pulmonary arterial temperature.

There are several **disadvantages**:

- The measurement requires the cooperation of the child. It is therefore not suitable for use in children less than 5 years of age, in some children with developmental delay, or in comatose or intubated patients.
- Hot baths, exercise, hot and cold drinks, and mouth breathing all influence the results. The site should not be used if patients have tachypnoea, which causes increased evaporative cooling of the oral cavity and therefore results in a misleadingly low temperature estimation [24].

Measurement of Temperature

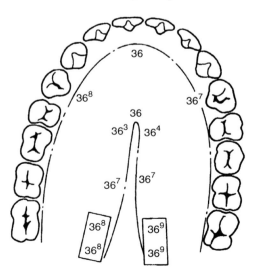

Fig. 4.6 Diagram of the floor of the mouth showing variations in temperature. The thermometer should be placed where the maximal temperature may be obtained

- There is variation in the temperature recorded from the sublingual area depending on exactly where the bulb of the thermometer is placed. Finally, oral laceration and mouth-to-mouth cross-infection may occur [25].

4.6.4
Rectum, Rectal Temperature (RT)

The method of measurement is:

- If a glass thermometer is used, ensure a minimum reading of mercury.
- Apply a sterile lubricant jelly on the bulb tip, or in case of an electronic thermometer, on the disposable probe.
- Following proper positioning of the child, the buttocks are separated and the thermometer is inserted without force to a distance of 5 cm into the rectum.
- The duration of measurement is 3 min.

The rectal route remained unchallenged for a century as the preferred site for the measurement of core temperature. In the 1960s, it began to be replaced by axillary and sublingual measurement.
Rectal temperature (RT) has the following **advantages**:

- It has been widely viewed as the gold standard for routine measurement of body temperature. RT measurement with a low reading thermometer is considered best clinical practice when dealing with potential hypothermia, that is, near drowning and neonatal cold injury.
- The site is not influenced by ambient temperature and its use is not limited by age.

There are numerous practical **disadvantages** to its routine use:

- It is frightening for small children and may be psychologically harmful for older children.
- The procedure may cause discomfort and is painful for patients with perirectal infection or irritation.
- The site is not hygienic and presents an infectious hazard. An outbreak of Salmonella cross-infection has been reported in newborn infants [26]. The transmission of human immunodeficiency virus through this route remains a concern. For the same reason this site should not be used in patients with neutropenia or other immunologic impairments. Oncology centers routinely avoid rectal temperature measurement.
- The measurement is time consuming, requires privacy, and has been reported to cause rectal perforation [27], calculated to occur in less than 1 in 2 million measurements [28].
- RT varies depending on how deeply the thermometer is inserted into the rectum, local blood flow, and the presence of stool and diarrhoea.
- RT may lag significantly behind a rapidly rising or falling core temperature because of relatively poor blood flow to the rectum. Even in a stable state, rectal temperature has been shown to differ significantly from pulmonary artery temperature [29]. When the body temperature is changing, the temperature in the rectum takes twice as long to

change as that in the pulmonary artery [30]. Therefore, rectal temperatures should not be used for patient monitoring during anesthesia. For the same reason, a misleadingly high temperature may be recorded after defervescence following antipyretic administration. In the presence of shock, perfusion of the bowel, including the rectum, may be markedly impaired, and rectal temperature will lag significantly behind a rapidly rising or falling core temperature.

In summary, it is questionable whether RT should be regarded as the gold standard for core temperature measurement.

4.6.5
Tympanic Thermometry

The method of temperature measurement is:

* A tympanic infrared thermometer is used with a disposable probe.
* The pinna is first gently retracted and the thermometer is inserted a few millimeters inside the left external ear canal until a beep indicates completion of the measurement.
* The measurement is repeated twice, and the highest reading is recorded.

The **basic principle** of infrared thermometry is as follows:

* Under normal conditions, 60% of total heat loss occurs via radiation in the form of infrared heat rays, a form of electromagnetic energy. This heat loss is increased during fever.
* As the tympanic membrane receives its blood supply from the carotid artery, its temperature may reflect that of blood flowing into the hypothalamus, thereby correlating closely with core body temperature.
* The thermometer measures the infrared rays emitted by the tympanic membrane.

There are many **potential benefits** to infrared ear thermometry:

* The technique is fast and easy to use without risk of cross-infection and is not influenced by environmental temperature. Parents and nurses rated tympanic thermometers as being more favorable in terms of ease, speed, cleanliness, and safety than oral or rectal thermometers [31]. A reduction in the numbers involved in a nosocomial outbreak of vancomycin-resistant enterococcus and clostridium difficile infection has been achieved by replacing rectal and oral thermometers with tympanic membrane thermometers [32].
* Tympanic thermometry (TT) is a practical method to measure body temperature in children in an emergency setting. It is more accurate than measurement taken by electronic axillary thermometer. It saves nursing time and is therefore cost effective since the measurement is 5 times faster than axillary measurements [33].

In recent years, tympanic thermometers have become very popular both with health professionals and at home. In the United States, 65% of pediatricians and 64% of family practice physicians regularly use infrared ear-based thermometer (IRET) [34]. As accuracy of body temperature measurement is particularly important in neutropenic children with cancer, IRET is suitable in providing high accuracy [35]. This group needs particular accuracy with regard to temperature measurement since intravenous antibiotics may be administered solely on the basis of a raised body temperature.

The main reason why the tympanic thermometer has yet to be regarded as the gold standard for body temperature measurement is that some studies have reported inaccuracies, mainly in children younger than 3 years of age [36]. These studies compared ear temperature with rectal or oral temperature as the reference standard. There is no evidence that either of these sites represents the core body temperature [13,37,38].

It has been known for about 40 years that the tympanic membrane can provide accurate measurement of core body temperature [39]. Recent studies (see next) have shown that tympanic temperature accurately reflects pulmonary artery temperature, even when the body temperature is changing rapidly. For this reason, infrared temperature has been found to be a reliable way of monitoring body temperature during anesthesia, during which the patient might be at risk of developing malignant hyperthermia or hypothermia [40].

4.7
Evidence-based Temperature Measurement

A search of all **evidence-based medicine (EBM)** reviews and systematic review studies (see Cochrane DSR, ACP Journal Club, DARE, and CCTR for systematic reviews 1991–2003: 39 articles; CINAHL 1982–2003: 83 articles; and PubMed 1980–2003: 582 articles on temperature measurements) was made for measurement of body temperature. There is universal agreement that AT is inaccurate and insensitive when compared to any core temperature technique (that is from the pulmonary artery, esophagus, or bladder) with the exception of afebrile neonates in neonatal units where the environmental temperature and humidity were maintained at optimum levels for neonates. A systematic review of 20 studies comprising 3201 children confirmed the inaccuracy of AT [41]. A systematic review of 44 studies comprising 5935 patients comparing TT and RT concluded that infrared ear-based temperature is not a good approximation of RT, although the mean differences between rectal and ear temperature measurements were small [42]. A third systematic review of the literature to determine optimal methods of temperature measurement in children concluded that RT is the optimal method until the child is old enough to cooperate with OT measurement [43].

The question remains: is the RT the satisfactory reference standard for core temperature? RT is reliable only if the body is in thermal balance and reacts slowly to changes in temperature. As there is consensus that the temperature of the pulmonary artery, esophagus, and bladder are representative of core temperature, a search of PubMed for all studies comparing TT with these sites was made, which is shown in Table 4.3. Most of these studies (which included febrile patients or patients who underwent cooling and re-warming during cardiac surgery) show TT to be accurate, including the three studies with children. Accuracy was defined as an ear-based thermometer measurement within 0.1 to 0.6°C or a high correlation ($r > 0.80$ of PA) [44–48].

Table 4.3 Outcome of comparison studies between core temperatures

No of Ref	No of patients	Core site	Other sites	Main outcome/conclusion
Group A				
40	15 C	PA/O	AT/RT	TT more accurate than RT
41	18 A	PA/O	AT/RT	TT second to OT, TT is the reading of choice
42	27 A	PA	RT	TT tracks PA closely
43	30 C	B	AT/RT	TT correlated relatively well with PA
44	38 A	PA/B	AT/OT	TT is relatively close estimate of PA
45	50 A	B	AT/OT	TT has good correlation with B
46	96 A	O	AT	No difference between TT and OT
47	51 A	PA	RT	Both TT and RT are accurate
48	128 A	PA	AT/RT	PA and TT were highly correlated
49	13 A	PA	AT/OT/RT	If RT contraindicated, OT or TT acceptable
50	9 A	PA	RT	PA and TT: not significantly different
51	20 C	PA	AT/RT	TT may be used instead of PA
52	32 A	PA	AT/RT	TT reflects PA more accurately than RT and AT
Group B				
53	15 A	PA/B	None	TT appears to give high readings
54	60 A	PA	AT	TT is clinically not reliable
55	102 A	PA	OT	OT is the most accurate
56	72 A	PA	OT	OT more accurate
57	32 A	PA	AT/OT	TT is not ideal
58	25 A	PA/B/O	AT/OT/FS	No noninvasive method is valid

(*PA* pulmonary artery; *O* oesophageal; *B* bladder temperatures) as a reference standard and ear-based temperature. *A group* Studies found TT to be accurate/or close to accurate. *B Group* Studies found TT to be less or not accurate. *CT* core temperature; *TT* tympanic temperature; *OT* oral temperature; *AT* axillary temperature; *FS* forehead skin temperature

4.8
Summary

Disagreement still exists as to the best anatomical site for temperature measurement. There is a consensus that

- AT does not provide accurate temperature measurements except in environments where the temperature is stable such as neonatal units and where the neonates are afebrile
- RT measurement is not favored by parents and nurses, and many hospitals such as ours have abandoned this method. The reluctance to take RT is cultural and is particularly widespread in Britain, Australia, and New Zealand. In all other countries, mothers usually take their babies' temperature rectally [59]. RT is contraindicated in neutropenic

oncology patients. This group needs particular accuracy with regard to temperature measurement since intravenous antibiotics may be administered solely on the basis of a raised temperature

* OT is not used in children less than 5 years of age and this is the group with the highest incidence of fever
* the tympanic site appears to be the most suitable for use in hospitals, GP surgeries, and at home. Evidence confirming the accuracy of the infrared ear-based thermometer is incomplete. This is probably because ear measurements were compared with rectal or oral measurements. Neither site represents the true core temperature

There remain a few unresolved issues. Error can potentially occur with TT if the probe is not directed towards the tympanic membrane. It is anticipated that in the future TT will include a visible signal (for example a green light) once the probe of the tympanic thermometer is correctly directed towards the tympanic membrane. There are only a few small trials comparing tympanic temperature with core temperature in neonates. Efforts should continue to find a suitable IRET for this age group. Once these concerns are taken into consideration, TT is likely to become the gold standard for all children.

References

1. Sarton G. Sarton on the history of science. Harvard University Press. Cambridge, Massachusetts. 1962
2. Musher DM, Dominguez EA, Bar-sela A. Edouard Seguin and the social power of thermometry. N. Engl J Med 1987; 316: 115–117
3. El-Radhi AS, Jawad MH, Mansor N, et al. Sepsis and hypothermia in the newborn infant: value of gastric aspirate examination. J Pediatr 1983; 103: 300–302
4. Baskin MN, O'Rourke EJ, Fleisher GR. Outpatient treatment of febrile infants 28 to 89 days of age with intramuscular administration of ceftriaxone. J Pediatr 1992; 120: 22–27
5. Miller G, Stein F, Trevino R, et al. Rectal-scalp temperature difference predicts brain death in children. Pediatr Neurol 1999; 20: 267–269
6. El-Radhi AS, Jawad MH, Mansor N, et al. Infection in neonatal hypothermia. Arch Dis Child 1983; 58: 143–145
7. El-Radhi AS. Hyperpyrexia in paediatric intensive care. Br J Intensive Care 1996; 6: 305–308
8. Lorin MI. Measurement of body temperature. Semin Pediatr Infect Dis 1993; 4: 4–8
9. Webb GE. Comparison of oesophageal and tympanic membrane monitoring during cardiopulmonary bypass. Anesth Analg 1973; 52: 729–733
10. Lilly JK, Boland JP, Zekan S. Urinary bladder temperature monitoring: a new index of body core temperature. Crit Care Med 1980; 8: 742–744
11. Chamberlain JM, Terndrup TE. New light on ear thermometer readings. Contemp Pediatr 1994: 1–8
12. El-Radhi AS, Carroll J. Fever in paediatric practice. Blackwell. Oxford. 1994, pp. 68–84
13. El-Radhi AS, Barry W. Thermometry in paediatric practice. Arch Dis Child 2006; 91: 351–356
14. Coffin LA. The taking of temperature. Pediatrics 1971; 48: 493–494
15. Bergeson PS, Steinfeld HJ. How dependable is palpation as screening method for fever. Clin Pediatr 1974; 13: 350–351

16. Banco L, Veltri D. Ability of mothers to subjectively assess the presence of fever in their children. Am J Dis Child 1984; 138: 976–978
17. Whybrew K, Murray M, Morley C. Diagnosing fever by touch. Br Med J 1998; 317: 321
18. Mayfield SR, Bahtia J, Makamura KT, et al. Temperature measurement in term and preterm infants. J Pediatr 1984; 104: 271–275
19. Haddock BJ, Merow DL, Swanson MS. The falling grace of axillary temperatures. Pediatr Nurs 1996; 22: 121–125
20. Kresh MJ. Axillary temperature as a screening test for fever in children. J Pediatr 1984; 104: 596–599
21. Scholefield JH, Gerber MA, Dwyer P. Liquid crystal forehead temperature strips. Am J Dis Child 1982; 136: 198–201
22. Ilsley AH, Rutten AJ, Runciman WB. An evaluation of body temperature measurement. Anaesth Intensive Care 1983; 11: 31–39
23. Dart RC, Lee SC, Joyce SM, et al. liquid crystal thermometry for continuous temperature measurement in emergency department patients. Ann Emerg Med 1985; 14: 1188–1190
24. Tandberg D, Sklar D. Effect of tachypnoea on the estimation of body temperature by an oral thermometer. N Engl J Med 1983; 308: 945–946
25. Shimoyama T, Kaneko T, Horie N. Floor of mouth injury by mercury from a broken glass. J Oral Maxillofac Surg 1998; 56: 96–98
26. McAllister TA, Roud JA, Marshall A, et al. Outbreak of Salmonella eimsbuettel in newborn infants spread by rectal thermometer. Lancet 1986; 2: 1262–1264
27. Smiddy FG, Benson EA. Rectal perforation by thermometer. Lancet 1969; 3: 805–806
28. Morley CJ, Hewson PH, Thornton AJ, et al. Axillary and rectal temperature measurements in infants. Arch Dis Child 1992; 67: 122–125
29. Hayward JS, Eckerson JD, Kemna D. Thermal and cardiovascular changes during three methods of resuscitation from mild hypothermia. Resuscitation 1984; 11: 21–33
30. Molnar GW, Read RC. Studies during open heart surgery on the special characteristics of rectal temperature. J Appl Physiol 1974; 36: 333–336
31. Barber N, Kilmon CA. Reaction to tympanic temperature measurement in an ambulatory setting. Pediatr Nurs 1989; 15: 477–481
32. Brooks S, Khan A, Stoica D, et al. Reduction of vancomycin-resistant enterococcus and clostridium difficile infections following change to tympanic thermometers. Infect Control Hosp Epidemiol 1998; 19: 333–336
33. El-Radhi AS, Patel S. An evaluation of tympanic thermometry in a paediatric emergency department. Emerg Med J 2006; 23: 40–41
34. Silverman BG, Daley WR, Rubin JD. The use of infrared ear thermometers in pediatric and family practice offices. Publ Health Rep 1998; 113: 268–272
35. El-Radhi AS, Patel S. Temperature measurement in children with cancer: an evaluation. Br J Nurs 2007; 16: 1313–1316
36. Peterson-Smith A, Barbar N, Coody DK, et al. Comparison of aural infrared with traditional rectal temperatures in children from birth to age three years. J Pediatr 1994; 125: 83–85
37. Iaizzo PA, Kehler CH, Zink RS, et al. Thermal response in acute porcine malignant hyperthermia. Anesth Analg 1969; 82: 803–809
38. Buck SH, Zaritsky AL. Occult core hyperthermia complicating cardiogenic shock. Pediatrics 1989; 83: 782–783
39. Benzinger M. Tympanic thermometry in surgery and anaesthesia. J Am Med Assoc 1969; 209: 1207–1211
40. Holdcroft A, Hall GM, Cooper GM. Redistribution of body heat during anaesthesia. Anaesthesia 1979; 34: 758–764

41. Craig JV, Lancaster GA, Williamson PR, et al. Temperature measured at the axilla compared with rectum in children and young people: systemic review. BMJ 2000; 320: 1174–1178
42. Craig JV, Lancaster GA, Taylor S, et al. Infrared ear thermometry compared with rectal thermometry in children: a systematic review. Lancet 2002; 360: 603–609
43. Duce SJ. A systematic review of the literature to determine optimal methods of temperature measurement in neonates, infants and children. DARE review 1994; 4: 1–124
44. Robinson JL, Seal RF, Spady DW, et al. Comparison of oesophageal, rectal, axillary, bladder, tympanic and pulmonary artery temperatures in children. J Pediatr 1998; 133: 553–556
45. Erickson RS, Meyer LT. Accuracy of infrared thermometry and other temperature methods in adults. Am J crit Care 1994; 3: 40–54
46. Summers S. Axillary, tympanic and oesophageal temperature measurement: descriptive comparisons in postanesthesia patients. J Post Anesth Nurs 1991; 6: 420–425
47. Schmitz T, Bair N, Falk M, et al. A comparison of five methods of temperature measurement in febrile intensive care patients. Am J Intensive Care 1995; 4: 286–292
48. Heidenreich T, Giuffre M, Doorley J. Temperature and temperature measurement after induced hypothermia. Nurs Res 1992; 41: 296–300
49. Morley C. Babies' rectal temperature: parents' reluctance reflects poorly on our culture. Br Med J 1993; 307: 1005
50. Robinson J, Charlton J, Seal R, et al. Oesophageal, rectal, axillary, tympanic and pulmonary artery temperatures during cardiac surgery comment. Can J Anaesth 1998; 45: 1133–1134
51. Shinozaki T, Deane R, Perkins FM. Infrared tympanic thermometer: evaluation of a new clinical thermometer. Crit Care Med 1988; 16: 148–150
52. Erickson RS, Woo TM. Accuracy of infrared ear thermometry and traditional temperature methods in young children. Heart Lung 1994; 23: 181–195
53. Erickson RS, Kirklin SK. Comparison of ear-based, bladder, oral and axillary methods for core temperature measurement. Crit Care Med 1993; 21: 1528–1534
54. Amoateng-Adjepong Y, Del Mundo J, Manthous CA. Accuracy of an infrared tympanic thermometer. Chest 1999; 115: 1002–1005
55. Klein DG, Mitchell C, Petrinec A, et al. A comparison of pulmonary artery, rectal and tympanic membrane temperature measurement6 in the ICU. Heart Lung: J acute Crit Care 1993; 22: 435–441
56. Milewski A, Ferguson KL, Terndrup TE. Comparison of pulmonary artery, rectal and tympanic membrane temperatures in adults intensive care unit patients. Clin Pediatr 1991; 30: 13–16
57. Romano MJ, Fortenberry JD, Autry E, et al. Infrared tympanic thermometry in the paediatric intensive care unit. Crit Care Med 1993; 21: 1181–1185
58. Chang Y, Ho L, Huang T, et al. Accuracy of infrared ear thermometry and traditional body temperatures for medical intensive care unit patients. J Nurs (China) 2000; 47: 53–63
59. Nierman DM. Core temperature measurement in the intensive care unit. Crit Care Med 1991; 19: 818–823

Fever in Common Infectious Diseases

5

Core Messages

> Infection of the respiratory tract is the most common reason for seeking medical advice and hospital admission in children. A viral upper respiratory tract infection (URTI) is the most common infection of the respiratory tract.

> In developing countries, acute respiratory infection remains a leading cause of childhood mortality, causing an estimated 1.5–2 million deaths annually in children younger than 5 years of age.

> In developed countries, viruses are responsible for most upper and lower respiratory tract infections, including pharyngitis and pneumonia.

> Although the degree of fever cannot differentiate between viral and bacterial diseases, high fever is associated with a greater incidence of serious bacterial diseases such as pneumonia or meningitis.

> Worldwide, diarrheal disease is the leading cause of childhood deaths under 5 years of age.

> If the fever does not have an evident source, urinary tract infection (UTI) should be considered, particularly if the fever is greater than 39.0°C and persists for longer than 24–48 h.

> Widespread vaccinations against bacteria causing meningitis, such as Hib, and vaccines against meningococci and pneumococci have dramatically reduced the incidence of meningitis.

> A child with fever and nonblanching rash should be promptly evaluated to exclude meningococcal diseases.

> Young children with malaria may present with irregular fever and not with typical paroxysms of fever, occurring particularly in early falciparum infection or as a consequence of previous chemoprophylaxis, which modifies the typical pattern of fever.

A.S. El-Radhi et al. (Eds.) *Clinical Manual of Fever in Children.*
Doi: 10.1007/978-3-540-78598-9, © Springer-Verlag Berlin Heidelberg 2009

5.1
Acute Upper Airway Infection

An upper airway infection is the most common infection in children, accounting for half to two-thirds of all childhood infections. This term includes viral URTI, tonsillopharyngitis, otitis media (OM) and epiglottic diseases.

5.1.1
Viral Upper Respiratory Tract Infection (URTI)

URTI is an exceedingly frequent infection characterized by nasal obstruction and discharge, fever, throat irritation, malaise, headache, and cough. The initial watery nasal discharge is followed rapidly by mucopurulent nasal discharge, which does not necessarily indicate bacterial infection. The combination of innate immunity and maternal immunoglobulin-G (IgG), transferred during the last trimester of pregnancy, provides some protection against the organisms causing URTI. It has been estimated that young children may have as many as 12 respiratory infections per year if he or she attends nursery, 9 infections per year if a sibling attends school, and 6 or 7 per year if the child and a sibling are not at school [1].

Well over 100 viruses are known to cause respiratory tract infection, such as rhinoviruses, influenza A and B, coronaviruses, parainfluenza 1, 2, and 3, adenoviruses, and respiratory syncytial viruses (RSV). Infection may result from inhalation, self-inoculation to the nasal mucosa, or airborne inoculation to the conjunctival mucosa. Children tend to have greater concentrations of viruses in the nasal secretion and shed them for longer periods of time than adults. Viremia is less common and the infection is usually restricted to the mucosa, including the sinuses and Eustachian tube.

Inflammatory mediators such as interferons (INF), rather than the virus itself, are responsible for many symptoms associated with cold. Injection of INF-α to volunteers has been found to cause fever, malaise, headache, and myalgia [2].

Fever in URTI has been studied [3,4], and the findings in affected children were:

* Fever was present in 50% of older children and in 90% of infants and young children.
* The degree of fever was not helpful in differentiating viral (mean degree 39.2°C) from bacterial infection (mean degree (39.3°C).
* A temperature greater than 39°C was recorded in 59%, 40°C or greater in 12%, and 40.5°C or greater in 3%.
* None of the children studied had a temperature exceeding 41°C, suggesting that a child with such a high degree of fever is likely to have another cause.
* High fever (>39.5°C) was associated with influenza A virus infections, occurring in more than 50% of children.
* Adenovirus infection caused fever exceeding 40°C in about 20%, while fever in rhinovirus infection was usually absent or mild.

- Fever associated with respiratory virus infection may last for 3–5 days. A prolonged duration of fever is, however, common. Fever lasting 5 days or longer occurred in 37% of children with this infection. The longest duration of fever (>7 days) may occur in association with adenovirus. The shortest duration of fever was associated with parainfluenza 2 viruses.

The knowledge that viruses can cause high and/or prolonged fever allows the physician to withhold antibiotic treatment and extensive investigations in children with prolonged fever who appear generally well, and common serious infections (e.g., UTI) have been excluded. In **differential diagnosis**, conditions mimicking URTI include the following:

- **Allergic rhinitis.** There is often a family history of atopy and a history of nasal symptoms with exposure to potential allergens, and the symptoms tend to be persistent. Nasal eosinophilia, increased serum IgE level, and the finding of possible allergens in skin prick tests or blood may confirm the diagnosis.
- **Streptococcal throat infection.** Children are usually older than 5 years. Fever tends to be higher than that in URTI. Nasal symptoms are usually absent.
- **Sinusitis** should be considered in a child with purulent nasal discharge and fever (usual range 38–39°C), localized pain and tenderness, mucosal erythema, and headache, whereas a higher fever with chills may suggest an extension of the infection beyond the sinuses.

For a febrile child with an URTI, the following recommendations may be useful:

- No specific therapy is indicated for most children.
- Symptomatic relief may sometimes be obtained with antipyretics in a febrile child with pain, excessive myalgia, or malaise. Paracetamol in a dose of 10–15 mg kg^{-1} may be administered at 4 h intervals.
- Antibiotics have no place in uncomplicated cases and should be avoided, as should antihistamines and cough suppressants.
- Nasal decongestants are rarely required, except perhaps for those infants with feeding or sleeping difficulty caused by the nasal obstruction.
- Vitamin C has been advocated for common cold, but its value is unproven.
- Amantadine is licensed for prophylaxis and treatment of influenza A but it is no longer recommended (see National Institute for Health and Clinical Excellence (NICE) guidance). Oseltamivir and zanamivir reduce replication of influenza A and B viruses by inhibiting viral neuraminidase. They are most effective for the treatment of influenza if started within a few hours of the onset of symptoms. Oseltamivir is licensed for use within 48 h of the first symptoms, while zanamivir is licensed for use within 36 h of the first symptoms. In otherwise healthy individuals they reduce the duration of symptoms by about 1–1.5 days. Oseltamivir is not licensed for use in children under 1 year because of concerns about neurotoxicity but it may be used under specialist supervision if the child is seriously ill. For further information on the treatment of influenza (see NICE guidance).
- There is limited data to suggest that antibiotics may reduce the duration of fever in children with Influenza. If there is any effect, this is likely due to a reduction in secondary bacterial infection. Figure 5.1 shows the proportions of children with virus infections who recovered with or without antibiotics.

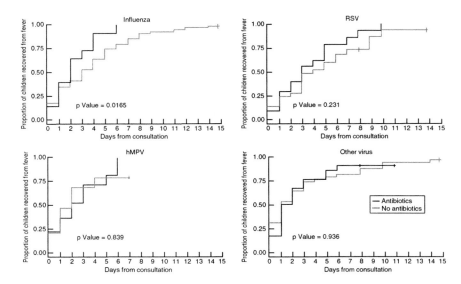

Fig. 5.1 Time to resolution of fever (days from consultation) according to virus detected and antibiotic prescribing. hmpv = human metopneumovirus, RSV = respiratory syncytial virus (obtained from *Arch. Dis. Child.* 2007; 92; 594–597; originally published online 16 Mar 2007; doi:10.1136/adc.2007. 116665)

5.1.2
Tonsillopharyngitis

Although most cases of tonsillopharyngitis are caused by viral agents, group A-β-haemolytic streptococci (GABHS) are the most common bacterial cause. Less common causes are pneumococci and other groups of β-hemolytic streptococci.

Streptococcal tonsillopharyngitis may begin abruptly with fever, malaise, sore throat, headaches, and abdomoinal pain. On examination, the tonsils are oedematous and hyperemic. There may be purulent exudates confined to the tonsils. The uvula is red and swollen, and the anterior cervical lymphnodes are enlarged and tender. There is usually an absence of conjunctivitis, coryza, or cough.

Cytokines, particularly interleukin-6 (IL-6) and tumor necrosis factor-α (TNF-α), play an important role in the pathogenesis of the inflammatory process of tonsillopharyngitis. High fever correlates with high levels of these two cytokines.

Diagnosis of streptococcal tonsillopharyngitis is established by throat culture and a more than twofold rise in antistreptolysin titers between two serum samples taken 2 weeks apart. Rapid antigen detection and polymerase chain reaction (PCR) tests are useful for providing rapid results.

The **differential diagnosis** of streptococcal tonsillitis is:

* **Scarlet fever** results from certain strains of haemolytic streptococci producing an erythrogenic toxin. The rash is an erythematous punctiform eruption that blanches on

pressure and spares the area around the mouth. Initially the tongue has a thick white cover, which develops in a few days into the typical strawberry tongue. Apart from the rash and the tongue, there is essentially no difference between streptococcal tonsillitis and scarlet fever. Fever in both conditions usually ranges from 39 to 40.5°C peaking on the second day of illness. Without treatment, the temperature usually subsides on the fifth day, whereas penicillin therapy causes a rapid normalization of temperature within 12–24 h.

- **Peritonsillar abscess** is a rare suppurative complication of tonsillitis causing a toxic appearance, fluctuant peritonsillar mass, and asymmetric deviation of the uvula.
- **Gingivostomatitis** is usually caused by herpes simplex infection in infants and small children. It is characterized by irritability, anorexia, and fever, which is usually in the range 38.5–39.5°C (rarely in the range of 40–40.5°C). The child has painful oral vesicles that soon rupture. Submaxillary lymphadenitis may occur. The disease is self-limited and lasts for about a week.
- Coxsakie viurs A may cause **herpangina**. The initial temperature ranges from normal up to 41°C; the temperature tends to be higher in younger children. Other features include headache and vomiting. Throat inspection reveals discrete punctuate vesicles, surrounded by erythematous rings on the soft palate, anterior pillars, and uvula.
- **Diphtheria**, which develops insidiously, has a grey, thick membrane that bleeds easily if removed. The associated fever in diphtheria is typically low grade. Frequently, there is a pharyngeal erythema and congestion (with or without tonsillar exudates). Anterior cervical adenitis is commonly present.

Penicillin eradicates streptococci from the throat, bringing the symptoms, including fever, rapidly under control and effectively preventing suppurative and nonsuppurative complications. Macrolides are adequate antibiotics in case of penicillin allergy. Paracetamol is used for pain and fever.

5.1.3
Otitis Media (OM)

OM is one of the commonest infections in children, particularly during the first 2 years of life, affecting about 60% of all children. At risk are those who attend day care centers and those whose parents smoke at home. The infection usually arises from a URTI, which spreads to the middle ear through the short and straight Eustachian tube. *Streptococcus pneumoniae* accounts for most of the bacteria recovered by tympanocentesis. In neonates and infants during the first 6 months of life, the most frequent bacteria are *E. coli*, Klebsiella, group B streptococci and *staphylococcus aureus*. Viruses are currently the most common cause of OM.

OM often presents with a sudden febrile illness characterized by:

- High fever, irritability, pain in the ear, and a prompt response to antibiotics. A temperature of <39°C occurs in about 25% and a temperature of >39°C in about 75%. The highest fever is recorded in children less than 2 years of age.

- History of or the presence of a URTI and sudden rise of fever.
- Rapid response of the fever following antibiotic therapy. Only 4% of children persist with fever lasting longer than 48 h. Persistent fever may suggest a viral cause, resistant bacteria, unsuitable antibiotic, or a complication of OM.
- High cytokine levels, which correlate with the degrees of fever. In OM and middle ear effusion, high levels of cytokines exist, including IL-1 and TNF-α.

The absence of fever suggests a more insidious variety of OM characterized by mild lassitude and irritability. Conductive hearing loss is often present with this variety.

Complications include perforation of the drum, mastoiditis, chronic otitis, cholesteatoma, facial paresis, increased intracranial pressure (causing bulging of the fontanelle in infants), meningitis, brain abscess, or lateral sinus thrombosis.

The use of antibiotics is controversial. The majority of cases of OM are caused by viral infection. If antibiotics are prescribed, Amoxicillin or a macrolide are sensible choices. The introduction of pneumococcal vaccines will help to further reduce the number of bacterial middle ear infections. The use of antihistamine, ear drops, or decongestant is controversial. Analgesics are often needed to reduce the pain. For a bulging tympanic membrane, or if the response to antibiotics is not prompt, myringotomy may rarely be considered for aspiration of fluid.

5.1.4
Infectious Mononucleosis

Infectious mononucleosis (IM) is an acute viral infection caused by Epstein–Barr virus (EBV). The symptoms, laboratory findings, and complications are shown on Table 5.1.

Table 5.1 Features and complications of clinical data of infectious mononucleosis[a]

Physical signs	%	Laboratory findings	%	Complication	%
Fever	100	EB-IgM	100	Pneumonia	3
Lymphadenopathy	80	Monospot test	98	Hemolytic anaemia	3
Pharyngitis	80	High transaminases	90	Agranulocytosis	0.1
Splenomegaly	50	>50% lymphocytes	50	Thrombocytopenia	0.1
Rash				Neurological	1.5
Palatal petechiae	50			Guillian–Barre syndrome	
Exanthem	10			Meningoencephalitis	
				Transverse myelitis	
Hepatomegaly	20				
				Other rare complications:	
Jaundice	5			Ruptured spleen	
				Myocarditis	
Airway obstruction	1–3.5			Pericarditis	
				Arthritis	
				Nephritis	

[a] Modified from [5] and [6]

A prodromal period of 3–5 days with malaise, fatigue, and headache may precede the onset of fever. Most (80%) patients will have fever symptoms pharyngeal and lymphadenopathy (pharyngeal form) and 20% present with fever alone (typhoidal form) [5]. Fever may last 4 days to 2 or 3 weeks (mean duration 1 week) peaking on the fifth day of illness [6]. The pattern of fever is frequently intermittent, with a usual range between 38.5 and 39.5°C, but rarely higher than 40°C. IM may presents as

- an asymptomatic infection occurring during early childhood;
- a typical IM triad of fever, pharyngitis, and lymphadenopathy occurring mainly in adolescents and young adults;
- a case of pyrexia of unknown origin (PUO), with fever as the only sign of the disease;
- a complication listed in Table 5.1;
- a cytomegalovirus mononucleosis characterized by prolonged fever and liver and haematological changes similar to those observed in Epstein–Barr infection. Heterophile antibodies are always absent. Pharyngitis is uncommon;
- Tonsillopharyngitis not responding to antibiotic administration or as an extensive rash following the use of ampicillin;
- EBV infection in association with a range of malignancies including Burkitt's lymphoma, nasopharyngeal carcinoma, and, in immunocompromised individuals, lymphoproliferative diseae [7].

Leukocytosis in the range of 10,000–20,000 is frequent. Absolute lymphocytosis (>50%) and atypical lymphocytes are usual findings. Tests to demonstrate heterophile antibodies (positive in more than 80%) have been superseded by several rapid slide tests (Monospot). IgM is positive in almost 100%. PCR for detection of EBV is now routine to aid diagnosis.

Therapy. IM is usually self-limiting, requiring only symptomatic treatment. Paracetamol is used to reduce the fever and pain. Steroids, usually given for two weeks, do not influence the extent or the duration of fever, and they are indicated mainly for impending airway obstruction. Hyperplasia of the lymphoid tissue in Walder's ring may occasionally cause severe airway obstruction and will respond to steroids. Emergency tonsillectomy and adenoectomy or tracheostomy are rarely required. Patients, particularly those with splenomegaly, should avoid excessive activity and trauma to minimize the risk of splenic rupture. Splenic rupture and neurological complications are rare but account for most fatalities.

5.1.5
Acute Upper Airway Obstruction

Viral croup (laryngotracheobronchitis) is a common cause of upper respiratory tract obstruction of the subglottic area. It is characterized by inspiratory stridor, cough, hoarse voice, and a variable degree of respiratory distress. Although symptoms often appear alarming, the infection is a benign, self-limiting illness, which usually persists for 2–6 days. Parainfluenza viruses account for about 75% of all isolates. Other pathogens include influenza A and B, adenovirus, and mycoplasma pneumonia. The attack rate is highest in the second year of life, and male children are predominately affected.

Onset is sudden (usually at night) with loud stridor and barking cough, preceded by a URTI. The severity of croup is assessed by a scoring system (Table 5.2).

5

	Mild–moderate	Severe
• Stridor	Minimal	severe
• Chest retraction	None	obvious
• Air entry	Normal	decreased
• Cyanosis	absent	present
• Level of consciousness	Normal	disorientated, drowsy

Table 5.2 Scoring system of severity for children with croup

Variable degrees of fever are present in about 40% the patients with croup, ranging between 38 and 39°C (mean 38.7°C). Children with spasmodic croup are usually afebrile. White blood cell count (WBC) and C-reactive protein (CRP) are often normal or slightly increased. Guidelines to manage a child with croup include:

• Most children with croup recover rapidly with minimal medical intervention. Children with mild croup and minimal or no respiratory distress can be managed at home. If hospitalization is required, the mother should, whenever possible, be with the child to minimize stress.
• Moderate to severe croup with stridor with or without respiratory distress may benefit from nebulized budesonide (2 mg), a single dose of parenteral or oral dexamethasone 0.6 mg kg^{-1} and oxygen if there is hypoxia (O$_2$-saturation <94%).
• Nebulized epinephrine (adrenalin) is effective in producing dramatic effects in alleviating the airway obstruction in severe croup.
• Although humidification is commonly used, trials have not shown this to greatly influence the clinical course of croup.
• Intubation is based on clinical grounds and supported by the presence of signs of respiratory failure as evident by hypercarbia.

Spasmodic croup is another entity of unknown etiology. Onset is always at night. The characteristic presentation occurs in a child who previously has been well without associated upper respiratory infection and who awakens at night with sudden dyspnea, croupy cough, and inspiratory stridor. Fever is usually absent.

Bacterial tracheitis is a bacterial infection (*Staphylococcal aureus* or *H. influenzae*) of the tracheal mucosa, often producing thick purulent exudates. This infection usually begins as a viral croup but progresses rapidly with high fever, toxicity, and worsening respiratory distress.

Epiglottitis is an acute bacterial infection characterized by marked swelling of the glottis and arytenoids area. Septicemia caused by *H. influenzae* type B is present in most cases. Epiglottitis is rarely seen nowadays following Hib vaccines. The infection has an abrupt onset with high fever, respiratory distress, dysphagia, drooling, irritability, restlessness, anxiety, and a thick muffled voice. In a report of 100 consecutive admissions of children with epiglottitis, fever was noted in 88, with a range from 39 to 40.5°C, [8] and a mean of 39.1°C.

Differentiating epiglottitis from viral croup may be difficult. Epiglottitis is now very rare. Patients appear very unwell, with higher degrees of fever and respiratory distress, and there is usually leukocytosis and high CRP.

5.2
Acute Lower Airway Infection

5.2.1
Bronchiolitis

A clear distinction between bronchiolitis and bronchitis in the first 2 years of life is difficult and of no therapeutic significance. Both are preceded by URTI. The diagnosis of bronchiolitis is made in the presence of a history of a URTI followed by acute onset of respiratory distress with cough, breathlessness, wheezing, tachypnea, and clinical signs of chest inflation, occurring during a winter epidemic of bronchiolitis. RSV is the most common etiological agent. Peak age is 4–6 months. Pre-existing chronic lung disease, congenital heart disease, immunodeficiency, prematurity, parental smoking, apnea, and infection in very early infancy predispose to severe illness and occasional death.

Information on the incidence of fever in bronchiolitis or on its relationship to clinical severity of bronchiolitis is limited. In a study of 90 children with bronchiolitis [9], fever (defined as a single recording of >38°C or two successive recording >37.8°C) was present in 28 infants (31%). Febrile children had a longer mean hospital stay and a more severe clinical course compared to those who were afebrile (Table 5.3).

In infants with bronchiolitis, hypoxia is common, and as many as 40% to 50% of cases require oxygen suppliment. A rise of body temperature results in an increase in energy expenditure of about 10% for each 1°C rise in temperature. These changes are accompanied by an increase in oxygen consumption of 10–12% for every 1°C rise in temperature [10]. The low incidence of fever in bronchiolitis may be due to low interferon production. Although interferon is known to be a potent endogenous pyrogen, this cytokine is significantly low during acute RSV bronchiolitis [11].

The mainstay of treatment is adequate oxygenation and hydration. Hypoxia, as measured by pulse oximetry, requires oxygen administration. Naso-gastric tube feeding or intravenous fluid is often required in moderate or severe cases to maintain fluid balance, to replace fluid loss from insensible sweating or tachypnea, and to minimize aspiration. Inhalation of a beta-2 agonist (salbutamol) or an anticholinergic agent (Ipratropium) is effective if there are signs of bronchospasms (wheezing or rhonchi on auscultation). Antibiotics are of no value unless the disease is complicated by bacterial infection. Corticosteroids, antihistamine, cough suppressants, and expectorants are also of unproven value. Ribavirin can be effective in reducing the shedding of virus and is used in immunocompromised patients.

Table 5.3 Summary of clinical data of 90 children hospitalized with bronchiolitis [9]

Group	Length of stay in days (Mean)	Clinical severity	
		Severe	Mild
Febrile (*n* = 28)	4.2 (1–13)	20 (71%)	8 (28.6%)
Afebrile (*n* = 62)	2.7 (1–10)	18 (29%)	44 (71%)
p-value	<0.005		<0.005

Palivizumab, an antibody directed against the virus, is recommended to prevent RSV in high risk individuals such as immunocompromised children.

5.2.2
Asthma

Asthma is defined as reversible obstructive airway disease characterized by bronchospasm, mucosal edema, and mucosal plugging. The airway obstruction is unevenly distributed throughout the lungs, leading to ventilation–perfusion imbalance and hypoxia. There is increased airway responsiveness to various stimuli, including respiratory viruses, house dusts, exercise, air pollutants, cigarette smoking, and drugs. Cytokines enhance eosinophil differentiation and maturation as well as endothelial adherence and activation. IgE synthesis is dependent on IL-4.

The clinical hallmarks of the disease are paroxysms of expiratory wheezing with prolonged expiratory phase, unproductive cough, and dyspnea. The predominant asthma type in school-age children (6–16 years) is the classic atopic variant that is associated with allergy problems as evidenced by the strong correlation with serum IgE levels and with skin-test reactivity to allergens. By contrast, asthma in children aged 1–5 years is characterized by recurrent, transient wheeze triggered by viral colds, a type previously termed as *wheezy bronchitis* and now as *preschool viral wheeze*. Physical examination reveals varying degrees of tachycardia, tachypnea, use of accessory muscles of respiration, and rhonchi on auscultation. Somnolence, fatigue, diminished wheezing, and breath sounds usually signal respiratory failure.

Markers of asthma severity include an admission to hospital in the previous 12 months, less privileged social class, parental smoking, and the frequency of prior and recent respiratory infections. Environmental factors such as climate and air pollution have been found to influence the prevalence and severity of asthma. Higher exposure rates to cockroaches and dust mites have also correlated with asthma severity. There are three stages of asthma severity:

- During early stage, hypoxia causes increased minute ventilation, a fall in Pco_2 and normal or elevated pH (respiratory alkalosis).
- Moderate asthma is associated with increased hypoxia, normal Pco_2, and pH.
- In severe asthma, hypercarbia, low pH, and respiratory/metabolic acidosis (respiratory failure) ensue as a result of respiratory muscle fatigue, hypoxia, and anaerobic cellular metabolism producing lactic acidosis.

Fever is not a frequent finding in acute exacerbations of asthma. It was recorded in only 18.8% on admission of 202 patients, mostly younger than 5 years of age (Table 5.4) [12]. Viruses are the most common cause of lower respiratory tract infection during the first few years of life and they can induce a febrile response.

The reasons why most asthmatic children are afebrile may be due to:

- Tachypnoea, which accompanies asthma, increases heat loss through evaporation.
- Reduced interferon production has been reported in children with bronchiolitis and asthma. Interferon is known to be a potent endogenous pyrogen capable of inducing fever.

Table 5.4 Clinical data of 202 children with asthma [12]

	Mean age in months (range)	Mean stay in days in hospital (range)	Asthma severity	
			Severe	Mild
<5 years				
Febrile = 27	24 (12–42)	1.7 (1–4)	1	26
Afebrile = 70	31 (12–58)	1.9 (1–9)	5	65
p-value	0.012	0.484	0.603	
95% CI	1.6–12.7	−0.3 to 0.7	n/a	
>5 years				
Febrile = 11	113 (78–172)	1.4 (1–2)	1	10
Afebrile = 94	118 (60–180)	2.2 (1–6)	18	76
p-value	0.700	0.065	0.688	
95% CI	19.1, 28.3	0.65, 15	n/a	

* Cytokines implicated in the pathogenesis of asthma, such as IL-5, IL-8, IL-4, and eosinophil cationic protein (ECP), are not known to be potent pyrogens, and their presence is unlikely to induce fever in asthma [13].

In this study [12], the severity of asthma was found to be inversely related to the degree of fever: children with severe asthma were usually afebrile, and mildly asthmatic children were often febrile. Similar observations were made at the turn of the last century when patients were noted to obtain a temporary relief of their asthma in association with fever. Subsequently various methods (diathermy) were used to treat fever [14]. It is possible that

* fever as a response to infection can limit the spread of infection by enhancing the host defense mechanisms to eliminate the viruses;
* as airway inflammation is a cardinal feature of asthma, cortisol, a potent glucocorticoid, is known to be elevated in febrile illness and could play a role as an endogenous anti-inflammatory agent [15].

Laboratory investigations such as full blood count, CRP and erythrocyte sedimentation rate (ESR) are of little value in asthma. Leukocytosis is common in the absence of bacterial infection. A chest X-ray is rarely indicated, unless the diagnosis is uncertain, in patients with fever >39°C and in case of severe asthma. Measurement of oxygen saturation is always indicated when a child is admitted to hospital. For older children, measurement of the peak flow is important and should be repeatedly performed. Allergy skin tests (to detect IgE antibody in the skin to inhalants such as pollens and house dust mites) and the radioallergosorbent test (RAST, detecting IgE to various allergens in the serum) are often performed, but they do not seem to be of great diagnostic or therapeutic value.

The most important principle of therapy is rapid reversal of the airway obstruction. Nebulized β-2 agonists remain the first line of treatment. Theophyllin may be added in severe asthma. Children with mild-moderate asthma who are not taking adequate fluids by mouth and all children with severe asthma should have intravenous (i.v.) fluid therapy. Corticosteroids are recommended for patients with acute severe asthma, but their effects are slow. Steroid therapy reduces symptoms and bronchial hyper-responsiveness and is currently widely used as an anti-inflammatory agent in asthma. Oxygen should be administered in all cases with hypoxia, delivered through a face mask to bring the oxygen saturation to >92%. Inhaled steroids are used prophylactically for patients who have more frequent asthma attacks and who have not improved on beta-2 agonist alone.

5.3
Pneumonia

In 1900, pneumonia, called by Osler "the captain of the men of death", was the most common cause of death, annually killing more than 200 people per 100,000 in the United States. By 1940, pneumonia was relegated to third, with approximately 70 deaths per 100,000 [16]. In children, pneumonia is common, but its true incidence is not established owing to the lack of an accepted clinical definition of pneumonia. Peak incidence occurs between 6 months and 5 years. Factors that increase the risk of pneumonia include malnutrition, parental smoking, immunosuppression, low socioeconomic status, and prematurity.

The lungs are not only involved in gas exchange but also in mediating host defense. This includes nonimmunological defense mechanisms (such as lysozyme secretion by macrophages) and immunological defense mechanisms (such as activation of macrophages and B and T lymphocytes). The alveolar macrophages respond to activation by exogenous pyrogens (such as endotoxin released by Gram-negative bacteria) by releasing potent inflammatory mediators, including IL-1, TNF, and IL-8. This leads to a febrile response, accumulation of neutrophils at the site of infection, and inhibition and repair of tissue injury. IL-8 is particularly important for neutrophil chemotaxis.

Diagnosis of pneumonia is based on the following features:

* Symptoms include fever, cough, dyspnea, tachypnea, grunting and nasal flaring, and referred pain. Lower lobe pneumonia may cause lower abdominal pain mimicking acute appendicitis. Upper lobe pneumonia may cause meningism (increased cerebrospinal fluid (CSF) pressure, but CSF is otherwise normal), causing suspicion of meningitis.
* Findings include inspiratory rales and bronchial breathing on auscultation. Tachypnea (>40/min aged >1 year, >50/min aged 2–12 m and >60/min aged <2m) is the WHO-defined criterion to diagnose pneumonia.
* Wheezing, cough and fever may occur with mycoplasma infection.
* Chest X-ray is diagnostic but is often of limited value in distinguishing bacterial and viral. The presence of effusion and/or lobar consolidation suggests bacterial etiology.

Isolation of the pathogens causing pneumonia is usually not possible in practice. Bacterial culture from the pharyngeal area or expectorated sputum is unreliable. However, pathogens can be identified by:

* blood culture (positive in 10% of cases with bacterial pneumonia);
* serum or urine counterimmuno-electrophoresis as a rapid and more sensitive technique than blood culture for the detection of bacterial antigens;
* culture of aspirated pleural effusion;
* high IgM, such as mycoplasma pneumoniae;

* respiratory secretion for rapid virus antigens (e.g., RSV, parainfluenza);
* serological tests showing fourfold rise of antibody titers;
* PCR, which is increasingly being used.

Marked leukocytosis, sometimes exceeding 40,000 mm^{-3} (leukomoid reaction) is very suggestive of bacterial pneumonia, particularly pneumococcal or *H. influenzae* pneumonia. Although inflammatory markers (WBC, CRP) are usually normal in viral pneumonia, mild leukocytosis with a left shift in the differential count may occur, particularly in influenza pneumonia.

Fever is the most common symptom of pneumonia in children older than 1 month of age. Reports [17, 18] on fever and pneumonia have indicated the following:

* Of the 100 febrile children with pneumonia, a temperature of >40°C occurred in 45, while the remaining 55 children had a fever of <40°C.
* Fever was present in all children with *H. influenzae* pneumonia, with a mean temperature on admission of 39.9°C (H. pneumonia is rarely seen nowadays).
* The onset of pneumococcal pneumonia was usually abrupt with a temperature of 39.5–40.5°C. The highest fever, however, tended to be with staphylococcal infection. (A temperature of 41°C is not an unusual finding.)
* The likelihood of pneumonia increased with increasing duration of fever longer than 3 days, that is, during a febrile URTI. A study of 711 children with pneumonia from 13 hospitals in England found that CRP, chest X-ray changes, or pyrexia were not associated with increased severity of the disease.
* In children <3 years old, a combination of >38.5°C, chest recession, and a respiratory rate of >50 per minute indicates pneumonia. Dyspnea is a more reliable sign of pneumonia in older children (The British Thoracic Society guidelines).

5.3.1
Pneumonia in Newborn Infants

Pneumonia during the neonatal period is usually caused by organisms acquired during or before delivery, mainly Group B streptococci. The amniotic fluid may be infected, or the mother is an asymptomatic carrier of these organisms. Predisposing factors are prolonged rupture of membrane, prolonged labor, or an infected, febrile mother. The infection by these bacteria is mainly due to low levels of opsonizing antibodies directed at the polysaccharides of the organism, impaired function of the lung macrophages, and polymorphonuclear leukocytes. Pneumonia may also accompany a generalized intrauterine infection by cytomegalovirus toxoplasmosis, listeria, or rubella virus. Chlamydia trachomatis is classically an afebrile pneumonia with a dry cough and increasing tachypnea. Conjunctivitis is present in about 50% of cases.

The newborn infant with pneumonia usually presents with signs of respiratory distress with tachypnea and grunting. Body temperature is often normal. If the mother has been febrile before delivery, an increased temperature may be detected in the infant in the first few hours of life owing to the constant temperature gradient between mother and infant during pregnancy.

5.3.2
Pneumonia at Age 1 Month to 4 Years

During this age, the rate of **viral pneumonia** is high, particularly in children around six months of age. RSV remains the most common cause of pneumonia in industrialized countries. **Febrile pneumonias** are commonly caused by RSV, influenza A and B, parainfluenza type B, and adenoviruses, while **afebrile pneumonias** are usually due to *C. trachomatis*, cytomegalovirus, or *Mycoplasma hominis*. Commonly, an URTI precedes the onset of pneumonia.

In developing countries, the causes and patterns of pneumonias are affected by malnutrition, poor housing, lack of early medical attention, and immunization. Pneumococci, streptococci, coliforms, *H. influenzae* and staphylococci are the more common causes of pneumonia with high mortality.

Staphylococcal pneumonia is a rather rare cause of pneumonia occurring sometimes as a complication of the influenza virus infection. Its presentation is with shaking chills and high fever >40°C, pallor, tachypnea, abdominal distension, and, rarely, cyanosis. The diagnosis should be suspected in any child younger than 1 year of age who appears ill and does not respond rapidly to conventional antibiotics such as penicillin and ampicillin. Chest X-ray shows multiple nodules, which undergo cystic formation (pneumatocele) and empyema.

5.3.3
Pneumonia at the Age of >4 Years

Pneumococcal and *Mycoplasma pneumonia* are the most frequently identified organisms, whereas viruses are less common at this age. In pneumococcal pneumonia, patients have often flu-like symptoms for several days before the onset of pneumonia, which begins by an abrupt onset of rigor and high fever. The cough becomes intense and is usually accompanied by chest pain. The sputum is classically rusty in color due to alveolar hemorrhage, but this is seldom seen nowadays in children.

Mycoplasma pneumoniae is characterized by insidious onset of fever, headaches, and abdominal pain, followed by cough. Transient skin rash is found in about 10% of cases. Mycoplasma pneumonia may also present with similar clinical and radiological features of pneumococcal and staphylococcal infection. In contrast to these infections, however, children with M. pneumonia appear well despite the extent of the X-ray lesions

Fever is present in more than 90% of patients. In a study of 66 children with mycoplasma infection [19], the temperature distribution was as follows: temperature <38°C was present in 22% of patients; 38.3–38.9°C in 30%; 39.4–40°C in 44%, and >40.6°C in 4%.

The diagnosis of M. pneumonia is difficult, but it may be made by a combination of the following:

* History of unresponsiveness to penicillin or amoxicillin
* A fourfold rise in antibody titer or a single titer of 128 or more
* IgM antibodies

* Serum cold-agglutinins in 50–70% of the cases
* Chest X-ray which is not diagnostic but commonly showing peribronchial and perivascular interstitial infiltrates
* A possibly high CRP or ESR and a normal WBC count.

About 5% may develop neurological complications, such as encephalitis, meningitis, cerebellar ataxia, focal neuropathy, or cerebral infarction. Other complications are hemolytic anemia, arthritis, rash (popular, vesicular, erythema multiform) myocarditis, pericarditis, and interstitial nephritis.

5.3.4
Pneumonia at Any Age

Aspiration pneumonia may occur subsequent to aspiration of secretion from the oropharynx in weak or neurologically impaired children (e.g., in preterm infants, cerebral palsy), in children with tachypnea (e.g., bronchiolitis), or following inhalation or accidental ingestion of kerosene or aspiration of gastric acid. The child presents with dyspnea, tachypnea, subcostal recession, cough, wheezing, and cyanosis. Children are usually afebrile with aspiration pneumonia, with possible exception of kerosene pneumonia, which is often associated with fever of 38–39.5°C. Chest X-ray shows infiltrates usually involving the right upper lobe in infants and right lower lobe in older children.

***Pneumocystis jiroveci* pneumonia** (Previously known as *Pneumocystis carinii*, the organism responsible for *Penumocystis carinii* pneumonia, PCP) occurs almost exclusively in patients who are immunocompromised, including those who are receiving immune-suppressive drugs for malignancy or organ transplantation, or HIV infection. About 85% of patients with HIV develop PCP during the course of their illness. Unlike most infectious complications in cancer patients, PCP may occur while the patient is in remission from the primary cause. Clinical manifestations include fever, cough, cyanosis, marked tachypnea with intercostals retraction and a paucity of physical signs of pneumonia. Among 1251 children with malignancies, PCP was identified in 51 (4.1%) [20]. Fever was the first sign of abnormality and occurred in almost all patients with, or shortly preceding, tachypnea. The extent of the fever varies from mild to severe.

The diagnosis is suggested by a chest X-ray showing a hazy, bilateral alveolar infiltration. Sputum examination and bronchoalveolar lavage (BAL) can identify PCP in most cases. The diagnosis is confirmed by detecting PCP by immunohostochemistry or PCR or by histological or cytological demonstration of thick-walled cysts, as obtained by BAL or from percutaneous transthoracic needle aspiration of the lung.

Antibiotic therapy of pneumonia depends on the age of the child and likelihood of the causative agent. Neonates are treated with penicillin and gentamicin. Older children respond to second and third-generation cephalosporins or co-amoxiclav. Suspected cases of staphylococcal pneumonia should receive anti-staphylococcal agent such as flucloxacillin. Patients with mycoplasma pneumonia usually respond well to macrolides. The treatment of choice for patients with PCP is trimethoprim-sulfamethoxazole (TMP-SMX) $20\,mg\,kg^{-1}$ per day.

5.4
Gastroenteritis

Worldwide, diarrheal disease is the leading cause of death under 5 years of age [21]. Data collected from 276 surveys on diarrhea in 60 countries between 1981 and 1986 have shown that one-third of all deaths in children below 5 years of age is caused by diarrhea. Approximately 1.5 billion diarrheal episodes and 4.6 million deaths in children occur per year (or 12,600 deaths per day), accounting for 21–29.3% of all childhood deaths [22,23]. In the absence of diarrheal diseases, the total infant and child mortality in developing countries would not differ significantly from that of developed countries [24].

In developing countries, bacterial (*Escherichia coli*, salmonella, shigella, campylobacter, and *Yersinia enterocolitica*) and parasitic (*Entamoebia histolytica, Giardia lamblia, Crptosporidium* species) pathogens are the major causes of gastroenteritis, particularly in summer months (Table 5.5). In Tanzania, diarrhegenic *E. coli* (35.7%) were the predominant enteropathogens [25]. In a recent study from Vietnam, stool pathogens were identified in 67.3%, of which rotavirus and diarrheagenic *E. coli* were the most common isolates [26].

In a study from the United States, 372 stool specimens from children with diarrhea grew bacteria in 176 (47%): Shigella toxin-producing *E. coli* (22.2%), *Salmonella* species (22.2%), *Campylobacter* species (14.2%), *Shigella* species (8%), and *Yersinia enterocolitica* (1.1%). Rotavirus was detected in 22.8% [27].

Fever or hyperthermia is common in both bacterial and viral gastroenteritis. High fever is commonly present in many bacterial causes (e.g., *Shigella, Salmonella, Shiga* toxin-producing *E. coli*). Fever is often absent or of low grade in other diseases (e.g., enteropathogenic *E. coli*, cholera). Other febrile conditions that cause diarrhea are shown in Table 5.6. Bacteria or viruses acting as exogenous pyrogens can cause fever by inducing endogenous pyrogens, which raises the hypothalamic thermoregulatory set point. Clinical and laboratory findings that can differentiate bacterial from viral etiology of acute gastroenteritis are shown in Table 5.7.

Dehydration, the most common cause of hyperthermia, leads to cutaneous vasoconstriction and decreased sweating, causing an increase in body temperature. In hypernatremic dehydration, an increase in sodium pump activity needed to offset the high extracellular sodium concentration may further raise the body temperature. High sodium levels may

Bacteria	Virus	Parasites
Salmonella	Rotavirus	*Giardia lamblia*
Shigella	Adenovirus	*Entamoebia histolytica*
E. coli	Other viruses	
Campylobacter jejuni		
Yersinia		
Vibrio cholerae		
Other bacteria		

Table 5.5 Major enteropathogenic agents in children with gastroenteritis

Table 5.6 Febrile non-enteritis diseases that cause diarrhoea

Conditions	Diagnostic clue
Intussusception	Intermittent, colicky abdominal pain, abdominal mass, cherry-red stoots
HUS	Bloody diarrhea, abdominal pain, renal failure, haemolysis
Appendicitis	young age of 1–3, predominately diffuse abdominal pain
Neuroblastoma	Abdominal mass
Primary Immunodeficiency	Associated recurrent infections
HIV-infection	Commonly associated with thrush, recurrent infections, weight loss
Kawasaki disease	Lymphadenopathy, conjunctivitis, rash, fever >5 days
Addison's disease	Diarrhea occurs in chronic adrenal insufficiency, abnormal electrolytes, pigmentation, adynamy
Crohn's disease	Associated weight loss, anaemia, high CRP

HUS hemolytic uremic syndrome

Table 5.7 Factors likely to predict the etiology of acute gastroenteritis

Bacterial etiology	Viral etiology
Fever >39°C	No fever or low-grade fever
Presence of bloody stools	No bloody stools
Summer months	Winter months
High CRP, WBC, IL-6	Normal or mildly elevated CRP, WBC, IL-6
Hyponatremia is common	Hyponatremia is uncommon
Increased WBC in stool	None to few WBC in stool
High serum TNF-α	Low serum TNF-α

CRP C-reactive protein; *WBC* white blood cell count; *IL* interleukin; *TNF* tumor necrosis factor.

also act directly upon the hypothalamus to increase the set point. For every 1°C increase of body temperature there is an increase in insensible water loss of 10%. Table 5.8 shows typical water losses based on caloric expenditure of 100 kcal kg^{-1} per day for an infant weighing 10 kg body weight.

5.4.1
Bacterial Gastroenteritis

Bacterial gastroenteritis is caused either by secretory pathogens (such as cholera, which causes watery diarrhea through colonization and adherence to the small bowel mucosa) or invasive pathogens (such as *Shigellae*, which cause inflammatory cell exudates in the distal bowel and/or colon). Secretory pathogens are likely to cause severe diarrhea. Invasive

Source of water loss	Approximate water loss (ml kg⁻¹ per day)
Insensible	
Skin	30
Respiratory	15–20
Sensible	
Stool	10
Urine	50–60
Total	105–120[a]

Table 5.8 Typical water losses per 100 kcal of energy expended for a healthy 10 kg child

[a] The above average calculation. The sum of insensible water loss (average 50 ml kg⁻¹per day) with 16 ml kg⁻¹ per day subtracted for endogenous water for oxidation produces 34 ml kg⁻¹ per day. The addition of 66 ml kg⁻¹ per day urinary loss would produce 100 ml kg⁻¹ per day fluid requirement

organisms may cause watery or grossly bloody diarrhea with cramps and tenesmus, but severe diarrhea is infrequent.

Salmonellae are Gram-negative rods with over 1400 known species. The most common serotypes are *S. typhimurium*, *S. enteritidis*, and *S infantis*. In industrialized countries non-typhoidal salmonellae (NTS) infection is more common. This is usually a self-limiting and benign disease, and invasion beyond the gastrointestinal tract occurs in only about 5% of patients. In many African countries bacteremia is a major cause of death, and NTS account for 20–50% of cases, ranking second only to pneumococcal pneumonia as the leading bacterial cause of child mortality [28]. In the United States it is between 800,000 and 3,700,000 [29]. Most human infections occur in late summer and early autumn and are caused by the ingestion of contaminated food (meat, poultry products, eggs) or water. Increased susceptibility to the infection occurs in children with sickle cell anemia, impaired cellular immunity, and achlorohydria.

About 12–48 h following ingestion of contaminated food, the onset is abrupt with nausea, fever, and crampy abdominal pain, followed by loose, watery diarrhea, occasionally containing mucus, blood, or both. The illness is indistinguishable from *Shigella* infection. Vomiting is a not a striking feature in salmonellosis.

Whereas salmonellosis in older children is usually a self-limiting disease requiring no antibiotic therapy, there is a significant incidence of bacteremia (range 15–45%) and meningitis in infants younger than 3 months. Bacteremia may occur in the absence of fever in this age group. The absence of fever usually excludes bacteremia in older children.

Endotoxin is a complex lipopolysaccharide structure that constitutes the outside portion of the cell wall of *Salmonella*. Endotoxin releases IL-1 from macrophage into the circulation, accounting for the fever and other systemic manifestations of the disease. Cytokines are responsible for the symptoms and development of the protective mechanisms in the disease. Mean serum concentrations of TNF-α, TNF-γ, and IL-12 were found to be increased during the acute phase of the disease and in those patients with early bacterial clearance compared with those of healthy controls and nonclearance patients [30].

In a study from Finland [31] comprising 102 children with salmonella gastroenteritis, 15 had a fever >40°C, 66 had a fever of 38–39.9°C, and 21 had a temperature of <37.9°C. There was a significant correlation between the degree of fever and the duration of organism excretion: a fever of >40°C had the shortest and no fever the longest duration of excretion (Table 5.9). Fever therefore appears to have a favorable prognostic influence on the duration of salmonella excretion. The gastrointestinal tract acts a major barrier against the potentially noxious substances, such as microbes. Immunological defenses include secretory IgA, macrophage, and activated T lymphocytes in the Peyer patches and lamina propria. Fever is beneficial to the infected host by enhancing macrophage and T-and B-cell activity.

Typhoid fever includes infection with *S. typhi* and *S. paratyphi* A, B and C, and rarely *S. choleraesuis*, *S. heidlberg*, and *S. typhimurium*. The incidence of typhoid fever in the United States is 0.2 cases per 100,000 population, with a case fatality rate of 1.3% [32].

Elevated proinflammatory pyrogenic cytokines, particularly TNF-α and IL-6, are responsible for the prolonged fever, which is characteristic of the disease. High serum levels of these cytokines have been linked to disease severity. A high level of IL-6 suggests poorer response to antibiotic therapy and its decline correlates with successful therapy. Vigorous antipyretic use may lead to shock.

In older children, presentation of a typical case follows the following steps:

Onset is insidious with fever (without shaking chills) present in all patients, and is associated with headache, cough, and abdominal pain.

Symptoms then gradually increase over 2–3 days. The child is often constipated, nauseated, and anorexic.

The temperature continues to rise in a stepwise fashion to reach 40–41°C. In young children the onset of fever is more often abrupt, then becoming sustained or intermittent. The stepwise pattern of fever is less common. In all ages, fever may continue for many days despite successful antibiotic therapy, and the child does not become afebrile until the end of the therapy. At the end of the first week, patients remain febrile with hot, dry skin, abdominal tenderness, hepatosplenomegaly, and relative bradycardia. Roseate spots may be detected in about 20–40%, characterized by a few discrete popular erythematous lesions confined to the anterior chest and abdomen. Delirium, convulsion, meningeal irritation, psychosis, and ataxia may be noted.

Table 5.9 Fever on admission and duration of bacterial excretion after salmonella gastroenteritis in 102 children [31]

Degree of fever (°C)	No of children	Duration of salmonella excretion (weeks)		
		Range	Mean	Mean (SD)
(A) >40 0	15	0–10	0	1.9 (2.9)
(B) 38–38.9	66	0–18	3	4.1 (4.0)
(C) <37.9	21	2–60	7	11.7 (15.1)

SD standard deviation.

p Value: (A) vs. (B), $p = 0.160$; (B) vs. (C), $p = 0.0011$; (A) vs. (C), $p = 0.0001$

If untreated with antibiotics, fever remains continuous at 39–40.5°C for 2–3 weeks before abating slowly.

By the end of 2 weeks, perforation or hemorrhage (in about 5%) may occur owing to typhoid ulceration and defects in coagulation. This serious complication is associated with 50% mortality.

Typhoid bacilli persist indefinitely in the bile passage in about 3–5% who recover from the infection.

Laboratory findings include leucopenia, anemia, thrombocytopenia, and increased serum aspartate transaminase (SGOT). Elevated agglutination titers of O and H antigens at 1:160 are significant. The diagnosis is based on isolation of *S. typhi* or other salmonella strains from blood or bone marrow culture.

Shigellae are gram-negative rods with worldwide distribution. Humans are the principal host for shigellosis (bacillary dysentery). Most patients are under 5 years of age; the infection is rarely seen in infants under 6 months of age.

Four serotypes are known: *Shigella flexneri*, *S. dysenteriae*, *S. sonnei*, and *S. boydii*. The first two species are more common in developing countries, whereas *S. boydii* and *S. sonnei* usually cause a self-limiting febrile illness in developed countries. Shigella must penetrate the mucosa in order to cause dysentery.

The disease onset is usually acute with fever and malaise, often progressing to dysentery consisting of cramps, tenesmus, and frequent stools composed largely of blood and mucosa. Severe dehydration is not a typical feature of the infection. High fever is common. Of 57 children with Shigella gastroenteritis, 27 (47%) had a fever greater than 40°C at presentation, 21 (37%) had a fever between 38 and 40°C, and the remaining 9 (16%) were afebrile [33]. In a recent study from Thailand, out of 80 children with shigellosis, the mean age of infection was 3.6 years. Fever was present in 77.6%, vomiting in 44.8%, and seizures in 27.6%. *Shigella sonnei* was the commonest species isolated (62.8%) [34].

Complications include toxic megacolon, protein-losing enteropathy, hyponatremia due to inappropriate antidiuretic hormone secretion, disseminated intravascular coagulation, renal failure, hemolytic uremic syndrome and bacteremia. Shigella bacteremia occurs in 4.0% of patients. Neurological symptoms, particularly convulsion, are among the most frequent extraintestinal manifestations of shigellosis occurring with or without evidence of the production of Shiga's toxin (neurotoxin). Death can occur in children with poor nutritional state.

Amoebic dysentery, caused by *Entameba histolytica*, may cause colitis simulating shigellosis. Virulence of *E. histolytica* depends on the trophozoites being able to bind to colonic epithelium. The infection tends to run a more chronic course with intermittent watery or semiformed diarrhea (containing blood and mucosa) without or with a low-grade fever. Young children tend to present with acute symptoms similar to cases with Shigella infection. Liver abscess may occur a few months after the intestinal infection, causing discomfort over the liver, intermittent fever with chills and sweats, and weight loss. Findings suggestive of amoebic liver abscess include an elevated right diaphragm, hepatomegaly, and a history of colitis. The diagnosis of amoebiasis is confirmed by demonstration of *E. histolytica* in a stool (motile trophozoites during the diarrhea, cyst if the diarrhea is not present) or in tissues. The indirect hemagglutination (HA) test and enzyme-linked immunosorbent assays (ELISA) are positive in almost all patients with amoebic liver abscess and in the majority of those with intestinal infection.

E. coli cause either non-bloody diarrhoea (e.g., enterotoxigenic *E. coli = ETEC*, entero-pathogenic *E. coli = EPEC*) or bloody diarrhea (e.g., Shigatoxin-producing *E. coli = STEC*, enteroinvasive *E. coli* = EIEC). Enteroaggregative *E.coli* (EAggEC) cause significant fluid loss and dehydration, but bloody stools are relatively infrequent.

* *ETEC* produce enterotoxins that cause copious watery diarrhea in developing countries. In its severe form, the illness resembles cholera, and is responsible for high mortality among young children. It is an uncommon cause of diarrhea in industrial countries, but it is the most common cause of traveler's diarrhea. EPEC infection was in the past a common cause of outbreaks of infantile diarrhea in industrialized countries, usually occurring in neonates and young children <2 years of age. Since the 1970s, the infection has been reported less frequently, and the severity of the illness has lessened in children of these countries. It can cause protracted diarrhea.
* *EIEC* and *STEC* produce Shiga toxins, causing a dysentery-like diarrhea and hemolytic uremic syndrome (HUS) by the strain 0157:H7.

Fever occurs frequently in the range of 38–40°C. Fever, very often low grade, is reported in only one-third of patients infected with EIEC and STEC. EPEC usually does not cause systemic manifestations because the organisms remain confined to the bowel lumen. Fever was found in only 5 of the infected 49 children from Addis Ababa [35].

Campylobacter enteritis is an important cause of enteritis in both developed and developing countries. *C. jejuni* is the most important species. The enteritis is a zoonosis, and a man-to-man transmission is unusual. Raw cow's milk and incompletely cooked poultry meat have caused most of outbreaks in the United Kingdom. Contaminated water is another cause of outbreaks particularly in developing countries.

Infection is usually self-limiting in industrialized countries, lasting 2–4 days, following an incubation time that averages 5 days. Children present with an acute illness accompanied by fever, diarrhea, and bloody stools in about 90% of cases. Abdominal pain occurs almost universally, but vomiting is mild and occurs in about 30%. In a study from Canada, all 32 children with this infection who were older than 12 weeks developed fever up to 40.5°C, whereas all 5 children who were younger than 12 weeks remained afebrile. In a study from Iraq (202 children with diarrhea; 13.86% detection rate of *C. Jejuni*), fever was detected in (82.14%) [36].

Yersinia enterocolitica is an anaerobic, Gram-negative bacillus that causes an infection mostly in cooler climates such as Scandinavia and Canada. Serotype O:3 is the most common isolate. Transmission of *Y. enterocolitica* to humans occurs from ingestion of contaminated foods (particularly contaminated pork), water, and milk.

Presentation is characterized by bloody diarrhea in about one-third of patients. The fever is usually mild, ranging between 38 and 39°C. The associated abdominal pain sometimes mimics appendicitis (pseudo-appendicitis). The disease is usually mild, although it can be prolonged (1 day to 3 weeks). A Canadian study of 181 children with Yersinia infection (45) reported that diarrhea occurred in 98%, fever in 88%, abdominal pain in 64.5%, and vomiting in 38% [37].

Rare complications are arthritis, erythema nodosum, intestinal perforation, diffuse ulceration, iliocolic intussusception, peritonitis, glomerulonephritis, meningitis, and perimyocarditis. The infection can occur as septicemia, and patients then have high fever, toxic appearance, and confusion.

5.4.2
Viral Gastroenteritis

Rotavirus infection is responsible for 30–60% of all cases of dehydration and diarrhea in young children (peak age 3–15 months) in both developed and developing countries. The infection is prevalent in winter months. Approximately 125 million cases of rotavirus diarrhea occur annually in developing countries, leading to an estimated 800,000–900,000 deaths a year and 25% of all deaths due to diarrheal diseases [38]. Although viremia is rare in healthy individuals, this was reported in 67% of immunocompetent children with rotavirus diarrhea [39].

Nosocomial acquired outbreaks of rotavirus have occurred in newborn nurseries and pediatric hospital wards. The virus can be detected in oropharyngeal aspirates with or without diarrhea. Spread occurs via the fecal–oral route. The virus is shed in feces in high concentration, which allows its easy identification by electron microscopy.

There is often a preceding or accompanying URTI or OM. Within 2 days of exposure, there is fever and vomiting, which last 1–3 days, and usually preceding the onset of watery diarrhea, which lasts 4–7 days. Dehydration occurs as a result of marked fecal fluid loss.

Most children with rotavirus diarrhea have fever. A study from Finland [40] reported that 14% of 336 infants had fever of 39–40.2°C and 65% had less than 39°C. Many cytokines, particularly IL-6, IL-10, and INF-γ, play an important role in the pathogenesis of as well as protection against rotavirus re-infection. IL-6 is elevated in children with fever. A vaccine is now available, although its use is not widespread as yet.

Enteric adenovirus. Several studies have shown that adenovirus is second to rotavirus as the most common cause of viral gastroenteritis, occurring commonly during the first year of life. The infection was identified in 8.6% of 900 pediatric inpatients with diarrhea, serotypes 40 and 41 being the most common isolates [41]. In contrast to enteric adenoviruses, other respiratory adenoviruses are not associated with diarrhea. Watery diarrhea is the most common presentation, usually followed by 1–2 days of vomiting. Illness typically lasts 5–12 days (mean 9 days). The duration of the diarrhea usually lasts longer compared to that caused by rotavirus. Severe dehydration is less common compared to rotavirus infection.

A low-grade fever for 1–3 days is commonly recorded with adenovirus enteritis. A Canadian study [42] of 127 children with adenovirus enteritis found that 41% of them had a rectal temperature of >38°C. The range of body temperature was 36.2–40.8°C (mean 38°C). The average duration of fever was 1.6 days (range 1–30 days).

The outcome of adenovirus gastroenteritis is generally good. Adenovirus is now more frequently diagnosed (due to PCR) in immunocompromised patients and is an important cause of mortality.

Other viruses. Norfolk virus and Norwalk-like viruses are major causes of small and large outbreaks of winter vomiting in older children and adults with or without diarrhea. These outbreaks occur commonly in recreational camps, communities, or schools in the United States. Presentation is similar to that of other types of viral gastroenteritis and includes anorexia, malaise, and fever and abdominal cramps, followed within 48 h by vomiting and watery diarrhea. Symptoms usually last 2–3 days, and full recovery is the usual outcome. Astrovirus can also cause gastroenteritis. The infection is frequently asymptomatic in the newborn infants.

Treatment. Breast milk is the best prophylaxis against gastroenteritis, and exclusively breast-fed children remain remarkably free of severe diarrhea in developed and developing countries.

The standard treatment of all diarrheal diseases is the replacement of fluid and electrolyte loss. This is best accomplished by oral rehydration solution (ORS), which has revolutionized the management of diarrheal diseases in developing countries. This is safe, cheap, convenient to use, and superior to i.v. fluids because it can be started early at home. The sugar–electrolyte mixture recommended by the WHO contains (mmol l^{-1} water) sodium 90, chloride 80, potassium 20, sodium bicarbonate 30, glucose 111; with an osmolality of 331 mosmol l^{-1}. A hypotonic solution with a sodium concentration of as low as 50–60 mmol l^{-1} and an osmolality of 224 mosmol l^{-1} has been shown in Finland to have clinical advantages over the standard ORS [43]. A systematic review found that rice-based ORS compared with standard ORS reduced the 24-h stool volume [44]. Intravenous electrolyte–glucose solution should be used for children with moderate to severe dehydration and persistent vomiting.

Antibiotic therapy is usually not required for patients with gastroenteritis because it does not affect the clinical course in most cases. Severe systemic manifestations associated with bacterial gastroenteritis (notably Shigella, campylobacter, Yersinia, and cholera) probably require antibiotics. Infants less than 3 months of age with salmonella gastroenteritis should be treated with an antibiotic, such as a third-generation cephalosporin or a quinolone depending on the regional resistance pattern. Patients with typhoid fever and *E. histolytica* should also receive antibiotic treatment.

5.5
Viral Hepatitis

Hepatitis occurs as a result of a variety of causes, including viruses (hepatitis viruses, EBV, cytomegalovirus), bacteria (leptospirosis), parasitic infection (amoebiasis), and drugs.

5.5.1
Hepatitis A

Hepatitis A (HAV) is a highly contagious infection, spreading mostly by fecal–oral contact from person to person.

The clinical features are usually mild, and most infected children have an anicteric illness with flu-like symptoms or gastroenteritis with lethargy, nausea, vomiting, abdominal pain, and anorexia. Clinical findings often reveal a tender and enlarged liver. Splenomegaly is present in about 20% of cases. About 99% of children recover completely from the infection. Fulminant hepatic failure may occur in the remaining 1%. Chronic hepatitis or cirrhosis is not part of the HAV infection.

Fever, usually low grade between 38 and 39°C, is found in about 40% of cases. The low incidence of fever in hepatitis is probably due to impaired production of IL-1, which increases slightly during the first week of illness, reaching a peak during the second and third week, and thereafter decreasing to a normal level. The impaired production of IL-1 does not appear to correlate with the severity of liver disease.

Diagnosis rests on detection of the specific IgM, which is a marker of recent infection. It is usually positive before the onset of jaundice, peaking at 1 week and is undetectable 4–8 weeks later. IgG anti-HAV indicates previous exposure and is detectable approximately 1 week later than IgM, and persists for years as a sign of immunity. High transaminase enzymes are characteristic of the disease. These enzymes are elevated during the anicteric phase of the illness and usually persist for a few weeks. Serum bilirubin and alkaline phosphatase are mildly or moderately elevated. Prothrombin time is usually normal.

Standard immunoglobulin preparations administered within 2 weeks of exposure have proved effective in preventing hepatitis A. Vaccine HAV is effective.

5.5.2
Hepatitis B Virus

Transmission of this virus usually occurs via the parenteral route or any bodily secretion or fluid. Children exposed to multiple blood transfusions are at high risk of contracting the virus. The incubation period for Hepatitis B (HBV) infection ranges from 6 weeks to 6 months (mean 90 days). The HB surface antigen (HBsAg) appears during the incubation period several weeks before clinical or biochemical illness develops, and is usually undetectable after 6 months. The core antigen (HBcAG) and e antigen (HBeAG) are other antigens of HBV associated with greater infectivity.

Neonates are at high risk if the mother has acute hepatitis or carries HbsAg (chronic carrier) at delivery. Viral acquisition may follow swallowing of maternal blood during delivery, rarely via the transplacental route, or through ingestion of breast milk. Most infants born to HBsAg-positive mothers remain asymptomatic for months and years.

Clinical manifestations are usually absent or mild without evidence of fever. The vast majority of children (>90%) infected with this virus develop a chronic carrier state, and less than 5% develop hepatitis. Children are at risk of developing hepatocellular carcinoma and should therefore be regularly monitored with serial ultrasound scan and serum α-fetoprotein. Patients have substantial abnormalities of cell-mediated immunity and cytokine production, including a decreased production of TNF-α.

In HBV infection in older children, prodromal symptoms may include urticaria and arthralgia, which precede a spectrum of clinical presentations ranging from acute viral hepatitis, severe or fulminant hepatitis, chronic persistent hepatitis, and chronic active hepatitis to the asymptomatic chronic carrier state .

5.6
Urinary Tract Infection

Urinary Tract Infection (UTI) is a common cause of an acutely febrile illness in children affecting 7% of girls and 2% of boys. The infection is mainly caused by ascending fecal bacteria from the perineum to the bladder. UTI is frequently the result of sepsis during the first three months of life, occurring more commonly in males. Known predisposing factors for UTI include maternal febrile UTI, congenital malformation of the urinary tract, urolithiasis, indwelling urinary catheter, constipation, and uncircumcised males. The principal sequence of UTI is vesico-ureteric reflux found in 30% of acute cases, which may lead to chronic renal failure and/or hypertension in adults.
The most common organisms are:

* Uropathogenic *E. coli*, which contain lipopolysaccharide, lipoprotein, and proteoglycan. By attachment of the bacteria to the urinary tract, these substances are capable of inducing an inflammatory response and fever.
* Less common etiological agents include *Proteus mirabilis, Klebsiella pneumoniae*, enterococci, and *Staphylococcus epidermidis*.

The proinflammatory cytokines IL-6 and IL-8 play an important role in the inflammatory process of UTI. Serum and urine IL-6 and urine IL-1β positively correlate with fever in UTI. UTI presents in one of the following ways:

* High fever, rigor, vomiting, meningism and abdominal discomfort, loin pain, and tenderness;
* Fever without apparent source (FWAS), occurring mainly in infants. The prevalence of UTI in FWAS varies between 4 and 13% (mean of 10%);
* As sepsis with or without fever, occurring in 30% of neonates, 21% of infants aged 1–2 months, and 5.5% of infants older than 3 months of age [45];
* Febrile seizure as the first symptom of an underlying UTI;
* Dysuria, frequency, urgency, or dribbling, occurring in older children, particularly in girls. The condition is usually afebrile, termed as *lower UTI*;
* Asymptomatic (without fever) bacteriuria is common in school girls (1–2%) but the infection is of little clinical or prognostic significance.

Diagnosis of UTI rests on the following findings:

* A febrile child without a focus whose urine may harbour the infection;
* Positive nitrite and leukocytes in the urine dipsticks, which are very suggestive of the diagnosis while the negative result of these two indicators virtually excludes it. A positive urinalysis is defined as 5 or more WBC per high power field;
* Urine culture as the ultimate tool to confirm or refute the diagnosis. UTI is diagnosed if the urine shows a colony count of 100,000 colonies per milliliter of a single bacterial species. Suprapubic puncture is important for accurate diagnosis during infancy. In older children midstream urine sample is sufficient;
* Leukocytosis > 15,000, high CRP (>40 mg l^{-1}) to support the diagnosis. CRP is particularly valuable when fever has been present for more than 12 h. IL-6 is a useful diagnostic tool for early recognition of UTI;

Once UTI is confirmed, recent guidelines suggest that a renal ultrasound scan should be arranged early in case of severe or recurrent infections. Micturating cystourography (MCUG) is currently less commonly performed than previously and should be reserved (along with DMSA isotope scan) for atypical presentation, or recurrent infections occurring in infancy.

Fever in UTI has the following significance:

- It is the leading complaint for seeking medical attention.
- High and prolonged fever is associated with high incidence of UTI.
- UTI is unlikely and insignificant without fever in children older than 2 months.
- In 1025 febrile children younger 2 months from the United States, uncircumcised male infants had a higher rate of UTI (21.3%), compared with female (5%) and circumcised males (2.3%). Infants with high fever $>39.0°C$ had a higher rate of UTI (16.3%) than those infants with lower degrees of fever (7.2%) [46].

Therapy. Systematic reviews of 23 studies (3295 children) showed no significant differences in persistent renal damage or duration of fever between oral antibiotics (a second-generation cephalosporin, cefixime, or co-amoxiclav) and short courses (2–4 days of i.v. therapy followed by oral therapy [47].

In conclusion, the diagnosis of UTI should be considered in every febrile child, particularly when the fever is without a focus and of a duration longer than 24–48 h. A delay in diagnosis and treatment increases the risk of scarring.

5.7
HIV Infection

By 2007, an estimated 33 million people are living with human immunodeficiency virus (HIV)/AIDS, with more than 2 million people newly infected and more than 25 million deaths since 1981 [48]. HIV is affecting millions of children worldwide. The vast majority of children are infected through vertical transmission from mother to child (about 95%). Typical presenting symptoms are fever, asthenia, failure to thrive, prolonged diarrhoea, recurrent infections, and lymphadenopathy.

Fever is very common in HIV infection, occurring in 85% (49%) and is caused by:

- The HIV infection itself
- Concurrent bacterial infection of gastrointestinal or respiratory system;
- Immune reconstitution syndrome (IRS). This is a transient deterioration or emergence of new manifestations (such as high fever, worsening of central nervous system (CNS) lymphadenitis lesions) of an opportunistic infection occurring after the initiation of antiretroviral therapy (ART). The syndrome also occurs after initiating anti-TB treatment in patients already on ART;
- Secondary infections (such as tuberculosis);
- Drug fever, commonly associated with ART;
- Unknown causes of fever, which may present as a case of pyrexia of unknown orgin (PUO).

The rate of concomitant secondary infections among the HIV-infected children has been estimated to be 3 times higher than the rate in the non-HIV-infected children [50]. The incidence of fever is higher with a co-infection such as TB. Children with fever >39.0°C are at high risk of bacteremia with S. pneumonia. Unexplained persistent and/or recurrent fever (>37.5°C intermittent or constant) for >1 month is considered as a moderately severe HIV (Clinical Stage 3, WHO HIV Criteria, August 2006).

In a study of 316 febrile children with advanced HIV disease [51], the diagnoses were

* disseminated mycobacteria avium complex (MAC) infection in 36%;
* tuberculosis in 16%;
* B lymphoma (6%);
* disseminated CMV infection (4%);
* extrapulmonary cryptococcosis (3.5%);
* cases presented as PUO (17%);
* other less frequent diagnoses such as drug fever, endocarditis, HIV primary infection, pancreatic abscess, *Pseudomonas aeruginosa* bacteremia, and visceral leishmaniasis.

Most of these patients (about 75%) were receiving cotrimoxazole prophylaxis with or without antiretroviral treatment.

Children with HIV infection often present with the following:

1. Fever without focal signs and duration <14 days in HIV (see Table 5.10);
2. Fever without focal signs and duration >14 days (see Table 5.11).

Evaluation of fever among patients with HIV infection requires a detailed history, focusing on:

* duration of fever;
* recent travel to an area of malaria or dengue disease;
* skin rash, cough, pain during swallowing, headache, diarrhoea, dysuria;
* weight loss;
* the last CD4 cell count (?) (normal CD count: 600–1000); and
* current treatment (e.g., ART) and adherence.

Examination should include routine physical examination focusing on areas likely to be involved in the infection, such as thorough palpation of the lymphnodes, neurological examination, and fundoscopy for cytomegalovirus (CMV) and TB.

Laboratory investigations should include the following:

* Blood tests: Complete blood count with differential counts; blood chemistry (transaminases, alkaline phosphatase, LDH); blood smear for malaria; serum cryptococcal antigen test = SCrAg); dipstick for malaria (rapid tests), if in endemic zone; viral load, CD4 count; dengue serology (if patient is living or have travelled to endemic areas);
* Urinalysis;
* Chest X-ray, abdominal ultrasound;
* Stool examination for bacterial culture and acid-fast bacilli (AFB);
* Lumbar puncture (Gram stain, Ziehl–Neelsen, of glucose/protein levels;
* Mantoux Test or INF-γ assay.

Table 5.10 Differential diagnosis of fever without focal signs and duration < 14 days in HIV infected children

Differential diagnosis	Diagnostic clues
Malaria	• Living or a history of visiting malaria area • Blood film/dipstick positive • The presence of anaemia, low platelets
Typhoid fever	• Seriously ill without apparent cause • Abdominal tenderness • Relative bradycardia in relation to body temperature • Maculopapular rash, often sparing palms
Urinary tract infection	• Dysuria, frequency, pyuria, tenderness in renal angles • Positive nitrate and WBC dipstick
Dengue	• Patient from areas at risk • Sudden onset of high fever with headache, pain behind eyes, joint and muscle pain. • Macular rash in 50% (centrifugal, itching) (In dengue haemorrhagic fever, there is in addition bleeding tendency, eg from the nose, bowel, fingers)
Septicemia	• Seriously ill with no apparent cause
Immune reconstitution Inflammatory syndrome	• Recent start of HAART • CD4% <10% at start of HAART • Rise in CD4⁺ lymphocyte count
Drug-induced fever	• Nevirapine, cotrimoxazole, dapsone, β-lactams, isoniazid, anticonvulsants, abacavir, efavirenz

HAART highly active antiretroviral treatment

Management of newly diagnosed children who present with PUO entails the following:

- A thorough search and adequate treatment of the secondary infections should be carried out prior to starting the antiretroviral therapy.
- The above investigations should be initiated prior to any treatment.
- Antibiotics to cover likely infections and particularly S. Pneumonia while waiting for results may be required.
- Patients with confirmed or probable TB (abnormal chest X-ray, positive gastric aspirate/sputum AFB, abdominal lymphadenopathy, positive INF-γ release assay) should start on antituberculosis treatment. This treatment is also indicated as an empirical therapy in cases of unexplained weight loss and fever in advanced AIDS.
- If a patient is not improving on anti-TB treatment, alternative diagnoses such as mycobacteria avium complex (MAC) should be considered.
- Patients responding to MAC therapy should continue until CD4 cells have adequately recovered. This may takes months/years.
- During the whole period of treatment, patients should repeatedly be re-evaluated for the appearance of new symptoms and signs, which may indicate additional infections.

Management of HIV patients with PUO while taking antiretroviral therapy should involve the following:

Table 5.11 Differential diagnosis of fever without focal signs and duration >14 days in HIV infected children

Differential diagnosis	Diagnostic clues
Disseminated TB	Advanced HIV/AIDS, with anemia AFB seen on sputum, gastric aspirate, CSF, pleural fluid and/or fine needle aspirate of lymph nodes Enlarged mediastinal or hilar lymph nodes, pulmonary infiltrates or miliary lesions on chest X-ray. Enlarged liver or spleen, or enlarged lymph nodes on abdominal ultrasound
Mycobacterium avium Complex (MAC)	Severe immunosuppression or WHO stage 4 disease Symptoms compatible with disseminated TB, but failing to respond to TB medicines Absence of peripheral lymphadenopathy Severe anemia and neutropenia
Cytomegalovirus (CMV)	Very low CD4 count (CD4 <50 cells mm^{-3} in children >5 years) or WHO stage 4 disease. Blind spots in one or both eyes, with signs of retinitis
Disseminated cryptococcal infection	Very low CD4 count (CD4 <50 cells mm^{-3} in children >5 years) or WHO stage 4 disease Headache, Molluscum-like skin lesions Positive serum cryptococcal antigen tests Isolation of the pathogen from CSF, lymph nodes, sputum, or skin ulcers (indian ink).
Visceral leishmaniasis	Splenomegaly, lymphadenopathy, pancytopenia Amastigotes seen in samples of tissue or body fluid under the microscope (Giemsa stain)
Bacterial endocarditis	Enlarged spleen, heart murmur petechiae on skin and mucosa, anaemia. Splinter hemorrhages in nail bed
Relapsing fever	Exposure to ticks or body lice Recurrent pattern of fever. Headache, muscle pain, enlarged liver and spleen, red eyes, and photophobia
Abscesses	Tender or fluctuant mass, often detected by ultrasound
Trypanosomiasis	Travel to or living in region with tsetse flies History of painful trypanosomial chancre at site of inoculation of the parasite. Bouts of high fever lasting several days separated by afebrile periods, lymphadenopathy, itching, and maculopapular rashes

AFB acid-fast bacilii; *CSF* cerebrospinal fluid; *WHO* World Health Organization.

- An associated skin rash should arouse the suspicion of drug fever. Nevirapine is a frequent cause of this. A common finding is elevation of liver transaminases. Abacavir is also a cause of hypersensitivity reactions and should never be used again, as it can be fatal.
- Patients who initially responded to treatment for opportunistic infections (OI) prior to the start of antiretroviral therapy, and then developed a worsening of the OI after the start of antiretroviral therapy (e.g. reappearing of fever), should be considered as having

5

IRS (if other obvious causes of fever are excluded). Patients should continue OI therapy and ART but steroids treatment should be considered.

5.8
Infection of the CNS

5.8.1
Meningitis

Meningitis remains one of the most important infectious causes of neurodisability and death in childhood. Newborn infants and children between 6 and 12 months of age are at greater risk of meningitis than older children; 90% of reported cases occur below 5 years of age. Congenital and acquired T- and B-cell defects, sickle-cell anemia, splenectomy, and malnutrition all predispose to meningitis. Definitions of the clinical variations of central nervous system (CNS) infection are provided in the Table 5.12.

The widespread use of vaccines against *Neisseria meningitides* and *H. influenzae* type B (Hib) has virtually eradicated the incidence of these forms of meningitis and their complications in well-immunized populations. The incidence of bacterial meningitis in the United States has decreased by 55% since the introduction of Hib vaccines in 1990 [52]. This has lead to an increase of the median age of patients with bacterial meningitis to 39 years. In developing world with low immunization rates, however, these types of bacterial meningitis still occur. The commonly used antibiotic prophylaxis of pregnant women for Group B streptococci and the recent introduction of vaccines against pneumococcal infection have the potential to reduce the incidence of this disease even further.

Meningitis occurs most commonly in the individual who bears the organisms as an asymptomatic carrier. Organisms enter the CNS through vulnerable sites in the blood–brain barrier (choroid plexus or cerebral microvasculature). The cell wall components of these organisms stimulate macrophage-equivalent brain cells (astrocytes, microglia). Once

Table 5.12 Definitions of meningitis, meningococcal disease, and encephalitis

• Confirmed meningitis: isolation of bacteria from CSF, blood or DNA detection through PCR from a patient with a CSF white cell count >10 cells mm^{-3}. Diagnosis is also accepted in case of postmortem diagnosis of meningitis or meningeal contrast enhancement on CT scan
• Probable meningitis: the presence of clinical symptoms and signs of bacterial meningitis in the absence of laboratory confirmation
• Meningococcal disease: a clinical condition caused by *Neisseria meningitidis* with purulent conjunctivitis, septic arthritis, and septicemia with or without meningitis
• Aseptic meningitis: the presence of CSF white cell count >10 cells mm^{-3}; CSF is negative for bacterial culture, occurring usually in summer months. Viruses are most common causes
• Encephalitis: an inflammation of the parenchymal tissue of the brain caused by an infection producing varying degrees of impaired consciousness

CSF cerebrospinal fluid; *PCR* polymerase chain reaction; *CT* computerized tomography.

bacteria reach the CSF, they are likely to survive because humural defenses, including immunoglobulin and complement and opsonic activities, are virtually absent. Meningitis may also result from hematogenous dissemination, or rarely by direct invasion from ear or sinus infection. Data suggest that several cytokines, particularly IL-1β, TNF-α, and IL-6, are increased in children with meningitis (Fig. 5.2).

5.8.2
Bacterial Meningitis

Neonatal meningitis is most common during the first week of life (early onset; beyond the first week of life it is termed late onset). The susceptibility of neonates to meningitis, particularly premature infants, is mainly due to immaturity of cell- and antibody-mediated immune mechanisms. The neonate is infected by bacteria from the maternal genital tract, the risk being higher after membrane rupture.

Gram-negative lipopolysaccaride or Gram-positive peptidoglycan
↓
Inflammatory mediators by CNS astrocytes, ependymal and glial cells
(IL-1, TNF-alpha, IL-6, IL-8, IL10)
↓
Fever, inflammatory changes, proteolytic products, toxic oxygen radicals
↓
Cerebral oedema, increased ICP, neuronal cell death by apoptosis
↓
Symptoms, including fever

Fig. 5.2 Pathogenesis of meningitis and fever

Table 5.13 Causes of bacterial meningitis

Neonate	
• Early onset	(Caused by vertical transmission)
	Group B streptococcus (GBS)
	Escherichia coli (*E. coli*)
	Listeria monocytogenes
	Coagulase-negative staphylococci
	H. influenzae
• Late onset	(caused by nosocomial or community spread)
	Gram negative enteric bacteria (GNEB)
	(*E.coli*, *klebsiella*, *enterobacter*, salmonella, proteus, pseudomonas)
	In developing countries: GNEB, *H. influenzae*
Older children	
	Neisseria meningitidis
	Streptococcus pneumoniae
	H. influenzae

A study of 274 neonates from England and Wales established an annual incidence of bacterial meningitis at 0.21 per 1000 births [53]. The overall case fatality rate was 6.6%. Group B streptococcus remains the leading pathogen (about 50% of cases, Table 5.13). In contrast to older children, the onset of neonatal meningitis is usually insidious. Infants present with the following:

- Symptoms such as failure to feed, lethargy alternating with irritability, seizures, vomiting, thermal instability (fever or hypothermia), cyanosis, apnea, jaundice; and respiratory distress;
- Signs such as an ill appearance, a tense or bulging fontanelle, pallor, and reduced capillary refill time. Neck stiffness and head retraction are not parts of the symptomatology.

Complications include hydrocephalus, ventriculitis, neurodisability, and seizures.

Meningitis in older children is mostly meningococcal (in combination with sepsis called *meningococcal disease*, MCD) or pneumococcal. Less common causes are *E. coli*, group B streptococci, staphylococci, Listeria, *Borrelia burgdorferi* (Lyme disease), TB, and fungi. Factors that increase the risk for bacterial meningitis include immunoglobulin deficiency (e.g., HIV infection), asplenia, neuro-surgical procedures (e.g., ventriculoperitoneal shunt), penetrating head injury, and cochlear implants (particularly for pneumococcal meningitis). Meningitis has a variety of presentations:

- In MCD, the nonspecific early symptoms (in the first 4–6 h) are fever, irritability, and decreased appetite. This is followed (at a median time of 8 h) by early symptoms of sepsis: leg pain, abnormal skin color, and cold hands and feet. Classic meningitis symptoms appear later (13–22 h): purpuric rash, impaired consciousness and meningism [54];
- Fever, vomiting, irritability or drowsiness, headache, and photophobia;
- Convulsive status epilepticus with fever.

Tuberculous meningitis compromises about 5–10% of extrapulmonary cases of TB. It often occurs within 6 months of the initial TB infection following hematogenous dissemination or a rupture of a subependymal focus into subarachnoid space. The incidence is highest in children aged 1–5 years. The three recognized stages are:

- conscious, with nonspecific symptoms (fever, night sweats, anorexia, weight loss, fatigue) and no neurological signs;
- onset of neurological signs: headache, confusion, drowsiness, neck stiffness; and
- stupor, deepening coma, focal neurological signs.

Fever in bacterial meningitis is:

- the most common presenting symptom in children beyond the neonatal age owing to the presence of inflammatory mediators, particularly IL-1 and TNF in blood or within the CNS. In MCD, fever was the first symptom in children younger than 5 years, and 94% developed fever at some point;
- uncommon in neonatal meningitis. It occurred in about 30% of 36 neonates with *E. coli* meningitis [55]. Neonates have a reduced capacity to produce cytokines, which may explain their frequent afebrile presentation;

* usually very high in older children. Temperatures between 40 and 41°C are common, with a mean degree of 39.2°C. The degree of fever varies depending on the age of the patient and the causative organisms. The incidence of fever was 71% with meningococcal infection, 88% with staphylococcal infection, and 90% with H. influenza type B. Children with TB meningitis have the highest incidence of fever with 97% [56];
* absent in rare cases of severe infection. Hypothermia carries a bad prognosis;
* short and often settles within 24–48 h in MCD. Its duration in pneumococcal infection is significantly longer than in other types of bacterial meningitis.

Fever is an important sign when monitoring the effect of treatment in bacterial meningitis; that is, normalization of fever is very suggestive of a good response and improvement. Non-responders may produce the following fever patterns:

* Persistent for 4–7 days
* Prolonged, more than 7 days
* Secondary fever (fever reappearing after at least one afebrile day).

The following considerations should be made in persistent or prolonged fever:

* The antibiotics or the doses used for meningitis therapy are inappropriate (e.g., penicillin administered for staphylococcal meningitis);
* The meningitis may be aseptic or TB meningitis;
* There are complications listed in Table 5.14;
* The child needs thorough re-evaluation to find out the cause of the fever;
* Morbidity and mortality are higher than in those cases who have responded to treatment.

Animal models of meningitis have provided substantial information on the pathophysiology of fever in the disease. Studies [57,58] investigating the influence of fever on experimental meningitis in rabbits concluded that high body temperature had a direct inhibiting

Table 5.14 Causes of persistent, prolonged, and secondary fevers

Persistent
• Causative organisms: *S. pneumonia* or *H. influenzae*, fungi
• Foci of the infection
• Nosocomial infection
• Subdural effusion
• Drug fever
• Phlebitis
Prolonged
• Causative organisms: *S. pneumonia* or *H. influenzae*, fungi
• Subdural effusion
• Drug fever
• Arthritis
Secondary
• Causative organisms: *S. pneumonia* or *H. influenzae*, fungi
• Nosocomial infection
• Subdural effusion
• Drug fever

effect on the growth rate of bacteria in the CSF. On the other hand, the lower the temperature, the faster was the rate of bacterial growth. Thus fever is likely to be a host defense in this disease. Similar results are available in human studies. The reported overall case fatality rate in 100 children with meningococcal infection (55 had meningitis) did not indicate a poor prognosis, but all children with hypothermia died [56].

In a study of 476 children with meningitis, 90% of patients with S. pneumoniae and N. meningitidis became afebrile within five days of the antibiotic therapy, compared to 72% of those with H. influenzae meningitis. The rate of persistent fever, prolonged fever, and secondary fever was 13, 13, and 16%, respectively [59]. Complications from meningitis including persistent and prolonged fever, have decreased following decreased incidence of meningitis due to routine H. influenza vaccination in 1992 and recently Pneumococcal vaccine, but still occur with other types of bacterial meningitis.

Laboratory findings include the following:

* Characteristic CSF findings (Table 5.15) and identification of the pathogens in CSF and/or blood cultures and/or PCR. In TB meningitis, additional positive findings are microscopy for AFB from CSF, gastric aspirate, sputum (ZN stain), tuberculin test >5 or 10 induration, history of TB contact, and radiological evidence in the CNS of tuberculoma and/or other changes, such as hydrocephalus;
* A polymorphonuclear leukocytosis and high CRP in the blood;
* High procalcitonin (PCT) level (>0.5 ng ml^{-1}). PCT is a precursor of calcitonin, which may be more valuable than CRP and IL-6 in differentiating bacterial from viral meningitis early. PCT is also higher in severe compared to mild disease.
* Other abnormalities are inappropriate secretion of antidiuretic hormone (ADH) with hyponatremia, water retention increased intracranial pressure and DIC. DIC manifests as thrombocytopenia, increased fibrin degradation products, and prolonged prothrombin (PT) and partial thromboplastin time (PTT).

Complications include seizures, neurodisability, paralysis of the cranial nerves, subdural collection, blindness, hydrocephalus, cerebral herniation, and deafness.

Table 5.15 Usual cerebrospinal fluid findings in normal and in various central nervous system, (CNS) infections

Normal	Cell mm^{-3}	Protein mg dl^{-1}	CSF/serum glucose ratio %
Normal	0–5 (lymphocytes)	20–40	>50
Bacterial meningitis	100–1000 (PMN)	100–500	<0.5
Tuberculosis	30–600 (lymphocytes)[a]	>100 up to 3 g	<0.5
Viral meningitis	100–2000 (lymphocytes)[a]	Normal to 200	Normal
Encephalitis	Normal to few hundreds	50–100	Normal
Abscess	10–100 (PMN per lymphocytes)	30–200	Normal

PMN polymorphonuclear cells

[a] PMN predominate initially with lymphocytes predominating after 48 h

Table 5.16 Treatment recommended for children with tuberculosis

Drugs	Daily dose Mg	Maximal daily mg kg⁻¹ per day	Major side effects
INH	10	300	Peripheral neuropathy
Rifampicin	10–20	600	Hepatitis
Pyrazinamide	25–35	2 g	Hepatotoxicity
Ethambutol	15–20	2 g	Optic neuritis
Streptomycin	40	1 g	Ototoxicity

Therapy consists of prompt i.v. administration of antibiotics. Neonates are treated with cefotaxime, penicillin (or ampicillin), and gentamicin for a duration of 2 (GBS and Listeria) or 3 weeks (Gram-negative bacteria). Older children are treated with third-generation cephalosporin cefotaxime or ceftriaxone. Treatment of TB meningitis is shown in Table 5.16.

Dexamethasone has been advocated for the treatment of bacterial meningitis. Early administration of dexamethasone has been shown to reduce the duration of fever, levels of cytokine concentration, and the incidence of hearing impairment. It is mainly beneficial for *H. influenzae* and *S. pneumoniae* meningitis if it is given with or before antibiotics.

Intravenous fluid should be restricted to minimize the effect of inappropriate ADH effect and the cerebral edema. Monitoring the electrolytes and body weight are important for the management of the fluid and electrolyte balance.

The presence of coma, shock, seizures, and hypothermia are associated with poor prognosis. Children with TB meningitis usually make full recovery if they are fully conscious at presentation, while those in coma have a high rate of neurodisability and deaths. The younger the child, the worse the prognosis.

Viral Meningitis

The true incidence of viral meningitis is unknown mainly because CSF with aseptic meningitis is often not examined for viruses. The incidence of proven viral meningitis is 0.05 per 1000 live births [53]. The most frequent etiological agents remain non-polio enteroviruses (echovirus and coxsackievirus). Mumps meningitis, which used to be the most common form of viral meningitis prior to the combined measles, mumps, and rubella (MMR) vaccination in 1988, has declined dramatically. Symptoms are similar to those of bacterial meningitis but they are usually mild and the children appear generally well. This infection affects mainly older children.

Fever varies usually between 38.5 and 39.5°C, rarely higher. Fever along with drowsiness and irritability are the major presenting symptoms. The incidence of fever is around 70%.

Of the various cytokines capable of inducing fever, INF-γ produced in the intrathecal space appears to be associated with the pathogenesis of viral meningitis, and the production of fever. CSF INF-γ levels correlate well with the severity of febrile episodes.

Laboratory findings include clear, or rarely opalescent, CSF (Table 5.15). CRP and WBC are usually normal. Procalcitonin is a useful marker to differentiate bacterial and aseptic meningitis.

Diagnosis requires isolation of the specific virus from the CSF and/or a fourfold rise in antibody titer to the virus. Rapid identification of the virus by immunofluroscent examination of the CSF is possible for many viruses. The prognosis is very good.

5.8.3
Acute Viral Encephalitis

This is an illness with an acute onset and rapid progression caused commonly by the herpes simplex virus (HSV). Other viruses include varicella, cytomegalovirus, EBV, coxackievirus, echovirus, poliovirus, mumps, measles and adenovirus. The annual incidence is 8.8 per 100,000 children younger than 16 years of age [60].

Clinical features vary depending on the nature of the causative virus, the age of the patient, and the severity of the infection. Commonly, the disease begins with an acute onset of fever, headache, and vomiting. Evidence of meningeal irritation and stiff neck is often lacking. Encephalitis is suggested by drowsiness, paralysis, coma, seizure (febrile seizure), ataxia, tremor, mental confusion, or hyperexcitability. Ataxia is common, particularly following varicella encephalitis.

Fever is common in viral encephalitis irrespective of the causative agent. It was present in 30% patients with mumps encephalitis, in 85% with coxackievirus B encephalitis, and in 90% of patients (a third had a fever greater than 39°C) with herpes encephalitis [61]. Fever, lethargy, and headaches may last 4–5 days before other symptoms (such as behavioral abnormalities) occur.

Laboratory diagnosis of herpes encephalitis mainly depends on PCR detection from the CSF, which is highly sensitive and specific. Electroencephalogram (EEG) commonly shows paroxysmal focal abnormalities (such as slow complexes every 2–3 s) over the involved temporal areas. A computerized tomography (CT) scan of the head may show characteristic low-density lesions in these areas, in addition to diffuse brain edema. Magnetic resonance imaging (MRI) is a superior investigation for showing lesions in the temporal areas, uni- or bilateral.

Therapy with acyclovir should be initiated to all cases with suspected encephalitis while awaiting laboratory confirmation.

Subacute sclerosing panencephalitis (SSPE) is a progressive inflammatory disease of the CNS caused by persistent, aberrant measles virus infection, characterized by progressive loss of intellectual function, with behavior and learning difficulty, often associated with abnormal myoclonic movements. High anti-measles antibody titers in serum and CSF confirm the diagnosis. The mean interval between measles and the onset of SSPE is about 10 years. The MMR vaccine has resulted in virtual elimination of SSPE. Fever is not part of SSPE.

5.8.4
Brain Abscess

Brain abscess is uncommon in children. It may occur as a complication of OM, mastoiditis, sinusitis or meningitis, or ventriculoperitoneal shunt infection, following trauma or surgery to the skull, or as a result of haematogenous dissemination in children with acyanotic congenital heart disease.

Fever was the most common clinical finding in a study [62] of 101 children with brain abscess, occurring in 80% of the children, followed by vomiting, headache, seizure, focal neurological abnormalities, and lethargy. Papilledema and meningeal signs were also common. Overall mortality was 30%. High fever, age less than 1 year, multiple brain foci, and the presence of meningism or coma have a poorer prognosis.

The most frequently encountered pathogens are *S. aureus*, streptococci and Gram-negative aerobic bacilli.

Laboratory findings in the CSF reveal that the CSF culture is usually negative unless there is rupture of the abscess into ventricles. A CT scan shows the characteristic finding of a ring-enhancing lesion.

Therapy consists of antimicrobial treatment (third-generation cephalosporin, vancomycin, and metronidazole) with or without surgical excision or aspiration.

5.9
Osteomyelitis and Septic Arthritis

(See also Chapter 12: Differential Diagnosis: Arthritis)

Infection of the bone may occur as a complication of septicemia or due to local trauma (e.g., wound, abrasion). Acute hematogenous osteomyelitis involves most commonly the rapidly growing metaphysis of the long bones. The femur and tibia are most commonly affected bones. Septic arthritis is usually hematogenously acquired or the result of an extension from an osteomyelitic lesion. The knee is most commonly involved. *S. aureus* is the most frequent bacteria causing the infection (accounts for 90%), followed by kingella kingae, *S. pneumonia*, *S. pyogenes*, and *P. aeruginosa*, which are less common causes. Children with sickle-cell anaemia and other hemoglobulinopathy are at high risk of osteomyelitis caused by non-typhi salmonella.

This infection presents:

* In neonates with irritability and tenderness when the affected area is touched and limited movement of the affected extremities (pseudoparalyis). Fever is either mild or absent;
* In older children with high fever, refusal to walk, bone pain, and limping (if the lower extremities are affected). Examination reveals localized pain, tenderness, warmth, and erythema of the affected area.

The diagnosis is based on the following criteria:

* The isolation of bacterial pathogens or positive PCR from blood (positive in 30–60%), bone, or joint. Needle aspiration of the soft tissue or incision and drainage of the bone may yield the organism. In septic arthritis, joint fluid aspiration usually reveal purulent exudates with $>50,000$ leukocytes mm^{-3}, Gram-positive cocci, and a positive culture. Leukocytosis and elevated CRP are usually present. CRP is a very reliable parameter to assess the effectiveness of the treatment and recovery.
* Radiological findings (soft-tissue swelling, bone rarefaction, periosteal elevation, bone necrosis) may not appear during the first two weeks of the infection. A nuclear bone scan (showing increased uptake of the isotope) is a valuable adjunct to the diagnosis and is often positive before the appearance of the lesion in the X-ray.

Fever is the most common presenting symptom of bone infection, occurring in 90% of admission with a mean temperature of 39.1°C [63]. Most of those who were afebrile on admission became febrile during the ensuing 48 h after admission. Normalization of fever is not usually achieved during the first week despite antibiotic treatment. High fever usually continues for 4–5 days after the treatment. Therefore the presence of persistent and high fever during treatment does not necessarily signify failure of antibiotic treatment.

Initial antibiotics are likely to include i.v. ceftriaxone with clindamycin, flucloxacillin, or Fucidin for 3–6 weeks.

5.10
Viral Exanthems

Viral exanthems are common causes of febrile illness in children. More than 50 viral agents are known to cause a rash. Historically, exanthems were numbered in the order in which they were differentiated from other exanthems. Thus the first was measles; second scarlet fever; third rubella; forth the so-called Filatov–Dukes disease (no longer recognized as an entity); fifth erythema infectiosum, sixth exanthema subitum. As more exanthems were described, numerical assignment became impractical.

5.10.1
Measles

The first written record of measles is credited to Rhazes, a Persian physician of the tenth century; before that measles was thought to be a mild form of smallpox. Sydenham in the seventeenth century drew an accurate clinical picture of the disease, including recognition of its complications. When the United States was swept by measles during the seventeenth and eighteenth centuries, the infection was still believed to be a sequel to smallpox. Measles virus was cultivated in 1938.

Prior to the present vaccine, the attack rate of measles worldwide was close to 100% and measles was an important cause of mortality. In the United States, in 1949, measles ranked seventh among the causes of death for ages 1–4 years, which were mainly due to pneumonia. Following routine vaccination in 1963, measles has been almost eliminated. In the United Kingdom, the mortality rate until 1950 was 1 per 1000 measles cases. Following routine vaccination in 1968, the mortality rate decreased to 1 per 5000 [64].

In developing countries without immunization, measles affects virtually all children by the age of 4 years, the highest incidence being in the second half of the second year. Mortality in the past has ranged between 15 and 25%. More recently, this mortality has decreased progressively in developing countries, for example, in India and Africa. The single most important factor affecting mortality is poor nutritional status, leading to deficiencies in cell-mediated immunity and often death due to giant-cell pneumonia, diarrhea, or inclusion body encephalitis.

Measles is caused by paramyxovirus, which spreads by droplets from person to person. The incubation period is about 11 days. The spreads of the virus occurs through the following steps:

* Virus enters the epithelium of the conjunctiva and upper respiratory tract;
* Viral antigens presenting cells of the mononuclear phagocytic system, followed by expansion of antigen-specific T lymphocytes;

- High affinity IL-2 receptors rise before the onset of the rash and remain elevated for several weeks;
- Following its spread by day 5 to the mononuclear phagocytes of the liver and spleen, the virus continues its spread by day 8 via the blood to its target tissue (eye, lung, and gut epithelial cells). During these stages, viral spread is limited by natural killer cells and cytotoxic T cells. B cells are primed to produce antibody.

Clinically, the infection progresses through the following steps:

- The pre-exanthem stage expresses like a common cold, with abrupt fever, sneezing, dry cough, and conjunctivitis. The temperature increases gradually to reach a level ranging from 39 to 40.5°C. About 24 h prior to the appearance of exanthema, Koplik's spots can be detected in about 80% of cases as tiny (about 1 mm) whitish spots in the buccal mucosa opposite the lower morals.
- The exanthem appears at the peak of symptoms with a temperature of about 39.5°C. The rash appears first behind the ears and spreads to the face, neck, trunk, and extremities. The rash begins to clear on the third day. During the exanthem period, the fever usually peaks on the second or third day, and then falls by lysis over a 24-h period. Fever that persists after the third day may signify bacterial complication. There are signs of pharyngitis, cervical lymphadenopathy, and occasionally a mild splenomegaly. Shortly after the rash appears, the child becomes anergic, with suppression of the delayed hypersensitivity to skin test antigens and reduced lymphoproliferation and lymphokine production in response to mitogenic stimuli. The infectivity decreases considerably with the onset of the rash.

Blood counts often show leucopenia and lymphopenia. Suppression of immune function is manifested *in vivo* by the loss of response to tuberculin skin test. On the other hand, there is an increased activation of lymphocytes and macrophages, plasma INF-γ and IL-2 receptors. The diagnosis of measles can be confirmed by measles complement fixation or hemagglutination antibody test.

Complications include pneumonia (viral or bacterial), OM, gastroenteritis, laryngitis, encephalitis, bronchiectasis, reactivation of tuberculosis, and SSPE.

Gamma globulin (0.25 mg kg^{-1}) within 5 days of exposure to measles virus prevents the disease. Oral vitamin A (400,000 U) can decrease mortality in children in developing countries.

5.10.2
Varicella

Varicella zoster virus is a member of the herpesvirus family. The eruption is often the first sign of the onset of varicella, particularly in young children. Older children and adults may have prodromal symptoms preceding the characteristic eruption by 1–2 days, which include fever in the range of 38–38.5°C (temperature up to 40.5°C may occur), malaise, headache, and abdominal pain. The characteristic eruption of macules and papules appears first on the back, then on the rest of the trunk, spreading within hours to the face and scalp. The lesions progress from macules to papules to vesicles and begin crusting within 8–10 h. Characteristically, these lesions are found simultaneously. The highest body temperature of up to 40.5°C occurs during the first 3 days of eruption and falls to a normal level on the fourth day.

When maternal varicella develops within 4 days of delivery, neonates develop severe varicella within 5–10 days postpartum. The disease is associated with a mortality of around 20% due to disseminated chickenpox, usually with severe pneumonitis. When maternal varicella develops 10–20 days before delivery, transfer of maternal antibodies causes a more benign illness.

Varicella is usually a benign disease. Complications include pneumonia in about 1% (affecting primarily adults and newborns), with a chest X-ray showing nodular infiltrates, secondary staphylococcal skin infection, thrombocytopenic purpura, cerebellar ataxia, and encephalitis. Secondary bacterial infection from *Staphylococci* and *Streptococci* can be fatal and will need urgent treatment. Varicella is severe and may be fatal in patients with impaired cellular immunity, such as those receiving cytotoxic drugs. Children with hypogammaglobulinemia recover normally from varicella.

Most patients require no special treatment. Aspirin should not be administered because of the risk of Reye's syndrome. Itching can be relieved by simple soothing lotions such as calamine and oral antihistamine. Patients with severe varicella or with complication should receive acyclovir. This antiviral drug promotes the cutaneous healing and reduces the duration of fever. A vaccine is now available and is increasingly being used to prevent this disease.

5.10.3
Rubella

Rubella virus may cause inapparent or severe infection. The infection is usually mild, and children usually present with sore throat, rash, lymphadenopathy (prominent in the posterior cervical area), and low-grade fever (rarely exceeding 39°C) for several days. Fever may persist for 1–2 days, rarely 3 days. In older children, particularly in females after puberty, the infection is more severe and prolonged. There are usually painful, with visibly enlarged lymph nodes involving postauricular, occipital, and posterior cervical nodes, with polyarthralgia or arthritis.

The infection with rubella virus is particularly important to pediatricians because of possible fetal–maternal transmission. Congenital infection (rubella syndrome) is highest in the early weeks of pregnancy, manifesting as eye disease (cataract, retinopathy, glaucoma), sensorineural deafness, heart lesions (patent ductus arteriosus, pulmonary artery stenosis, aortic stenosis, coarctation of the aorta or ventricular septal defect), neurological abnormalities, or thrombocytopenic purpura. Prevention of maternal rubella used to be through routine immunization of all girls of 11–14 years of age and women of child-bearing age, but the use of the MMR has been more successful in reducing rubella syndrome by preventing transmission of the virus from children to pregnant mothers.

5.10.4
Erythema Infectiosum

Erythema infectiosum (EI) or the fifth disease is an acute, benign communicable disease with a characteristic eruption. It usually affects children aged 5–15 years. The infection is caused by parvovirus B19, which also can cause a transient aplastic crisis in patients with hemolytic anemia and hemoglobulinopathy, and an arthritis similar to rheumatoid arthritis. The mean incubation time is 9 days (range 4–14 days).

The eruption is generally the first and only diagnostic clinical manifestation of the disease, occurring in 100% of cases. It starts on the face with a "slapped cheeks" appearance, resembling scarlet fever. The rash spreads to the trunk and extremities in 1–4 days after the onset of the facial rash. The rash is erythematous maculopapular and tends to assume a reticular or lacy pattern, which last for 4–6 days. Common associated clinical findings are pruritis, arthralgia/or arthritis (mainly in adults), and headache. Fever is observed in about 23% of cases. Encephalitis is a very rare complication.

5.10.5
Exanthema Subitum

Exanthema subitum (ES) is caused by human herpes virus 6 (HHV-6), and was identified in 1988. The virus is recognized as a major of febrile illness with viremia and a high temperature (mean 39.7°C), sometimes with rash. Occasionally the virus can cause an inapparent infection without fever, a rash without fever, or a fulminant hepatitis and death.

ES is the most common febrile exanthem in children under the age of 3 years. Approximately 30% of children develop this disease eventually. Ninety percent of all cases occur in children aged 6–24 months. The incubation period is between 5 and 15 days.

Before the onset, children may have a short period of irritability and malaise. Onset of fever is abrupt (sometimes triggering a febrile seizure) and characteristically continuous (or less commonly intermittent), often as high as 40–41°C. The fever persists for 3–4 days in about 75% and for 5–6 days in the remaining 25%. There is usually no focus to explain the presence of fever except often a mild pharyngitis, suboccipital or posterior cervical lymphadenopathy. The temperature usually drops by crisis over a period of a few hours, coinciding with the appearance of the rash (Fig. 5.3). The rash appears predominately on the neck and trunk, lasting 24–36h. Characteristically, the child becomes well and afebrile when the rash erupts.

When fever is intermittent, the temperature is normal or slightly elevated in the morning, only to rise to 40–40.5 by early evening. Fever may fall by lysis over a period of 24–36h.

Laboratory findings commonly show leukocytosis of 12,000–20,000 with a slight increase in neutrophils.

5.11
Tropical Diseases

5.11.1
Tuberculosis

Tuberculosis is a major cause of morbidity and mortality throughout the world. Although reported cases have declined, particularly in developed countries, 1–3 million still die annually from the disease. The number of TB cases in the United States has declined from 6036 in 1962 to 1261 in 1985; 80% of them occurred in the minority groups living there

5

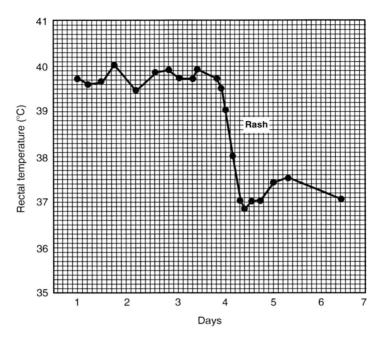

Fig. 5.3 Continuous fever pattern seen in erythema subitum, with a drop in temperature by crisis

[65]. However, after four decades of steady decline, the annual case rate leveled off in 1985 and has increased worldwide during the past two decades. Children acquire the infection from adults who have active disease and are expectorating tubercle bacilli. Children themselves are noncontagious. Therefore, every effort should be made to identify the adult source for eradicating the source.

When TB bacilli are inhaled, only the fine particles containing one to three tubercle bacilli reach the alveolar macrophages of the lung. Although macrophages are able to eliminate tubercle bacilli, they must be activated by T lymphocytes, especially INF-γ, in order to do so.

Neonatal TB occurs through transmission of infection from mother to infant via the placenta or amniotic fluid. Neonates present with feeding difficulty, failure to thrive, jaundice, respiratory distress, or hepatosplenomegaly. Fever is usually absent. Chest X-ray shows bronchopneumonia. The disease often runs a fulminant course with rapid multiplication of tubercle bacilli and minimal giant-cell formation.

In older children, *primary infection* (refers to infection in a person with no prior immunity) is asymptomatic in most cases. Occasionally there is low-grade fever (38–38.5°C). Radiologically, a parenchymal lesion is usually not visible, but hilar adenitis is prominent and may cause compression of the adjacent soft bronchus, causing wheezing and nonproductive cough. With increased compression, or following perforation of an infected lymphnode into the bronchus, segmental atelectasis may ensue. Other presentations are erythema nodosum, phlyctenular conjunctivitis (as a result of hypersensitivity reaction), or TB pneumonia, which resembles radiologically bacterial pneumonia with high fever, cough, and dyspnea.

Miliary TB in children usually presents with no specific symptoms and signs. Fever is present in about 75% of cases, with anorexia, weight loss, night sweats, and dyspnea. Ophthalmoscopy may detect typical choroidal tubercles in the retina. Almost one-third of the children with active TB may have extrapulmonary manifestations, such as adenitis (frequently as a nontender, firm-tender, firm cervical lymphadenitis, or TB meningitis (see Section 5.8.1).

The diagnosis of TB is established by:

* History of contact with an infectious case;
* Symptoms: persistent, unremitting cough, persistent fever and fatigue, night sweating, chest pain, and weight loss;
* Identification of the mycobacteria (positive in about 30–40% of cases), from sputum, gastric fluid, pleural fluid, CSF, or other tissues, or by PCR. Acid-fast smear is positive in 10–20%;
* X-ray findings, often in the form of "unresolved pneumonia", with enlarged mediastinal lymphadenopathy;
* Positive tuberculin test, performed by using 5 tuberculin units of purified protein derivative (PPD). A positive reaction is 5 mm or more induration present after 48–72 h;
* Detection of Mycobacterium tuberculosis specific antigens (IFN-γ release assay).

Fever in TB may occur in the following situations:

* In pulmonary (e.g. miliary TB) and extrapulmonary TB as a leading manifestation of the disease. Children with combined intrapulmonary and extrapulmonary TB have a higher peak and a longer duration of fever than those with intrapulmonary TB alone [66];
* In any form of TB as a persistent sign for several months, even after appropriate therapy has been instituted. Fever in excess of 38.8°C often correlates with persistent fever for more than 2 weeks, and sometimes up to several months. Persistent fever is mostly due to the disease itself;
* In HIV as a coinfection, often present as unresolving pneumonia. This carries a high mortality despite adequate anti-TB and HIV therapy;
* In hypersensitivity to anti-tuberculous drugs (usually appearing between the third and fifth day of treatment). This should be considered in any patient with persistent fever after initiation of therapy. Such a drug reaction should be suspected if the fever becomes higher than it was prior to therapy and when other manifestations of hypersensitivity such as rash or eosinophilia appear;
* In adult TB-infected patients in about 40%, usually low-grade and appearing insidiously.

Drugs used for treatment of TB are shown in the Table 5.16. A 6-month regimen for drug-susceptible TB with isoniazid (INH) and rifampicin and pyrazinamide for the first 2 months followed by INH and rifampicin for the remaining 4 months is recommended. If drug resistance is possible, initial treatment should include ethambutol, streptomycin, amikacin, or ciprofloxacin until drug susceptibility result becomes available. Shorter regimes using four drugs in the initial phase are increasingly being adopted.

5.11.2
Malaria

Malaria is caused by a protozoan of the genus *Plasmodium* transmitted by anopheles mosquitoes. The four species that commonly infect man are *P. malariae* (benign quartan malaria), *P. vivax*, *P. ovale* (benign tertian malaria), and *P. falciparum* (malignant tertian malaria). Whereas *P. vivax* invades mostly the youngest erythroblast and *P. malariae* invades primarily the older erythrocytes, in both no more than 1–2% of erythrocytes are infected at a time. *P. falciparum*, on the other hand, invades all ages of erythrocytes indiscriminately, resulting in a very high infection rate. The number of malaria cases and deaths is estimated at 200–300 million and 2–3 million, respectively. Over 50% of childhood deaths in many parts of Africa are attributed to malaria. Most cases of imported malaria to the United Kingdom are *P. falciparum* and *vivax*.

Patients with *P. falciparum* infection have elevated TNF-α, soluble IL-2 receptors, and natural killer cell activity, but a decrease in the CD4:CD8 lymphocyte ratio. The level of TNF correlates with the severity and mortality rate in patients with this infection. Changes in the TNF also correlate with the rise and fall in temperature during *P. vivax* paroxysms.

Infected children present with fever, lethargy, headache, cough, anorexia, nausea, vomiting, diarrhea, abdominal pain, and dehydration. Physical examination reveals splenomegaly (detected in almost 100%) and commonly hepatomegaly. Nephrotic syndrome may occur with *P. malariae* infection. The presenting clinical signs of cerebral malaria are severe headache, irritability, delirium, coma, hyperpyrexia, convulsion, and meningism.

In endemic regions, malaria is a major cause of fever, occurring in virtually 100% of cases. Classical periodicity of fever may not occur in children during the first few years of life: intermittent, continuous, or remittent patterns may all occur.

A child with fever caused by malaria may present with the following:

- A typical tertian paroxysm (*P. vivax* and *P. ovale*) in a nonimmune child (usually in the afternoon or evening) with shivering and rigor, lasting 1–2 h. The skin is cold and pale. The next stage is marked by high fever, up to 41°C, lasting 2–4 h. The skin is dry and warm and the patient feels hot and has usually headache. The last 2–4 h are characterized by a drop in body temperature to normal with sweating. In tertian infection, the paroxysm recurs at 48 h intervals (Fig. 5.4) while in quartan infection the paroxysm recurs at 72 h intervals (Fig. 5.5). Early in the infection with *P. falciparum* the fever may be irregular or continuous. A significant correlation exists between heavy parasitemia of 2% or greater and high grade temperature.
- Malaria is the most common cause of febrile seizure (FS) worldwide.
- Blackwater fever is a state of acute intravascular hemolysis accompanied by hemoglobulinuria, as a complication of *P. falciparum*.
- Human parvovirus B19 infection adds to the severity of anaemia. The virus is highly erythrotropic, infecting erythroid progenitor cells.
- Associated diseases as a complication of malaria are, for example, pneumonia, or anemia.

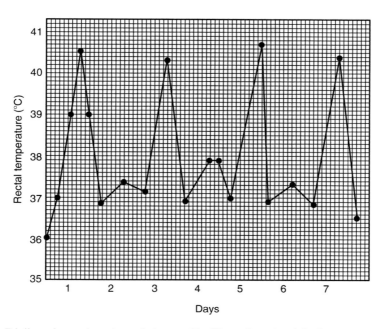

Fig. 5.4 Febrile cycle seen in tertian malaria caused by *Plasmodium vivax* infection

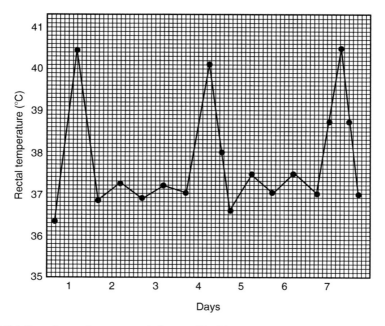

Fig. 5.5 Febrile cycle seen in quartan malaria caused by *Plasmodium malariae* infection

Table 5.17 Drugs used for prophylaxis and therapy of malaria[a]

	Dose	Adverse reaction
Prophylaxis		
Chloroquine	5 mg base/kg/weekly	Retinal damage
Fansidar	125–750 mg (according to the age)	Severe mucocutaneous reaction
Therapy		
Chloroquine	10 mg kg^{-1}; followed by 5 mg kg^{-1} in 6 h, then 5 mg kg^{-1} Twice daily for 2 days	Gastrointestinal upset, visual disturbance, rash
Quinine	25 mg kg^{-1} per day three times for 10–14 days	Tinnitus
Primaquine	0.3 mg base kg^{-1} once daily for 14 days	Methaemoglobulinemia, haemolytic anemia (in G6PD)

[a] Treatment of malaria varies considerably around the world and advice about antimalarials will depend upon the location and expert advice

- The pattern of fever is irregular (and not with typical periodic fever). This may occur in young children in early falciparum infection or as a consequence of previous chemoprophylaxis, which modifies the typical pattern of fever.
- PUO is present, with fever as the only sign of malaria without anemia or splenomegaly.
- Recurrent fever months after treatment of falciparum malaria persist owing to relapsing *vivax* or *ovale* infection if the child initially had a mixed infection [67].

Diagnosis is easy when children present with typical paroxysms of fever. Definite diagnosis is made by a Giemsa-stained blood smear (thick smear increases the yield). A rapid diagnosis can be obtained by utilizing ribosomal ribonucleic acid (rRNA) of the parasite. Laboratory findings include anaemia, with Hb concentration of 5–11 g dl^{-1} and leucopenia. Thrombocytopenia, hyponatremia, and hypoglycemia may also occur.

Therapy. Hospitalization for any child with suspected or confirmed malaria is always indicated to assess severity and extent of severity. Paracetamol is commonly used for fever management. Paracetamol has been reported to prolong parasitemia, although the evidence for that was found to be insufficient [68]. Chemoprophylaxis and therapy are shown in the Table 5.17. Chloroquine remains the treatment for choice for benign malarias, while quinine is given for falciparum malaria. Children receiving iron therapy may be at increased risk of fever associated with severe parasitemia (see the section on anaemia in Chapter 6)

5.11.3
Brucellosis

Brucellosis is primarily a zoonotic infection caused by small, nonmotile, Gram-negative coccobacilli of the genus *Brucella*. There are four important species pathogenic to humans: *B. melitensis* (Malta fever, found primarily in goats and sheep), *B. abortus* (abortus fever, in cattle), *B. suis* (swine), and *B. canis* (dogs). The infection is transmitted to humans through direct contact with infected animals or their products, and through consumption of infected milk, milk products, or meat. More than half a million cases per year occur worldwide.

The clinical features of brucellosis depend largely upon the infected species of organism. Infection with *B. melitensis* produces more severe symptoms and signs than other species, with fever, arthritis, arthralgia, backache, anorexia and weight loss, tender hepatosplenomegaly, and lymphadenopathy.

Fever is a prominent feature in brucellosis, which manifests:

* in almost every patient (90–100% of cases);
* often insidiously over the course of several days;
* sometimes suddenly with chills, rising sharply to a peak up to 40.5°C and swinging considerably;
* as a remittent pattern, falling usually to a normal level;
* as periodic fever, with symptoms lasting a few days or weeks followed by symptom-free intervals that last weeks and months. During this period patients feel tired and may run a low fever in the evening; and
* as PUO, particularly in endemic areas.

Complications include spondylitis, osteomyelitis, granulomatous reaction of the eye, meningitis, or meningo-encephalitis. *B. endocarditis* is rare and may be responsible for most death due to the disease

Laboratory findings include anemia, leucopenia, lymphopenia, and raised liver enzymes. The diagnosis is established by positive culture of brucella organisms from blood or bone marrow aspirate, or positive serological tests (agglutination titer of >1:80).

Several antibiotics are recommended. In a multicenter therapeutic study of 1100 children with brucellosis in Kuwait (101), the most effective treatment in young children was a combination Co-trimoxazole for 3 weeks and gentamicin during the first 5 days. In children older than 8 years, a combination of doxycycline (or tetracycline) is given for three weeks and gentamicin during the first 5 days. Rifampicin has also been used successfully in combination with streptomycin in the treatment of brucella endocarditis.

5.11.4
Lyme Disease

Lyme disease (LD) is a multisystem inflammatory disease caused by the spirochete *Borerlia burgdorferi*. It is transmitted by the deer tick (*Xodides dammini*). LD is the most common vectorborne illness in the United States. *B. burgdorferi* is a potent inducer of IL-1 from peripheral blood mononuclear cells.

Lyme disease has been divided into three stages:

* The first one consists of a flu-like illness with a characteristic annular skin rash (erythema migrans), which develops at the site of the tick bite in approximately two-thirds of patients. Antibiotics at this stage may prevent subsequent stages.
* The second stage follows 2–12 weeks after the tick bite and is characterized by disseminated infection causing aseptic meningitis and cranial neuritis (most commonly

presenting as Bell palsy) and carditis (most commonly presenting as atrioventricular block or myocarditis).

• The third stage is characterized by oligoarticular arthritis and acrodermatitis chronica atrophicans from 6 weeks to 2 years after the tick bite in 50–80% of patients.

IL-1 and IL-1 receptor antagonist, both produced by monocytes and macrophages, may influence the course of arthritis. High concentration of IL-1 receptor antagonist and low concentration of IL-1 may indicate rapid resolution of arthritis, whereas the reverse pattern of cytokine concentration may indicate recovery.

Fever is often an early of the disease, occurring with other flu-like manifestations. Fever is usually intermittent and low-grade and has been reported in about 50% of children. Fever, however, can be as high as 40°C and persistent, which can cause PUO.

Diagnosis of LD depends on characteristic clinical features, in particular the appearance of erythema migrans. Specific IgM antibodies against *B. burgdorferi* appear 3–4 weeks after the infection and peak after 6–8 weeks. Specific IgG antibodies usually become detectable in the second month after the onset of infection.

Uncomplicated cases of LD are treated with oral penicillin or amoxicillin divided into three doses for 21 days. For children older than 12 years, doxycycline twice daily for 21 days or tetracycline for the same duration is effective. For arthritis, antibiotic therapy should continue for 4 weeks and often includes a third-generation cephalosporin. For meningitis, penicillin G/cephalosporin is given intravenously for 2–3 weeks.

5.11.5
Leptospirosis

Leptospirosis is a zoonosis caused by the genus *Leptospira*. Human infections occur through contact with water (e.g., flood water) or soil contaminated with infected animal's urine. The incubation period is usually between 6 and 12 days. The disease is characteristically biphasic:

• The primary phase manifests as an influenza-like illness lasting 5–7 days with abrupt onset of chills and fever 39.5–40.5°C lasting 3–7 days. This phase reflects the presence of leptospiremia.
• In the second phase, lasting 4–30 days, specific antibodies begin to appear. Fever is not prominent in this phase, but may occur as a result of aseptic meningitis mediated by antigen–antibody reaction.

Clinically, the patients presents in one of the following three forms:

• The mild and more common form of the disease is characterized by headache, myalgia, arthralgia, abdominal pain, and conjunctival suffusion. Fever lasts longer than 5 days in two-thirds of cases.
• In the more severe and potentially fatal form, patients present with jaundice, hemorrhage, anemia, disturbance of consciousness, and renal dysfunction.
• PUO may occur in about 10% of cases.

Laboratory findings include leukocytosis, hyperbilirubinemia, and intravascular hemolysis. Leptospirochets may be cultured from the blood (dark-field microscopy), urine, and CSF.

IgM-ELISA test may confirm the diagnosis. Penicillin is the treatment of choice and should be given during the first phase of illness to prevent complications.

5.11.6
Leishmaniasis

Of the three clinical forms of leishmaniasis, cutaneous, mucocutaneous, and visceral, only the latter form is associated with febrile episodes. The disease is transmitted to humans by bite of infected sandfly *Phlebotomus*. It is the second most fatal parasitic disease after malaria. Coinfection with HIV has been reported [69].

The visceral form (also known as kala azar, black fever) is caused by the protozoan *Leishmania donovani*. The infection produces the following clinical course:

* Following the invasion of the blood stream, the organisms settle in the reticuloendothelial system and viscera, where they multiply within the cell's cytoplasm despite being engulfed by mononuclear cells. Eventually, the mononuclear cells rupture and release many organisms, which are subsequently engulfed by other phagocytic cells.
* A few months after the initial bite, the patients develop symptoms manifested by varying degree and patterns of fever (see below), emaciation, massive hepatosplenomegaly, lymphadenopathy, profound weakness, and pancytopenia. The weakness is mainly caused by anemia and chronic infection. The pancytopenia is caused by a combination of invading the bone marrow by leishmania, hypersplenism, and autoimmune process. Thrombocytopenia may be severe enough to produce bleeding. Leukopenia causes secondary bacterial infections, such as pneumonia.
* Death occurs within 1–2 years in 80–90% of untreated patients.

All infected children have fever (Table 5.18), which manifests in protean patterns:

* In young children, it increases gradually to a peak within 2 weeks from the onset (40–41.1°C), becoming then intermittent (temperature returning to a normal level within the same day) or continuous (fever fluctuates by less than 1°C) and resolving usually by lysis.

Clinical findings	%
Fever	100
Splenomegaly	96
Hepatomegaly	91
Abdominal distention	89
Respiratory distress	50
Diarrhea	13
Jaundice	3
Associated septicemia	2
Hemorrhage	1

Table 5.18 symptoms and signs of kala azar in 100 children, admitted to Baghdad's University Hospital

- In older children, with more chronic presentation, fever may be continuous initially but is usually low grade.
- Classically fever is double quotidian (two spikes within 24 h or a 12 h cycle).
- PUO may occur with a duration between 1 and 18 months [70], with a median duration of fever of 4–5 weeks.

Pathogenesis and fever are related to the interaction of T-helper cells and various cytokines. INF-γ, IL-6, and IL-4 are involved during active disease [71]. IL-10 is known to suppress the macrophages, which may explain the paucity of cytokines secreted by these cells. Diagnosis is by identifying the parasite from bone marrow or splenic aspirate. Treatment is presently with Miltefosine, orally 2.5 mg kg^{-1} per day for 4 weeks. Pentavalent antimony compounds and liposomal amphotericin B are also used. Defervescence usually occurs after a median of 6 days of treatment.

5.11.7
Fever and Malnutrition

It has been estimated that 10.6 million children are still dying yearly, mostly due to pneumonia, diarrhea, neonatal causes and, in sub-Saharan Africa, malaria [72]. Malnutrition was an underlying cause in over 50% of the deaths. These children are particularly susceptible to measles and tuberculosis. Chronic infections, on the other hand, may lead to loss of nutrients and malnutrition.

Protein-calorie malnutrition (PCM) has been divided into severe (kwashiorkor, marasmus, and intermediate cases), moderate severe (nutritional, dwarfing, or stunting and wasting), and early (clinically detectable only by anthropometric measurement). In developing countries, the severe form of malnutrition is common as a result of several factors, including severe dietary imbalance. Marasmus results from deficiency of all nutrients, whereas kwashiorkor is due primarily to protein deficiency. In developed countries, PCM may result from debilitating chronic diseases.

Patients with PCM are susceptible to infection and fever for a variety of reasons:

- Delayed mononuclear cell release from the bone marrow
- Impaired T-cell-mediated immunity, deficiency in circulating levels of the complement system and interferon
- Normally, reduced secretary IgA (B cells and circulating immunoglobulins)
- Impaired acute-phase response

Fever in a malnourished child is usually the result of infection. Respiratory infection, for example, pneumonia, TB, and intestinal infection are most common. In severe malnutrition, fever may be absent, and instead hypothermia may occur in response to infection signifying a poor prognosis for survival.

Malnourished children who are febrile are at increased risk of paracetamol-induced hepatotoxicity. Reduction in calorie or protein intake in association with multiple doses of paracetamol may have profound effects on sulfate and glucuronide. The combination of malnutrition and HIV is particularly devastating.

References

Acute URTI

1. Dingle JH, Badger GF, Jordan WS. Illness in the home. Press of Western Reserve University. Cleveland, Ohio 1964
2. Scott GM, Secher DS, Flowers D, et al. Toxicity of interferon. Br Med J 1981; 282: 1345–8
3. Putto A, Ruuskanen O, Meurman O. Fever in respiratory virus infection. Am J Dis Child 1986; 140: 1159–63
4. Wright PF, Ross KB, Thompson J, et al. Influenza A infections in young children: Primary natural and protective efficacy of live-vaccine-induced or naturally acquired immunity. N Engl J Med 1977; 296: 829–34

Infectious Mononucleosis

5. Shurin S. Infectious mononucleosis. Pediatr Clin North Am 1979; 26: 315–26
6. Rapp CE, Hewetson JF. Infectious mononucleosis and the Epstein-Barr virus. Am J Dis Child 1978; 132: 78–86
7. Auwaerter PG. Recent advance in the understanding of infectious mononucleosis: Are prospects improved for treatment or control? Expert Rev Anti Infect Ther 2006; 4: 1039–49

Acute Upper Airway Obstruction

8. Davis HW, Carter JC, Galvis AG, et al. Acute upper airway obstruction: Croup and epiglottitis. Pediatr Clin North Am 1981; 28: 859–80

Bronchiolitis & Asthma

9. El-Radhi AS, Barry W, Patel S. Association of fever and severe clinical course in bronchiolitis. Arch Dis Child 1999; 81: 231–4
10. El-Radhi AS, Carroll J. Fever and hyperthermia. In: Fever in paediatric practice. Blackwell. Oxford 1994, p.19
11. Issac D. Production of interferon in respiratory syncytial virus bronchiolitis. Arch Dis Child 1989; 64: 92–5
12. El-Radhi AS, Patel S. The Clinical Course of Childhood Asthma in Association with Fever (Unpublished)
13. El-Radhi AS, Hogg CL, Bungre JK, et al. Effect of oral glucocorticoid treatment on serum inflammatory markers in acute asthma. Arch Dis Child 2000; 83: 158–62
14. Philips K, Shikany S. The value of hyperpyrexia in the treatment of asthma. South Med J 1935; 28: 801–12
15. Nickels DA, Moore DC. Serum cortisol responses in febrile children. Pediatr Infect Dis J 1989; 8: 16–20

Pneumonia

16. Levin S. The atypical pneumonia syndrome. J Am Med Assoc 1984; 251: 945–8
17. McCarthy PL, Tomasso L, Dolan TF. Predicting fever response pf children with pneumonia treated with antibiotics. Clin Pediatr 1980; 19: 753–60
18. Clark JE, Hammal D, Spencer D, et al. Children with pneumonia: How do they present and how are they managed?. Arch Dis Child 2007; 92: 394–8
19. Copps S, Allen V, Sueltmann S, et al. Community-outbreak of mycoplasma pneumonia. J Am Med Assoc 1968; 204: 121–6
20. Hughes WT, Price RA, Kim HK, et al. Penumonitis in children with malignancies. J Pediatr 1973; 82: 404–15

Gastroenteritis

21. William CH, Robert HG, Robert EB, et al. Effects of nutritional status on diarrhea in Peruvian children. J Pediatr 2002; 140: 210–6
22. Kosek M,Bern C, Guerrant RL. The global burden of diarrhoeal disease, as estimated from studies published between 1992 and 2000. Bull World Health Organ 2003; 81(3): 197–204
23. Bhutta ZA, Belgaumi A, Abdur Rab M, et al. Child health and survival in the Eastern Mediterranean region. Br Med J 2006; 333: 839–42
24. Glaeson M, Merson MH. Global progress in the control of diarrhoeal diseases. Pediatr Infect Dis J 1990; 9: 345–55
25. Vargas M, Gascon J, Casals C, et al. Etiology of diarrhea in children less than five years of age in Ifakara, Tanzania. Am. J. Trop. Med. Hyg. 2004; 70(5): 536–9
26. Vu Nguyen T, Le Van P, Le Huy C, et al. Etiology and epidemiology of diarrhea in children in Hanoi, Vietnam. Int J Infect Dis 2006; 10: 298–308
27. Klein EJ, Boster DR, Stapp JR, et al. Diarrhea etiology in a Children's Hospital Emergency Department: A prospective cohort study. Clin Infect Dis 2006; 43(7): 807–13
28. Kariuki S, Revathi G, Kariuki N, et al. Characterisation of community acquired non-typhoidal Salmonella from bacteraemia and diarrhoeal infections in children admitted to hospital in Nairobi, Kenya. BMC Microbiol. 2006; 6: 101
29. Chalker PR, Blaser MJ. A review of human salmonellosis: Magnitude of salmonella infection in the United States. Rev Infect Dis 1988; 10: 111–23
30. Stoycheva M, Murdjeva M. Serum levels on INF-gamma, IL-12, TNF-alpha, and IL-10, and bacterial clearance in patients with gastroenteric Salmonella infection. Scand J Infect Dis 2005; 37: 11–14
31. El-Radhi AS, Rostila T, Vesikari T. Association of high fever and short bacterial excretion after salmonellosis. Arch Dis Child 1992; 67: 531–2
32. Ryan CA, Hargrett-Bean NT, Blake PA. Salmonella typhi infections in the United States 1975–1984: Increasing role of foreign travel. Rev Infect Dis 1989; 11: 1–9
33. El-Radhi AS, Newcombe T, Ghalli A. Effect of pyrexia on Shigella and Salmonella gastroenteritis (unpublished)
34. Hiranrattana A, Mekmuullica J, Chatsuwan T, et al. Childhood shigellosis at King Chulalongkorn Memorial Hospital, Bangkok, Thailand: A 5-year review (1996–2000). Southeast Asian J Trop Med Public Health. 2005; 36(3): 683–5
35. Thoren A, Wolde-Mariam T, Stintzing G, et al. Antibiotics in the treatment of gastroenteritis caused by enteropathogenic Escherichia coli. J Infect Dis 1980; 141: 27–31

36. Mohammed HF, Hassan MK, Bakir SS. Campylobacter jejuni Gastroenteritis in children in Basrah, Iraq. Med J Basrah Univ 2004; 22(1–2): 1–5

37. Marks MI, Pai CH, Lafleur L, et al. Yersinia enterocolitica: A prospective study of clinical, bacteriologic, and epidemiologic features. J Pediatr 1980; 96: 26–31

38. Cook SM, Glass RI, Le Baron CW. Global seasonality of Rota virus infection. Bull World Health Organ 1990; 68: 171–177

39. Blutt SE, Matson DO, Crawford SE, et al. Rotavirus Antigenemia in Children Is Associated with Viremia. PLoS Med. 2007; 4: e121

40. Ruuska T, Vesikari T. Rotavirus disease in Finnish children: Use of numerical scores for clinical severity of diarrhoeal episodes. Scand J Infect Dis 1990; 22: 259–267

41. Brandt CD, Rodriguez WJ, Arrobio JO, et al. Adenovirus and pediatric gastroenteritis. J Infect Dis 1985; 151: 437–43

42. Grajden M, Brown M, Petrasek A, et al. Clinical features of adenovirus gastroenteritis: A review of 127 cases. Pediatr Infect Dis J 1990; 9: 636–41

43. Rautanen T, El-Radhi AS, Vesikari T. Clinical experience with a hypotonic oral rehydration solution in acute diarrhoea. Acta Paediatr 1992; 81: 1–3

44. BMJ Publishing Group.Clinical evidence. BMJ Publishing Group. UK 2000; 4th Issue, pp. 373–9

UTI

45. Ginsburg CM, McCracken GH. Urinary tract infection in young children. Pediatrics 1982; 69: 409–12

46. Zorc JJ, Levene DA, Platt SL, et al. Clinical and demographic factors associated with UTI in young febrile infants. Pediatrics 2005; 116: 644–8

47 Hodson EM, Willis NS, Craig JC. Antibiotics for acute pyelonephritis in children. Cochrane Database Syst Rev 2007; no 4p. CD003772

HIV

48. Steinbrook R. Message from Toronto-Deliver AIDS treatment and prevention. N Engl J Med 2006; 355: 1081–4

49. Greenberg AE, Dabis F, Marum LH, de Cock KM. HIV infection in Africa. In, Pizzo PA, Wilfert CM (Eds). Pediatric AIDS. The challenge of HIV infection in infants, children and adolescents. 3rd Edition. Lippincott. Philadelphia. 1998; pp. 23–46

50. Andiman WA, Mezger J, Shapiro E. Invasive bacterial infections in children born to women infected with human immunodeficiency virus type 1. J Pediatr. 1994; 124: 846–52

51. Ruiz-Contreras J, De Jose MI, Ciria L, Mellado MJ, Ramos JT, Clemente J, Rodriguez-Cerrato V. Fever of unknown origin in HIV infected children. Int Conf AIDS. 1998; 12: 44 (abstract no. 12165)

Infection of the CNS

52. Dery MA, Hasbun R. Changing epidemiology of bacterial meningitis. Curr Infect Dis Rep 2007; 9: 301–7

53. Holt DE, Halket S, de Louvois J, et al. Neonatal meningitis in England and Wales: 10 years on. Arch Dis Child Fetal Neonatal Ed 2001; 84: F85–9
54. Thompson MJ, Ninis N, Perera R, et al. Clinical recognition of meningococcal disease in children and adolescent. Lancet 2006; 367: 397–403
55. Heckmatt JZ. Coliform meningitis in the newborn. Arch Dis Child 1976; 51: 569–73
56. Wong VK, Hitchcock W, Mason WH. Meningococcal infection in children: A review of 100 cases. Pediatr Infect Dis J 1989; 8: 224–7
57. Small PM, Täuber MG, Hackbarth CJ, et al. Influence of body temperature on bacterial growth rate in experimental pneumococcal meningitis in rabbits. Infect Immun 1986; 52: 484–7
58. Sande MA, Sande ER. The influence of fever on the development of experimental Streptococcus pneumoniae meningitis. J Infect Dis 1987; 156: 849–50
59. Lin TY, Nelson JD, McCracken GH. Fever during treatment for bacterial meningitis. Pediatr infect Dis 1984; 3: 319–22
60. Rantala H, Uhari N. Occurrence of childhood encephalitis: A population-based study. Pediatr Infect Dis 1989; 8: 426–30
61. Koskiniemi M, Vaheri A. Acute encephalitis of viral origin. Scand J Infect Dis 1982; 14: 181–7
62. Saez-Liorens XJ, Umana MA, Odio CM, et al. Brain abscess in infants and children. Pediatr Infect Dis 1989; 8: 449–58

Osteomyelitis

63. Ceroni D, Requsci M, Pazos J, et al. Acute bone and joint infection in children: How much attention should be paid to persistent fever during IV antibiotic therapy. Rev Chir Orthop Repar Appar Mot 2003; 89: 250–6

Viral Exanthems

64. Miller CL. Current impact of measles in the United Kingdom. Rev Infect Dis 1983; 5: 427–38

Tropical Diseases

65. Snider DE, Rieder HL, Combs D, et al. Tuberculosis in children. Pediatr Infect Dis J 1988; 7: 271–8
66. Lin YS, Chering HY, Yin CL. Clinical characteristics of tuberculosis in children in the North of Taiwan. J Microb Immun Infect 2005; 38: 41–6
67. Brabin JB Ganley Y. Imported malaria in children in the UK. Arch Dis Child 1997; 77: 76–81
68. Meremikkwu M, Logan K, Garner P. Antipyretic measures for treating fever in malaria. The Cochrane Database Syst Rev 2000, Issue 2. Art. No.: CD002151. D0I: 10.1002/14651858. CD002151
69. Mathur P, Samantaray JC, Vajpayee M, et al. Visceral leishmaniasis/HIV co-infection in India. J Med Microbiol 2006; 55: 919–22

70. Mathur P, Samantaray J, Chauhan NK. Evaluation of a rapid immunochromatographic test for diagnosis of kala azar and post kala azar dermal leishmaniasis at a tertiary care centre of north India. Indian J Med Res 2005; 122: 485–90
71. Ansari NA, Saluia S, Salotra P. Elevated levels of INF- , IL-10 and IL-6 during active disease in Indian kala azar. Clin Immunol 2006; 119: 339–45

Fever in Malnutrition

72. Bryce J, Boschi-Pinto C, Shibuya K, et al. World Health Organisation estimate of the causes of death in children. Lancet 2005; 365: 1147–52

Fever in Non-infectious Diseases

6

Core Messages

> Fever is commonly found in children with haematological disorders, of which sickle cell anaemia is the most common.

> An important cause of febrile illnesses in children with haemolytic disorders is infection with human parvovirus B19 (HPV B19).

> Children with cancer are often neutropenic and any associated fever needs urgent medical attention because of possible underlying serious bacterial infections, which may be responsible for 50% of deaths

> Fever in children with cancer may be due either to the disease (neoplastic fever) or to infection. The diagnosis of neoplastic fever should only be considered after exclusion of infection.

> Early administration of antibiotics to children with febrile neutropenia prior to confirming the infection has improved the survival in these children.

> In rheumatology, children with juvenile idiopathic arthritis have the highest incidence of fever. Children may present with persistent fever of unknown origin and are often subjected to intensive investigations, including many trials of antibiotics and occasionally laparotomy.

> In Kawasaki disease, fever has diagnostic and prognostic importance: higher temperature during days 10–13 of the disease and its continuation for more than 14 days is a risk factor associated with coronary involvement.

> Fever following vaccination is common and usually trivial. It is not a contraindication to further doses of vaccines.

A.S. El-Radhi et al. (Eds.) *Clinical Manual of Fever in Children.*
Doi: 10.1007/978-3-540-78598-9, © Springer-Verlag Berlin Heidelberg 2009

6.1
Haematology

6.1.1
Haemolytic Anaemia

Sickle Cell Anaemia

Children with haemolytic anaemia have the highest number of febrile reactions among all patients with anaemias. Sickle cell anaemia (SCA) is by far the most common single type of anaemia associated with fever.

SCA is an autosomal recessive defect in haemoglobin characterized by the following:

* Substitution of valine for glutamic acid at position 6 of the beta-chain, leading to production of a defective form of haemoglobin known as HbS
* HbS, which is less soluble than the normal HbA, causing RBC to sickle at low O_2
* RBCs that are too fragile to withstand the mechanical trauma of circulation, leading to haemolysis. Life span of SCA RBCs is 10–20 days; normal RBC life span is 120 days.
* An electrophoresis demonstrating mostly HbS, with a variable amount of HbF

The disease mostly affects those of African ancestry and people of Mediterranean and Middle Eastern descent. About 0.3% of Blacks in the USA are affected. Anaemia and crisis do not occur in the heterozygous state (SC trait).

Clinically the disease is characterized by recurrent episodes of painful, vasoocclusive crisis, occurring either spontaneously or precipitated by infection. Clinical manifestations include fever, vomiting, headache, bone pain, splenomegaly, pallor and jaundice. Episodes of fever, symmetrical swelling of the hands and feet (hand–foot syndrome or dactylitis) or abdominal pain are often the first symptoms.

Complications are numerous and life-threatening (Table 6.1):

* Susceptibility to overwhelming bacterial infections, e.g., septicaemia and meningitis, caused primarily by *Streptococcus pneumoniae* (400–600-fold increased risk, compared with normal children) [1], *H. influenzae* type B (invasive HiB infections have greatly decreased through vaccination), and *Salmonella osteomyelitis*, which presents insidiously with multiple and symmetrical bone involvement. This enhanced susceptibility results from deficient opsonizing and complement activities and defective splenic phagocytic function (functional asplenia), beginning as early as 3 months of age. Without prompt administration of antibiotics these infections are associated with high mortality.
* Acute splenic sequestration may cause circulatory collapse and rapid death as a result of pooling of blood in the liver and spleen.
* Acute chest syndrome is a combination of fever, and clinical and radiological evidence of pneumonia. It is the most common reason for hospitalization and perhaps mortality. Infection is predominately due to *S. pneumoniae*, *Mycoplasma pneumoniae* or *Chlamydia pneumoniae*.

Table 6.1 Summary of the complications of SCA

Complication	Presentation
Infection	Sepsis, pneumonia, osteomyelitis, meningitis
ASS	Enlargement of spleen, drop of haematocrit
Dactylitis	Swelling of the hands and feet, symmetric
Aplastic crisis	Parvovirus B 19 infection, drop of Hb
ACS	Gram- and + bacteria, atypical bacteria, viruses fat emboli
Stroke	Infarct of internal carotid/cerebral arteries
Hepatic	Cholelithiasis, cholecystitis, cholestasis, pancreatitis
Renal	Reduced urine concentration, enuresis, haematuria, chronic renal failure
Priapism	Painful penile erection, its persistence leads to Ischaemia and impotence
Leg ulcers	Deep venous thrombosis
Heart/lung	Myocardial ischaemia, pulmonary emboli

ASS acute splenic sequestration; *ACS* acute chest syndrome; *GBD* Gallbladder diseases

* Recurrent UTIs and vasoocclusive episodes causing medullary ischaemia, with a loss of renal concentrating ability and acidification that may lead to chronic polyuria manifesting as enuresis and renal failure.
* Infection with *Plasmodium falciparum* remains the commonest cause of sickle-cell crisis and a leading cause of death in Africa (although HbS tends to protect against malaria).
* Infection with human parvovirus B19 (HPV B19) selectively infects erythroblasts, leading to an arrest of erythropoiesis in bone marrow for 7–10 days. In immunocompetent individuals, this virus is the cause of erythema infectiosum, acute symmetric polyarthritis or hydrops fetalis. In patients with chronic haemolytic anaemia, the virus causes transient erythroblastopenia, which manifests clinically as a further drop of Hb. In patients with SCA, HPV B19 is the leading cause of acute erythroblastopenia as well as a cause of mortality. Fev er was found in 90% of patients with the infection, followed by pain and acute splenic sequestration [2].
* Priapism, a prolonged and painful penile erection, is often precipitated by sexual activity, with fever and/or dehydration being the next most common precipitating factors.

The majority of febrile episodes in SCA show no evidence of bacterial infection, and the fever is assumed to be caused by vasoocclusive crisis, atypical or viral organisms. Fever caused by vasoocclusive crisis is probably related to an inflammatory response resulting from avascular necrosis of the bone. The elevated temperature in children with only vaso-occlusive crisis is:

* commonly less than 39°C, and
* subsides within 1–2 days following rehydration and analgesia.

These episodes tend to increase in number until patients reach their third decades and then the episodes decline. Their frequency was found to correlate with clinical severity of the anaemia and early death in 3,578 patients followed at multiple centers in the USA [3]. In contrast, fever caused by infections is:

- usually greater than 39°C (especially fever greater than 40.0°C);
- unresponsive to rehydration and analgesics;
- associated with a more ill appearance than without infection;
- associated with a higher risk of deaths in children younger than 2 years; and
- usually associated with leukocytosis >20,000 and high CRP.

Bacterial infections in children with SCA occurred in 38% of febrile children [4]. If the cause of the fever is unclear (vasoocclusive or infection), it is imperative to commence prompt antibiotic therapy. Patients should be informed of the high risk of serious infections and they should be urged to visit medical facilities promptly for any illnesses associated with fever greater than 38.5°C (101.3°F).

Laboratory findings during vasoocclusive crisis are characterized by normocytic, hypochromic anaemia (usual Hb 6–10 g, RBC 2–3 million), leukocytosis, thrombocytosis, hyperbilirubinaemia and hyperplastic bone marrow. The marrow may become aplastic during sickling crisis or severe infection.

Management includes the following:

- Fluid therapy in the form of glucose–saline solution.
- Medications: analgesics (paracetamol and narcotics) are used to control the pain. Aspirin should not be given because of its adverse reactions, including the acidifying tendency. Children with high fever and who appear seriously ill irrespective of the degree of fever should be promptly treated with intravenous antibiotics (such as Ceftriaxone). Prophylactic penicillin reduces morbidity and mortality. Hydroxyurea, daily orally, reduces the painful crises by 50%. Deferasirox is an effective oral iron chelator to treat transfusional iron overload.
- Transfusion for anaemia. Regular transfusion reduces the risk of stroke and acute chest syndrome.
- The combined use of polyvalent pneumococcal vaccine and blood transfusions, which are required for serious complications such as acute sequestration syndrome and aplastic crisis. Regular blood transfusion for only anaemia is generally discouraged. Splenectomy may be indicated in sequestration crisis and hypersplenism.
- Allogeneic stem cell transplantation and gene therapy. However, these are not available for the majority of patients.

Homozygous Beta-Thalasaemia (Thalasaemia Major)

Homozygous beta-thalasaemia, the most severe form of the thalasaemia syndrome, is a chronic haemolytic anaemia characterized by a defective production rate of the beta chain of haemoglobin, which leads to hypochromic, microcytic anaemia, with HbF as the predominant Hb.

Clinical features are the consequence of the following:

- Anaemia with pallor, jaundice, splenomegaly, and decreased growth
- Expanded bone marrow, causing thickening of the cranial bones and maxillary hyperplasia
- Transfusional and absorptive iron load, causing cardiomyopathy and liver cirrhosis

Characteristic laboratory findings include hypochromic microcytic anaemia, with a large number of nucleated erythroblasts, target cells and basophilia.

Fever may occur subsequent to complications, including the following:

* Cardiac, such as pericarditis, lasting a few weeks with a tendency to recur. Patients present with fever, cough, chest pain and dyspnoea. Occasionally, fever is the only presenting sign. There is usually either a friction rub detected clinically or pericardial effusion found by an ultrasound.
* Unexplained fever (range, 39–40°C), associated with severe anaemia. This is often caused by HPV B19. The fever responds to antipyretics and blood transfusion.
* Infections in splenectomized children. Patients are highly susceptible to fulminating bacterial infection, particularly meningitis and bacteraemia, caused by *S. pneumoniae* and *H. influenzae* type B (very rare in immunized children). These infections are more frequent during the first 5 years of life, and therefore splenectomy should be deferred beyond this age. Oral penicillin, and pneumococcal and H. influenza vaccines have led to marked reduction in these infections. Bone marrow transplantation after the first year of life is curative and is recommended for children with this disease.

Other Haemolytic Anaemias

Several forms of congenital haemolytic anaemia (erythrocyte enzyme disorders such as glucose-6-phosphate dehydrogenase (G6PD) deficiency, cell membrane structure abnormalities such as hereditary spherocytosis, and acquired haemolytic anaemia such as autoimmune haemolytic anaemia), which may manifest clinically as haemolytic crises during febrile illness, and is caused by HPV B19 infection. The accompanying fever is usually mild and reflects the infection. The antigen that causes the haemolysis is phagocytosed by macrophages, inducing a febrile response. Fever occurs in about two thirds of cases, and may be associated with:

* Warm autoimmune haemolytic anaemia, with the antibody being directed against the rhesus (Rh) erythrocyte antigen. This antigen–antibody reaction has a maximal activity at 37°C.
* Cold autoimmune haemolytic anaemia occurring in an idiopathic form or in association with febrile infectious mononucleosis, Hodgkin's disease or underlying collagen vascular disease. The autoantibody agglutinates RBCs at a temperature below 37°C. In addition, patients have anaemia with splenomegaly. A positive direct Coombs' antiglobulin test and a high cold agglutinin titre confirm the autoimmune diagnosis.

6.1.2
Iron-Deficiency Anaemia

Iron deficiency (ID) is the most common cause of anaemia in children, due to diminished iron intake, decreased absorption or increased iron loss or requirement.

6

Clinical findings include irritability, tiredness, poor weight gain due to anorexia, glossitis and pica. In advanced cases there may be dysphagia or kiolonychia.

Diagnosis is established by the following findings:

* Microcytic and hypochromic anaemia
* Reduced serum ferritin (<10 ng ml^{-1}; normal concentration, 30–300 ng ml^{-1}), reduced serum iron concentration (<30 µg dl^{-1}; normal range, 70–140 µg dl^{-1}) in association with increased iron-binding capacity (>350 µg)
* Demonstration of a rise in reticulocytes (normally $<1\%$) and Hb concentration following a therapeutic trial with iron

Although fever is not a common finding in iron-deficiency anaemia, children may present with fever in the following conditions:

* Common childhood febrile illnesses. In tropical countries, ID is often caused by malaria, hookworm infection, schistosomiasis or HIV infection. ID may impair the cell-mediated immunity and the bactericidal activity of neutrophils, thus predisposing children to infection. Iron supplement may reduce these infections. Conversely, some studies have shown that ID may be an important defence mechanism in preventing bacterial growth (nutritional immunity). For example, the administration of iron to ID children was found to increase their susceptibility to malaria [5]. However, systematic reviews of randomized controlled trials concluded that iron supplement does not significantly increase the risk of overall infection [6].
* Infection by HPV B19. Although this infection mainly affects patients with chronic haemolytic anaemia, patients suffering from decreased production, increased destruction or loss of blood red cells are also at risk of developing aplastic crisis. Patients present with 2–3 days of fever due to viraemia, followed by a sudden onset of anaemia.
* As a rare side effect of iron treatment, along with increased sweating.

6.1.3
Megaloblastic Anaemia

Megaloblastic anaemia is uncommon in children but may occur as a result of the following:

* Deficient or defective utilization of folic acid (intestinal malabsorption, tropical sprue, long-term anticonvulsant therapy, anti-metabolite such as methotraxate, and antimicrobials such as trimethoprim-sulphamethoxazole).
* Increased demand of folic acid, e.g., in chronic haemolytic anaemia.
* Vitamin B$_{12}$ deficiency, which is less common than folic acid deficiency. Congenital deficiency of the intrinsic factor (a product of parietal cells of the gastric mucosa that transports the vitamin across the intestinal mucosa) and autoimmune diseases that lead to gastric mucosal atrophy are the main causes of vitamin B$_{12}$ deficiency.

Clinical signs of folic acid deficiency are those of anaemia. In contrast to vitamin B$_{12}$ deficiency, neurological manifestations do not occur. Patients with vitamin B$_{12}$ deficiency may present with glossitis, intermittent diarrhoea and constipation, weight loss and neurological involvement (peripheral neuropathy, ataxia, loss of vibratory and position senses).

Laboratory findings of megaloblastic anaemia include macrocytosis (mean corpuscular volume >90 beyond the first few days of life), reticulocytopenia and hypersegmentation of the granular leukocytes. The smear shows anisocytosis and poikilocytosis, basophilic stippling of the RBCs and Howell-Jolly bodies (a remnant of the nucleus). Diagnosis is established by low folic acid (serum level <5 ng ml^{-1}) or low vitamin B$_{12}$ (serum level <150 pg ml^{-1}).

Fever may occur with megaloblastic anaemia. It was present in 40% in one study [7], and 46% in another [8] of patients with either folic acid or vitamin B$_{12}$ deficiency. The elevation of temperature was usually minimal but sometimes exceeded 40°C, and was usually associated with a more severe anaemia. No cause for the fever is usually found, and temperature subsides once the patients are treated with folic acid or vitamin B$_{12}$.

6.1.4
Neutropenia (see also 6.2.1:Fever in Neoplastic Diseases)

Neutropenia, defined as a polymorphonuclear leukocyte concentration of less than 1,000 mm^{-3}, results from either impaired cell production of the bone marrow or increased peripheral utilization. If the concentration is less than 500 mm^{-3}, the neutropenia is considered severe. About two thirds of cases do not show a focus of infection. The main causes of neutropenia are shown in Table 6.2. The principal risk of neutropenia is infection, e.g. bacteraemia. Table 6.3 lists high- and low-risk factors leading to infection.

Table 6.2 Main causes of neutropenia

Causes	Diseases
Impaired cell production	
Congenital	Fanconi syndrome, associated with pancreatic insufficiency (Shwachman-Diamond- syndrome)
Acquired	
Viral infections	Human herpes-6, rubella
Bacterial	Typhoid and paratyphoid, brucellosis
Antibiotics	Sulfanamides, chloramphenicol
Other drugs	Antithyroid, anticonvulsants, Phenothiazines
Autoimmune diseases	SLE
Anaemia	Advanced megaloblastic anaemia
Cyclic neutropenia	(see text)
Storage diseases	Glycogen storage disease
Bone marrow failure	Malignancy, cytotoxic therapy (see next section)

Table 6.3 High and low risk factors for infections in patients with neutropenia

High risk factors for infection	Low risk factors for infection
• Neutropenia $<500\,mm^{-3}$	• Viral-induced
• Neutropenia >10 days	• Solid tumours
• Defects in humoral or cellular immunity, eg low CD4	• No underlying disease
• History of splenectomy	• With normal mucosal immunity
• Bone marrow transplantation	
• Indwelling catheter	
• High fever >39°C, chills	
• Hypotension or shock	

Specific symptoms of neutropenia are lacking. Children may present with the following:

- Painful ulceration of the mouth and perirectal area, or recurrent pneumonia.
- Fever (often high with rigors) without a focus of infection (Chap. 1) in about two thirds of cases. Bacteraemia is detected in about a third of cases. Fever can be suppressed by therapeutic medications, such as steroids and nonsteroidal anti-inflammatory agents.
- Rarely hypothermia, which carries a poor prognosis.

Cyclic neutropenia is a sporadic or familial disorder, characteristically recurring every 3 weeks, each episode lasting 3–6 days. The condition is caused by mutations in the gene encoding neutrophil elastase (ELA2). Recurrent bouts of fever accompanying cyclic neutropenia are associated with the appearance of an endotoxin-like material in the blood, presumably resulting from the escape of endotoxins across the bowel wall. Prophylactic antibiotics and granulocyte colony-stimulating factor (G-CSF) are effective treatments.

Although endogenous pyrogens responsible for fever induction were thought to originate in the polymorphonuclear cells, patients with marked neutropenia can develop high fevers, suggesting that these endogenous pyrogens are also produced by sites other than neutrophils, such as monocytes and macrophages (Chap. 3).

6.1.5
Febrile Reactions to Blood Transfusion

Febrile and afebrile reactions to blood transfusion may occur (Table 6.4):

- **Haemolytic reactions** of the recipient's or the donor's RBC (usually the latter) may occur during or after the administration of blood or blood products because of incompatibility. An infusion of as little as 20 ml of incompatible red cells can trigger the haemolysis. These reactions occur in 1:7,000 transfusions, causing a mortality of around 10% [9]. The most severe reaction results in intravascular destruction of the donor RBCs in the receipt's plasma. Clinical manifestations include immediate onset of fever, chills, headache, dyspnoea, chest pain and possibly signs of shock. After the

Table 6.4 Blood transfusion reactions and their management

Reactions	Management
Febrile	
Haemolytic reactions	Discontinue the transfusion and commence plasma expander or normal saline. Mannitol and frusemide may be considered
Non-haemolytic	Antipyretic (paracetamol), transfusion may continue
Bacterial	Discontinue the transfusion. Antibiotic after BC is taken
Non-cardiogenic	Discontinue the transfusion
Post-transfusion	Prevention through appropriate laboratory tests
Non-febrile	
Urticaria	Antihistamine. Transfusion may continue
Anaphylaxis	Discontinue the blood transfusion

BC blood culture

acute phase, signs of renal failure may occur in some patients. The most common cause of haemolytic reactions is human error (e.g. mislabeling, mixing up the samples, and incorrect identification of blood group) or antibodies against blood group antigens other than A, B, O or Rh.

- **Febrile reactions without haemolysis** are most common reactions. One in every 200–500 transfused blood units causes these reactions. These are characterized by chills, fever with a rise of temperature of at least 1°C within 4 h of blood transfusion (usually within a few minutes) and defervescence within 48 h. Occasionally, headache, shock or cyanosis is observed. These reactions are primarily due to antileukocyte antibodies in the recipient, which react to antigens of transfused WBCs. The resulting antigen–antibody complement complexes may activate recipient macrophages to release IL-1. Cytokines such as IL-6 and IL-8 may also play a role. The use of WBC-reduced blood components is an effective way to prevent these febrile reactions. Premedication with an oral antihistamine and an oral antipyretic agent may also modify these reactions.

- **Bacterial febrile reactions** could be due to bacterial antigens or endotoxin in the carrying solution or the tubing. The latter complications have been almost eliminated by using disposable transfusion sets. In most blood transfusion services, donor blood is cooled to 4°C within 6 h of blood collection to minimize bacterial multiplication. Platelet concentrates are most often implicated as a source of bacterial contamination. Fever (in 80%), chills, tachycardia, vomiting, shock, disseminated intravascular coagulation and acute renal failure may rapidly occur. Bacteria (such as pseudomonas) are usually introduced into blood products during collection, processing and transfusion. *Yersinia enterocolitica* is one of the few human pathogens that can grow at 4°C and may contaminate blood products, but the risk is low. Fever and shock may occur immediately after the infusion has been started. About one third of all patients with this complication die.

6

- **Non-cardiogenic pulmonary oedema** occurs in one in 5,000 transfusions. Donor anti-leukocyte antibodies form complexes with the recipient's granulocytes, which become trapped in the pulmonary vasculature. Clinical symptoms include dyspnoea, chills and fever. A chest X-ray confirms the diagnosis of this reaction.
- **Post-transfusion-transmitted infections**, such as hepatitis B and C viruses, HIV type 1 and 2, human T-cells lymphotropic virus type 1 and 2, cytomegalovirus, malaria and toxoplasmosis, remain a serious threat to the recipient of a transfusion. In contrast to bacterial contamination, these viral and protozoal infections manifest clinically days to months after the transfusion and the donor is always the source of infection. Laboratory tests screen most of these diseases, and therefore the chances of contracting one of these diseases are low (about 3 in 10,000 blood transfusions).
- **Allergic reactions** may commonly occur as a result of hypersensitivity of the patient to various proteins in donor plasma. The reaction is very common with the administration of fresh frozen plasma and may also occur with intravenous IgG infusions. The manifestations include urticaria pruritis, oedema, dizziness and headache. Anaphylaxis, though a rare reaction, may occur particularly in patients with hereditary IgA deficiency. Common complaints are dyspnoea, chest and abdominal pain and shock. Fever is characteristically absent.

Box 6.1 summarizes the important aspects of fever discussed in Sect. 6.1.

Box 6.1 Summary Points of Febrile Children with Haematological Disorders

> Fever is common in haemolytic diseases and SCA is the most common single cause of fever among haemolytic anaemias.

> Fever may be the first sign of a serious bacterial infection, such as septicaemia, and so it is essential for the parents to know what to do when their child is feverish.

> Although bacterial infections are not confirmed in the majority of cases with SCA, prompt administration of antibiotics are indicated if the aetiology of fever or the presence of vasoocclusive crisis is uncertain.

> An acutely febrile child with a sudden decrease of Hb should be suspected and screened for infection by human parvovirus B19 (HPV B19).

> Fever caused by bacterial infection is usually greater than 39 oC, does not respond to rehydration and analgesics, and is associated with an ill appearance, a leukocytosis > 20,000 and a high CRP. Children younger than two years are at particular risk for bacterial infection. .

> If the temperature is >39°C the child should immediately seek medical attention. If it is <39°C for over 24 h, your GP should be consulted.

> If the temperature is <39°C and the child is well with signs of an upper respiratory tract infection, a simple antipyretic, e.g. paracetamol, is offered and the temperature is checked in an hour's time. An increase in temperature above the first measurement indicates the need for medical attention.

> If the child is unwell (irrespective of the temperature level), pale, has a rapid breathing or more than mild pain, medical attention should be sought immediately.

6.2
Neoplastic Diseases

6.2.1
Fevers in Neoplastic Diseases (Febrile Neutropenia)

Fever with or without associated infection is common in patients with cancer who are often neutropenic. It is arbitrarily defined as a single temperature measurement exceeding 38.5°C or a 38.0°C recorded on two occasions 1 h apart.

In general, the incidence of fever is higher in children than in adults, occurring most commonly with leukaemia and Hodgkin's disease (HD). Fever may be due to either the disease (neoplastic fever) or infection. The differential diagnosis can be difficult, and therefore the diagnosis of neoplastic fever is only likely after exclusion of infection. Table 6.5 shows the difference between the two causes. Screening tests for infection, such as WBC and CRP, are helpful, particularly if the results are highly abnormal.

Most fevers in patients with cancer are non-infectious in origin or an infection cannot be confirmed. Neoplastic fever of non-infectious origin may be caused by:

* Cells of certain tumours, e.g., leukaemia, renal carcinoma and HD, releasing IL-1 spontaneously, which acts upon the hypothalamus to produce fever. The necrosis of tumours may also be pyrogenic.
* Certain neoplasmas, which are capable of increasing metabolic rate.
* Complications occurring during the course of the disease, e.g., haemolytic anaemia or haemorrhage into the brain or adrenal glands.
* Psychogenic fever, leading to a mild fever, which is abolished by sedatives.
* Treatment with chemotherapy, e.g., bleomycin, duanorubicin and interferon (INF).
* Irradiation of the tumour mass (radiation fever).
* Blood transfusion (see earlier text).
* An absent or delayed antibody production, leading to persistence of certain viruses in bone marrow. This occurs particularly during chemotherapy. Parvovirus B19 is the classical example of these viruses.

Table 6.5 Factors that are in favour of either neoplastic or infection fever

	Infection fever	Neoplastic fever
Fever	>39.5°C	38–39.5°C
Rigor	Yes	No
Relative bradycardia	Yes	No
Ill looking	Often	Usually non-toxic
Neutropenia	Main cause	No
Response to antipyretics to naproxen	Yes	No response, but responds
WBC, CRP, ESR	Elevated	Mildly elevated or normal

6

Classically the neoplastic fever is intermittent, as suggested by the German physician Wunderlich in 1856. Sustained, hectic or remittent fevers may also occur. Fever usually does not respond to common antipyretics (such as paracetamol or aspirin) but it does respond to indomethacin or naproxen. Naproxen causes a prompt and complete lysis of neoplastic fever with sustained normal temperature while receiving this therapy (**Naproxen test**). This drug is therefore useful in the differential diagnosis between neoplastic and non-infectious fevers. During the first 24 h of naproxen therapy, patients with lymphoma may develop hallucination and hypotension. Steroid therapy is usually associated with striking but transient antipyretic effect in both neoplastic and infectious fevers.

Fevers in patients with cancer are frequently caused by infections, which are the leading cause of death in these children. High fever (>39.5°C), particularly if it is associated with chills, is suggestive of infection. Factors that increase the susceptibility of oncology patients to infections are:

* Marked and prolonged neutropenia.
* Underlying cancer, particularly leukaemia and advanced-stage lymphoma
* The use of high-dose chemotherapy (cytosine arabinoside) and stem cell transplantation.
* Malnutrition, which affects lymphocyte function, neutrophils, monocyte cells, and complement system.
* Indwelling catheter or tubes.
* Associated defects of humoral and cell-mediated immunity, causing increased susceptibility particularly to encapsulated bacteria (*S. pneumoniae, H. influenzae, N. menigitidis*), listeria, salmonella and viruses.

Table 6.6 shows the main causes of fever and infection in neutropenic patients.

Table 6.6 Main pathogens, causing infections in children with cancer

Gram-positive
  • Staphylococcus aureus, S. epidermidis
  • Alpha-haemolytic streptococci
  • Enterococci
  • Listeria

Gram-negative
  • Enterobacteriae, eg E. coli, Klebsella
  • Pseudomonas aeruginosa

Viruses
  • Herpes simplex
  • Herpes zoster
  • EB virus

Fungi
  • Candida species
  • Aspergillus

Protozoan
  • Pneumocystis carinii
  • Toxoplasma gondii

Patients with febrile neutropenia should be rapidly evaluated and treated with antibiotics without awaiting culture results. Any delay in antibiotic treatment may lead to uncontrolled progression of infection and death. Figure 6.1 shows an algorithm for antibiotic treatment. Table 6.7 shows frequently and empirically used antibiotics while waiting for culture results. In children with neutropenia and persistent fever refractory to antibiotics invasive fungal infection should be considered. Liposomal amphotericin (AmBisome) is an effective treatment.

Granulocyte colony-stimulating factor (G-CSF) has been used to promote neutrophil recovery after cytotoxic chemotherapy or for patients with cancer undergoing bone marrow transplantation. The administration of this growth factor is frequently associated with the development of fever, which occurs during or shortly after the end of infusion. The fever induction by GM-CSF may be partly mediated through prostaglandin pathways since it is blocked by premedication with ibuprofen. A recent systematic review [10] concluded that the role of treatment with this growth factor remains uncertain. It shortens hospitalization and fever duration but there was no evidence for a shortened duration of neutropenia.

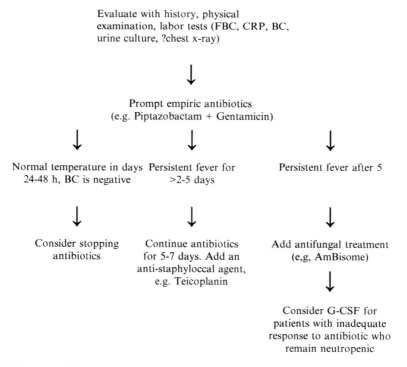

Fig. 6.1 Summary of the management of a febrile child with cancer without a focus of infection

Febrile non-neutropenic patients with cancer remain susceptible to infection because of associated lymphocyte dysfunction. These patients should be evaluated with CRP, BC, urine and chest X-ray. If they do not have an indwelling catheter, antibiotics are rarely indicated.

Leukaemia

Leukaemia is the most common form of malignancy in children, occurring in about four per million children. Peak incidence occurs in the age group of 2–6 years (mean age, 4 years). Of the 2,000 cases diagnosed in the USA each year, three quarters of the cases are acute lymphoblastic leukaemia. The cause of leukaemia is largely unknown. Ionizing radiation and chemotherapy are the only established factors predisposing to leukaemia. Symptoms and signs of leukaemia are shown in Table 6.8. These features are mainly caused by bone marrow infiltration and extramedullary spread.

Findings associated with poor prognosis include high initial leukocyte count, severe thrombocytopenia, lymphoblasts of L2 or L3 subtypes, massive organomegaly and lymphadenopathy, patients younger than 2 years or older than 10 years, CNS involvement at diagnosis and failure to achieve complete remission after 4–6 weeks of induction therapy.

Fever occurs in around 60% in children, being frequently neoplastic in origin. In contrast, the fever of adult leukaemia is largely due to infection. Pyrogenic cytokines involved in fever generation include the following:

- IL-1 and IL-2 production is elevated in many patients, which may play an important role in the immunological response to the leukaemic cells.
- Tumour necrosis factor (TNF), which is usually high at presentation and reaching undetectable levels after remission.
- High IL-6 levels, which significantly correlate with fever and acute-phase proteins such as CRP. IL-6 may stimulate the release of prostaglandin E2 (PGE2) into the blood, which reaches and increases the hypothalamic set-point. Il-6, in support of IL-3, may also induce the differentiation and proliferation of leukaemic blast cells.

Table 6.7 Commonly used antibiotics for patients with cancer and febrile neutropenia

Drug	Dose (mg kg^{-1})	Frequency	Route
Piperacillin/tazobactam	90	4	IV
Ceftazidime	100–150	4	IV
Gentamicin	6–7.5	Once daily	IV
Teicoplanin	10	Twice daily for 3 doses, then once daily	IV
AmBisome	1	Once daily	IV

Table 6.8 Clinical data in children with leukaemia

Symptoms/signs	%	Laboratory findings	%
Hepatosplenomegaly	68	Leukocytes	
		<10,000	53
Splenomegaly	63	10,000–49,000	30
Fever	61		
Lymphadenopathy	50		
Bleeding (purpura)	48		
Bone pain	23		
CNS involvement	5		

Fever due to infection is more frequently present during the neutropenic and terminal stages in lymphoblastic leukaemia. In acute myelogenous leukaemia, fever caused by infection in patients with neutropenia occurs in the majority of instances during the induction of remission and during relapse. In both types of leukaemia, infections are responsible for death in at least 50% of children.

Treatment of acute lymphoblastic leukaemia consists of induction therapy with vincristine and prednisolone, which induces remission in 85% of cases, while the addition of L-asparginase or anthracyclines (especially doxorubicin), or both, increases the rate to 95%. CNS prophylaxis of radiotherapy is no longer recommended. Five doses of intrathecal methotraxate are given. Maintenance therapy is best achieved with methotraxate once or twice a week and 6-mercaptopurine daily. Intermittent pulses of vincristine and prednisolone are added to prolong remission.

Children with neutropenia and fever are best treated with third-generation cephalosporins and aminoglycoside. The addition of gammaglobulin may shorten the duration of fever.

Hodgkin's Disease

Hodgkin's disease is a malignant neoplasm of lymphoreticular cells of unknown aetiology. Reed-Sternberg cells are the malignant cells of the disease. The cell lines secrete TNF, macrophage, colony-stimulating factor and PGE2. The currently accepted staging classification of HD is summarized in the Table 6.9.

Most children with HD present with cervical lymphadenopathy, involvement of the mediastinal and/or hilar masses, which may be discovered on routine chest X-ray. Systemic

Stage	Involvement
I	Single lymph node
II	Two or more lymph nodes
III	Lymph node region
IV	Disseminated involvement of one or more

Table 6.9 Stages of Hodgkin's disease

manifestation of HD includes fever, weight loss, anorexia, pruritis and night sweats. Tumour cell lines spontaneously synthesize and release IL-1, TNF, macrophage, colony-stimulating factor and PGE2. Some constitutional symptoms, termed B-symptoms (fever, weight loss and night sweats) are mediated by IL-1.

Fever is a frequent and important manifestation of HD for the following reasons:

* It occurs in about 30% of cases at presentation and in about 60% during the course of illness. The pattern of fever was found to be remittent in 67%, intermittent in 20% and relapsing in the remaining 13% [11]. Only a small number of patients during the course of fever have the relapsing Pel-Ebstein fever (high fever for about 10 days, regularly alternating with an afebrile period of similar duration). This pattern was described in 1887 and was thought at that time to be diagnostic of HD.
* The commonest cause of fever is the disease itself (neoplastic fever). Fever may also be due to increased susceptibility of patients to viral, bacterial and fungal infections as a result of impairment of T-lymphocyte-mediated immunity or chemotherapy.
* There is a positive correlation between the fever and the clinical stage of HD. Fever occurs more frequently in the advanced stage owing to increased incidence of infection. As survival is related to the clinical stage of the disease, fever is more frequently encountered at terminal stages (similar to leukaemia).
* The presence of fever at the time of diagnosis was found to be a bad prognostic sign, and febrile patients in stages IIb and III lived significantly shorter than afebrile patients [11].

Mild to moderate leukocytosis, lymphopenia, eosinophilia, thrombocytosis, and anaemia, and increased inflammatory markers (ESR, CRP) are common findings. Investigations include FBC, ESR, CRP, liver and renal function tests, chest X-ray, thoracic CT-scan, lymphangiogram (or abdominal CT), biopsy of lymph nodes and liver and bone marrow aspiration (demonstrating Reed-Sternberg cells).

Treatment includes full mantle irradiation (all lymph nodes above the diaphragm) for stages I and II. Such treatment cures 85–90% of patients. A combined regimen of radiotherapy with chemotherapy (mechloroethamine, vincristine, procarbazine and prednisolone (the MOPP programme)) are used for stages III and IV. This regimen cures about 75% – 50% of patients in stages III and IV respectively. Others recommend surgical treatment of all patients with a negative bone marrow biopsy in order to limit the toxicity of radiation, such as sterility and the risk of a second malignancy. Patients with HD who receive radiation therapy are also at risk of thyroid disease (hypothyroidism, Graves' disease, thyroid cancer).

Neuroblastoma

Neuroblastoma originates in the neutral-crest cells of the sympathetic nervous system, mostly from the adrenal medulla. It is the most common extracranial solid tumour of childhood, accounting for 7% of all cases. Over two thirds of cases occur during the first 5 years of life (median age, 2 years).

Children may present with the following features:

* An abdominal mass arising from adrenal medulla may extend beyond the mid-line of the abdomen. An abdominal plain X-ray or ultrasound scan may detect stippled calcification in the adrenal gland. Intravenous urography (rarely used nowadays) may show inferior displacement of the kidney without distortion of the pyelocalyceal system.
* Metastasis into the skull (producing signs of increased intracranial pressure and lytic lesions), tubular bones (producing pain and tenderness), the liver (causing rapidly growing abdominal mass), the orbit (causing proptosis) or skin as the subcutaneous nodules may occur during the neonatal period.
* Horner's syndrome (meiosis, ptosis, enophthalmia, anhydrosis) may be seen.

Fever may be a feature of these localized tumours. Children with disseminated neuroblastoma, usually involving bone marrow, often present with fever up to 40°C, irritability and weight loss. Because of the absence of localized features, children may be evaluated for pyrexia of unknown origin.

Diagnosis is suggested by the radiological appearance of the tumour and confirmed by biopsy, by increased levels of catecholamines and their metabolites in the urine (vanillylmandelic acid and homovanillic acid) or by bone marrow aspiration in cases with disseminated neuroblastoma. Increased uptake of Tc diphosphate is often positive before the bony lesions can be detected radiologically.

Young children aged less than 1 year have the best prognosis and can generally be cured regardless of their disease stage. Other children with advanced disease and metastasis have a poor prognosis (less than 20%). The DNA content of tumour cells and the presence of chromosome 1p abnormalities are also of prognostic value. Mass screening of urine for increased catecholamine is feasible and can further improve the prognosis.

Treatment consists of tumour excision at stages I and II. Localized but unresectable tumours can be treated with a 4-month course of cyclophosphamide and doxorubicin. Treatment with disseminated neuroblastoma may also benefit from this combination, with or without cisplatin and etoposide.

Nephroblastoma (Wilms' Tumour)

This is the second most common malignant retroperitoneal tumour in children, occurring at a rate of 7.5 cases per million children in the USA. The tumour commonly presents as an abdominal mass in a young child (median age, 3 years), often detected by a parent (in over 80% of cases). Other presentations include fever (reported incidence, 23–50% of cases), haematuria and hypertension (caused by rennin secretion). Cough and dyspnoea may occur because of pulmonary metastasis.

Fever is not a usual part of the symptomatology. However, children may occasionally present with fever, abdominal pain and vomiting. A rapidly enlarging flank mass, with hypertension, anaemia and fever may result from massive haemorrhage into the tumour.

Diagnostic features include intravenous urography, showing characteristic distortion and displacement of the pyelocalyceal system, and abdominal ultrasound scan. A chest X-ray is required to exclude pulmonary metastasis.

Therapy consists of excision of the tumour, radiation therapy and chemotherapy.

6.2.2
Tumours of the Central Nervous System (CNS)

Most children with tumours arising from the CNS present with headache, vomiting, ataxia, visual defects, hemiparesis, double vision, lethargy or irritability. Fever is not a common finding in these patients. Fever, however, may occur:

- In hypothalamic tumours (mostly astrocytoma), which affect the thermoregulatory centres. Hypothermia may also occur. There may be emaciation with marked loss of subcutaneous tissue despite a normal or increased appetite, excessive sweating, diabetes insipidus, precocious puberty and hypogonadism.
- In astrocytomas, which are relatively benign tumours of the CNS, and known to produce IL-1, mediating the induction of fever. Within the CNS, IL-1 may be involved in immunological processes and haemorrhage. Despite the production of IL-1, patients with astrocytomas do not often have fever.
- In the highly malignant medulloblastoma. This tumour requires chemotherapy and/or radiation therapy to the brain and spine. As a result, bone marrow suppression (causing anaemia, leucopenia and thrombocytopenia) is common, predisposing patients to infection and fever.
- With immunotherapy. This therapy uses several cytokines such as lymphokine-activated killer cells, IL-2 and INF-α and -β, to treat intracranial tumours, particularly astrocytomas. These cytokines commonly produce fever as an adverse reaction. A combination of lymphokine-activated killer cells and Il-2 can induce tumour regression by lysing malignant glioma cells while sparing normal brain tissue. The use of this approach is limited owing to the toxicity of IL-2 and the higher success rate of alternative forms of therapy.

Hyperthermia has been used as a treatment. Multiple microwave sources were implanted to raise the patient's temperature above 43°C. This technique has not gained wide use.

6.3
Rheumatic Diseases and Vasculitis

Fever has important diagnostic, therapeutic and prognostic values and remains a challenge to the paediatricians and rheumatologists despite the advance made in the field of medical diagnosis and technology. Fever can be the initial symptom of a rheumatic disease or its flare, of an infectious complication or of therapeutic failure.

6.3.1
Rheumatic Fever (RF)

RF is an inflammatory disease occurring subsequent to infection with group A strepto-cocci. Protein M and lipoteichoic acid (antigenic fragments of Gram-positive bacteria) are the chief virulence factors of this group. Antibodies (e.g., cross-reacting antibodies) may cross-react with cardiac myocytes, (causing carditis), joint cartilage (causing arthritis) and thalamic and subthalamic nuclei of the CNS (causing chorea). The pathogenic feature is the Aschoff body, which is a granuloma with localized areas of fibrinoid swelling of collagen and perivascular infiltration. An altered response to streptococcal antigens has been implicated in the pathogenesis of RF. These antigens may stimulate the secretion of IL-2 from lymphocytes, which causes an increased natural killer cell cytotoxicity and the pathological changes in RF.

The diagnosis is established by criteria of two major manifestations or one major plus two minor criteria in addition to an evidence of increasing titres of antibody to streptococcal antigens (Table 6.10).

Carditis occurs in ~90% of children with RF who are younger than 3 years and in about 40% of older children. The most common manifestation is an apical murmur of mitral regurgitation. Severe carditis may manifest as cardiomegaly or congestive cardiac failure. If carditis does not occur in the initial attack of RF, the heart is usually not involved in subsequent attacks. A child with carditis may have tachycardia disproportional to the degree of fever (relative tachycardia).

Fever <39°C occurs in 70%, > 39.5°C in 25% and no fever in 5%. It is one of the minor criteria and is not of great value in assisting in the diagnosis. In addition:

* fever is present in the majority of cases, but its absence does not exclude RF.
* the fever of RF has no characteristic pattern. Diurnal variations are common but large daily swings, as seen commonly with rheumatoid arthritis, are not observed. Relative bradycardia is common with conduction defects.

Table 6.10 Accepted Jones criteria of RF

Criterion	Presentation
Major	
Carditis	Tachycardia, gallop rhythm, cardiomegaly, intractable cardiac failure
Polyarthritis	Migratory polyarthritis, often persists for weeks if untreated, but respond n 12–24 h to aspirin
Chorea	Abrupt aimless movement, emotional instability
Erythema marginatum	Transient erythematous rash over the trunk, with later occurring blanching in the centre
Subcutaneous nodules	Non-tender, pea-sized nodules on the extensor surface of the joints
Minor	Fever, arthralgia, grade 1 heart block (ECG) In addition to: Supporting evidence of recent streptococcal infection

- a high degree of fever is mainly found when the clinical manifestations occur acutely. With a more insidious onset, low-grade fever is detectable only in the afternoon, with a tendency to persist for several weeks.
- during the acute attack, fever subsides in a few days even without medication.
- high fever characteristically responds abruptly to aspirin treatment, unlike the fever in rheumatoid arthritis.
- children with chorea are usually afebrile.

During the acute phase of RF, both the ESR and CRP are high. A rise of ASO titre greater than 320 is evident within 1–2 weeks after the streptococcal infection, reaching a maximum level in 3–5 weeks after the infection. A rise of ASO titre has a better diagnostic value than a positive throat culture. Two-dimensional echocardiography is an important diagnostic tool for evaluation of cardiac lesions.

Bed rest is advisable for febrile children with acute symptoms of RF, and should be strict for cases with carditis. Penicillin (orally, 250 mg qds) is used for treatment for 10 days and bd to prevent recurrences of the RF. Salicylate alone is used to treat cases uncomplicated by carditis. Symptoms, such as polyarthritis and fever, respond markedly to salicylate therapy, and the diagnosis of acute RF is in doubt if patients treated with salicylate are not improved substantially within 48 h. Rebounds of inflammatory activity may occur when aspirin therapy is tapered off or discontinued. Steroids (prednisolone, 2 mg kg^{-1} per day) are more effective in controlling symptoms of carditis.

The most effective prophylaxis consists of 1.2 million units of monthly benzathine penicillin injection or oral penicillin (250 mg bd). For patients with carditis this prophylaxis should continue for life.

6.3.2
Juvenile Idiopathic Arthritis

Juvenile idiopathic arthritis (JIA) is a childhood disease (before the age of 16 years) characterized primarily by arthritis, which lasts al least 6 weeks and in which no other cause has been found. The cause of JIA remains obscure. Different arthritogenic stimuli (exogenous infection or endogenous antigens) may activate the immune response seen in this type of arthritis. Antigen-presenting cells (macrophage or dendritic cells) in the synovial membrane ingest, process and present these antigens to the lymphocytes, which initiate a cellular immune response and stimulate the differentiation of B lymphocytes into plasma cells that secrete antibodies. In addition, cytokines (IL-1, IL-6, TNF-α and GM-CSF) are present in large quantity in the synovial fluid, which participate in the inflammatory process of the joint, such as increasing production of collagenase and PGE2. Only a small quantity of T-cell products, such as IL-2 and INF-γ, are present.

IL-1 is a powerful stimulus of bone and cartilage resorption. It induces the acute phase-response and fever and also potentiates chronic inflammation of arthritis by induction of lymphocyte growth factors, such as IL-2 and its receptors. IL-1 receptor antagonist, which is produced by the same cells that produce IL-1 (monocytes and macrophages), is greatly increased in the synovial fluid in patients with JIA. This antagonist competes with IL-1α

and IL-1β for binding to IL-1 receptors. The relative amount of IL-1 and IL-1 receptor antagonist in JRA may influence whether the inflammation remains active or suppressed.

There are three major presentations of JIA:

* About a quarter of all patients with JIA present with systemic JIA (Still's disease) characterized by high fever and other systemic manifestations. Arthritis may occur during the course of the disease. Males and females are equally affected, with a mean age of 4 years. The rash characteristically is fleeting, salmon-coloured, macular or maculopapular, occurring particularly when the temperature is elevated. Other features include lymphadenopathy, splenomegaly, leukocytosis, anaemia, myocarditis and pericarditis.
* The polyarticular onset or adult type occurs in about half of the patients, with an abrupt or insidious arthritis of several joints (more than 4 joints). Occasionally, patients present with systemic manifestation such as low-grade fever, lymphadenopathy and recurrent rash. This type of onset occurs in females more than males, with a mean age of 12 years. Essentially this presentation is the classical version of JIA.
* In the remaining cases, presentation involves monoarthritis or pauciarticular arthritis. There are further subdivisions of these groups for classification purposes. Knee, ankle or hip joints are usually involved. Systemic manifestations are usually absent or mild. Iridocyclitis is an important sign.

Fever is a prominent feature in Still's disease:

* It has been found in 84% of cases in one study and has been noted in 24–90% of nearly 1,000 cases reported in the literature since 1958 [12].
* The commonest pattern of fever is intermittent, often hectic, with a daily rise in the evening, then falling to normal in the morning (Table 6.11). As the fever continues, the pattern may become double quotidian (Fig. 6.2). Other encountered febrile patterns include continuous and periodic fever.
* Chills frequently precede the febrile episodes.
* Fever is usually high, ranging from 39.5°C to 41.2°C, which is usually associated with the occurrence of rash, generalized lymphadenopathy and splenomegaly, whereas these manifestations are usually absent with no fever. Pericarditis may occur more frequently in the presence of high fever, accompanied by rash and leukocytosis.
* Fever may precede articular manifestations by weeks, months and even years (mean, 3.5 months) in about one third of the patients with JIA. Children who present with only fever are considered as having persistent fever of unknown origin (PUO) and are subjected to intensive investigations, including many trials of antibiotics and occasional

• Intermittent, hectic, higher in the evening
• Double quotidian, often follows the above pattern
• Continuous, with little or no variation
• Periodic fever, occurring every few days
• Pyrexia of unknown origin, lasting many weeks

Table 6.11 Variety of fever pattern observed in patients with JIA

6

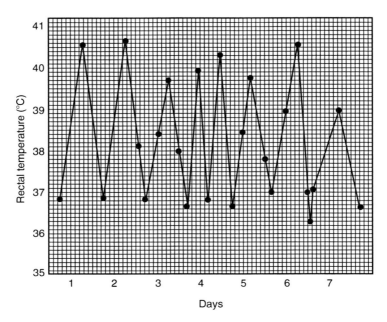

Fig. 6.2 A temperature chart of a child with juvenile idiopathic arthritis, showing a high fever that shows a double quotidian pattern on the fourth day of hospital admission

laparotomy. The appearance of the characteristic rash is an important sign in suggesting the diagnosis.

- The fever of the Still's type of JIA tends to be higher than that of RF, and the swings are more pronounced. It does not respond to antibiotics and does not respond promptly to salicylate therapy.

Common laboratory findings include leukocytosis, increased ASO titres (noted in as many as 40%), antinuclear factors (present in 30%) and positive rheumatoid factor (in 10–30%). The concentration of IL-1β correlates with clinical and laboratory disease activity.

The basic treatment regimen consists of non-steroidal anti-inflammatory drugs, mainly ibuprofen (10 mg kg^{-1}) or diclofenac (1 mg kg^{-1}) three times daily. Intra-articular steroid injection is a first line of treatment in oligoarthritis. Immunosuppressive agents (methotrexate, cyclosporine) are often first line therapy in polyarthritis. Immunomedulatory (TNF antagonists), and a supportive programme such as physiotherapy are also used. Antibodies directed against the early phase of the immune response, such as anti-IL-2-receptor antibodies, anti-CD4 antibodies and antithymocyte globulin have been tried with limited success.

6.3.3
Systemic Lupus Erythematosus (SLE) and Other Connective Tissue Diseases

SLE (systemic lupus erythematosus) is an acute inflammatory connective tissue disorder of unknown aetiology. Autoantibodies are important for the diagnosis and are responsible for many of its clinical manifestations. Beyond the neonatal age, females account for 90% of cases, although during infancy and old age the male and female prevalence are more similar. Antinuclear antibodies, including anti-DNA, are usually present, suggesting that SLE is an autoimmune disease. Clinical features of SLE are shown in Table 6.12.

Neonatal SLE: is characterized by cutaneous lesions with or without congenital heart block. Fever is not a sign of neonatal SLE. Manifestations of neonatal SLE are caused by transplacental transfer of maternal IgG antibody to the fetus (particularly anti-Ro antibodies). Mothers of affected children may be asymptomatic at the time of delivery. Approximately 40% of the mothers have active SLE or Sjogren syndrome.

In older children, clinical features related to fever include the following:

* SLE may present abruptly with fever, simulating an acute infection, or may develop over months with only episodes of fever, malaise, arthralgia and weight loss.
* Fever, which ranges from moderate to high degree, occurs in about 80–85% of cases, accompanying the facial erythematous rash in about 40% of cases.
* Fever is more common in childhood SLE than in adult SLE [13]. A close correlation usually exists between the degree of fever and serum concentrations of INF, rather than IL-4.
* Active SLE is often associated with a raised ESR but normal CRP. This serves as a clue that infection is not a cause of the fever.

Fever, mild to moderate arthritis, pleuropericarditis and lymphadenopathy usually respond to non-steroidal anti-inflammatory drugs or a low dose of prednisolone. Aspirin (80 mg kg^{-1}) is now rarely used. Interestingly, it frequently causes hepatotoxicity in lupus patients. High fever associated with severe arthritis, active glomerulonephritis, severe thrombocytopenia, severe haemolytic anaemia and neurological abnormalities may require prednisolone (0.5–1 mg kg^{-1} per day) for 4–6 weeks before being tapered off. The patients are maintained at the lowest possible dose that will control clinical and laboratory abnormalities. An intravenous bolus of 500 mg of methylprednisolone may be required for initial control of active SLE.

Dermatomyositis is a systemic connective tissue disease, characterized by inflammatory and degenerative changes of the muscles and skin. There is evidence of immune-mediated microangiopathy underlying the pathogenesis of childhood dermatomyositis. The most common finding is a symmetric, dusky erythema of the face and extensor surfaces of the

Table 6.12 Main clinical findings in SLE

Neonatal Lupus	Lupus rash, congenital heart block heart failure, hepatosplenomegaly, petechial
Older child	
Skin	Malar rash, discoid lupus
Mouth	Ulcers
Joints	Non-erosive polyarthralgia/arthritis
CNS	Headache, confusion, psychosis, seizure due to vasculitis, high fever
Renal	Lupus nephritis (nephritic/nephrotic syndrome
Cardiac	Pleuro-pericarditis
Other	Fatigue, malaise, fever, Hughes (antiphospholipid) syndrome
Laboratory findings	High ESR, normal CRP, lymphopenia, thrombocytopenia, haemolytic anaemia ANA, dsDNA, antiphospholipid antibodies

6

extremities. Periorbital oedema with a heliotrope hue is characteristic. The skin rash may be slightly elevated, smooth or scaly, with associated atrophy and telangiectasia in the V-shaped area of the face and upper chest. In contrast to the adult form, dermatomyositis in children is not associated with malignancies.

Symmetrical proximal muscle weakness may appear insidiously as difficulty in raising the arms above the shoulders or rising from sitting position. A more acute onset occurs in approximately one third of patients.

The fever associated with dermatomyositis is

* generally in the range of 38–39°C in 50–75% of patients, with 5–10% having high spikes (usually associated with the acute fulminant form of this disease).
* the second most common presenting sign (after muscle weakness) of the disease; its onset often follows the development of the weakness.
* more likely in individuals who have specific autoantibodies for myositis such as the anti-synthestase antibodies [14].

The ESR, CRP and muscle enzymes are usually elevated. Electromyography shows spontaneous fibrillation, positive sharp potentials and polyphasic short potentials during voluntary contraction. Muscle biopsy may show necrosis, phagocytosis and lymphocytic infiltrations.

6.3.4
Other Connective Tissue Diseases

Fever can also be a part of a number of other connective tissue diseases such as Sjogren's syndrome and scleroderma. However, these are not common in childhood.

Progressive systemic sclerosis is characterized by fibrosis, degenerative changes and vascular abnormalities. T-cell hyperactivity may correlate with disease activity. Vascular injury could be mediated by cytokines, including IL-2, -4 and -6.

Clinically, the most common presentation is tightening and swelling of the extremities, particularly the fingers, Raynaud's phenomenon and polyarthralgia. Subcutaneous calcifications often develop later. Progressive systemic sclerosis is rare in children, and fever is not often present on presentation or during the course of the disease.

6.3.5
Macrophage Activation Syndrome

Macrophage activation syndrome (MAS) has been reported in association with many rheumatic diseases, connective tissue diseases, or malignancy, but most commonly with systemic-onset JIA (SOJIA). High-grade fever (spiking and intermittent), pancytopenia, encephalopathy, coagulopathy and elevated transaminases are the common presenting manifestations. MAS is a serious complication of childhood systemic inflammatory disorders that is caused by activation and proliferation of T lymphocytes and macrophages. Measurement of the serum ferritin level may assist in the diagnosis and may be an indicator of disease activity. MAS is related to the haemophagocytic syndromes and may be fatal. It is differentiated from SOJIA by its persistent fever (the fever in SOJIA is quotidian – febrile episode with a spike occurring daily), the presence of encephalopathy and pancytopenia.

6.3.6
Kawasaki Disease

Kawasaki disease (KD) is an acute inflammatory disease that principally affects infants and young children, 85% being less than 5 years of age with a peak incidence at 1–2 years. Initially described by Kawasaki in Japan, where KD is endemic, the condition has been recognized worldwide.

The disease is a form of vasculitis of unknown origin. Speculation as to aetiology ranges from infectious causes to hyperimmune response. The production of most acute-phase reactants, such as IL-1, IL-6, TNF-α and CRP is increased. The circulating B cells are increased while the T cells are decreased.

The diagnosis is established on the criteria shown in Table 6.13. Features include the following:

* Bilateral conjuntival inflammation without exudates. Anterior uveitis is frequently present, usually beginning shortly after the onset of fever and lasting as long as 2 weeks.
* Mucosal changes, including erythema, cracking and peeling of the lips, strawberry tongue and erythema of the oropharyngeal mucosa.
* Cervical lymphadenopathy with a minimum of one lymph node of at least 1.5 cm in diameter, involvement being usually unilateral without suppuration.
* The rash appearing within 5 days of onset of fever and consisting of morbiliform maculo-papular, scarlatiniform erythroderm or an urticarial rash, mainly on the trunk.
* Changes of the hands and feet, including erythema and/or firm induration. Characteristic finger and toe desquamation begins in the periungual regions and typically develops 10–20 days after the onset of fever.

Other less specific features include arthritis/arthralgia, aseptic meningitis, hepatic dysfunction, hydrops of the gall-bladder, vomiting, diarrhea, abdominal pain and pneumonia. The most serious features are those affecting the cardiovascular system:

* Myocarditis occurs in about 25% of cases, with the findings which include tachycardia, gallop rhythm, and non-specific ST-T wave changes on the ECG. Myocarditis generally resolves completely.

Table 6.13 Diagnostic criteria of Kawasaki disease

Fever persisting for at least 5 days plus at least four of the following five:
1. Bilateral, painless conjunctival inflammation without exudates
2. Changes of the oropharynx mucosa, cracking lips, strawberry tongue
3. Acute unilateral non-purulent cervical lymphadenopathy >1.5 cm
4. Polymorphous rash, primarily truncal
5. Changes of peripheral extremities: oedema and/or erythema of hands and feet

- Mild self-limiting pericardial effusion may develop toward the second week.
- Coronary artery aneurysm (CAA) is the major feature affecting the otherwise excellent prognosis. Dilatation may be noted as early as 6 days after the appearance of fever, with the peak of detection by echocardiography at 2 weeks. New lesions are rarely identified beyond 4 weeks after the onset of fever. CAAs occur in 15–20% of cases. Aneurysms may also occur in other arteries, such as renal, axillary and iliac arteries. The prognosis for resolution of aneurysms is good unless the aneurysm is giant.

Echocardiography is usually performed 14, 21 and 60 days after the onset of illness. Fatality may occur in about 2% and is usually the consequence of myocardial infarction secondary to thrombosis in the CAAs.

Several risk factors associated with coronary involvement include the following:

- Higher temperature during days 10–13 of the disease, prolonged more than 14 days [15].
- Age under 1 year.
- Anaemia, high platelet count, WBC greater than $30\times109\,L^{-1}$, prolonged elevated ESR or CRP.
- Aneurysms in other arteries.
- High Il-6 and IL-8 levels may predict coronary artery formation.

Fever is always present in KD and reflects elevated levels of proinflammatory cytokines, particularly IL-1 and TNF, which are mediating the vascular inflammation. KD should be considered in any child with prolonged and unexplained fever. Fever is generally hectic and high (39–41°C), spiking and often remittent daily for 5 days to as long 4 weeks. It is minimally or not responsive to antipyretics and remains above 38.5°C during most of the illness. Untreated fever usually last 5–17 days, with a mean duration of 8 days [16]. Fever usually resolves within 1–2 days after initiation of aspirin and gammaglobulin treatment.

Laboratory findings are not diagnostic, but characteristically include leukocytosis with increased neutrophils, mild to moderate normocytic normochromic anaemia, almost universally increased ESR and CRP and thromocytosis, which begins in the second week and peaks at about 3 weeks (mean count, $800,000\,mm^{-3}$). Less characteristic findings include raised aspartate and alanine aminotransferase, increased ASO titre, IgG, IgA and IgM, and pyuria and proteinuria.

Aspirin is recommended in a dose of 30–50 mg kg^{-1} per day, divided into four doses. After the resolution of the acute symptoms (usually after 14 days), aspirin dose is reduced to 3–5 mg kg^{-1} per day in a single dose for its antithrombiotic effect. Aspirin is continued for 3–4 months if there is no CAA, until CAA resolves (coronary aneurysm <8 mm) or indefinitely if the coronary aneurysm persists (CAA >8 mm). If the patient cannot take aspirin, dipyridamole (persantin) is recommended.

Intravenous immune gammaglobulin (IVIG) plus aspirin reduces the incidence of coronary artery abnormalities. A large single dose of gammaglobulin (2 g kg^{-1} body weight) infused over 10 h is more effective than the previously recommended regimen of four smaller daily doses. In addition, children treated with a single infusion regimen had a lower mean temperature while hospitalized, as well as shorter mean duration of fever. The mechanisms by which gammaglobulin prevents the coronary vasculitis are unclear, but the effect of IVIG in vitro is to decrease the percentage of B cells and increase that of T cells. If there is no defervescence within 48h, a repeat IVIG and pulse methylprednisolone (600 mg m^{-2}) twice daily for 3 days should be considered.

6.4
Unclassified

6.4.1
Postoperative Fever (See also Chap 12, Sect. 12.16)

Postoperative fever is defined as a temperature greater than 38°C on two consecutive postoperative days, or 39°C on any postoperative day. Fever during the postoperative period is common, occurring in 25–50% of cases. The magnitude of fever is correlated with the extent of the surgery; i.e., minor surgery is rarely associated with fever.

The importance of postoperative fever exists in the possibility of infection, which can lead to death if not properly treated. Serious infection may exist in the absence of fever, e.g., during the neonatal period and in immunosuppressed children.

Early postoperative fever (within 48h postoperatively) is often caused by the trauma of surgery and involves pyrogenic cytokines, such as IL-1β, IL-6 and TNF-α. IL-6 is the main mediator of acute phase response and fever.

Infection is the cause of fever in about 10–25% of febrile postoperative patients, usually occurring after 48h. Fever associated with an ill appearance, the finding of a source of infection (e.g. wound infection) or abnormal laboratory tests such as leukocytosis, elevated ESR or CRP also suggest an infectious source.

Factors that increase the likelihood of infection include:

* Long postoperative stay in hospital
* Major and/or long operation
* Fever commencing on the third postoperative day or later and fever over 39°C that persists or has a hectic pattern
* The presence of intravascular catheter, the prolonged use of nasogastric or endotracheal tube, indwelling urinary catheter or shunt

Table 6.14 shows the main infectious and non-infectious causes of postoperative fever.

Physical examination should focus on sites most likely to be the cause of fever, including the operative site, abdomen (for distension, tenderness, absence of bowel sounds), upper respiratory tract for infection and lung auscultation.

The extent of investigation required to elucidate the cause of fever depends on the results of detailed history, such as pre-existing diseases, and findings on examination that may be related to infection. Investigations that are frequently performed in the absence of a clear cause of fever include full blood count, liver function tests, blood and urine cultures, chest X-ray and occasionally viral studies. A CT scan, ultrasonography or both are sometimes required for detecting intra-abdominal abscess.

Infectious causes	Non-infectious causes
Wound infection	dehydration
Peritonitis	haematoma
Intravenous line infection	pulmonary atelectasis
Viral infection	transfusion reaction
Pneumonia	drug reaction
Urinary tract infection	warm ambient temperature
Infectious diarrhoea	
Bacteraemia	
Osteomyelitis	

Table 6.14 Main causes of post-operative fever

6.4.2
Fever Following Vaccination

The current UK childhood immunization programme has been revised so that the children should receive:

* Three doses of combined DTaP/IPV/HIB vaccine and two doses of pneumococcal vaccine and meningococcal C vaccine by 4 months
* A booster dose of HIB, meningitis C and pneumococcal vaccine and first dose of MMR by 14 months
* A fourth dose of DTaP/IPV and second dose of MMR by school entry
* A fifth dose of Td/IPV before leaving school

The immune response forms the basis of an adequate vaccination, hence fever is common. Vaccine, like other antigens, activates antigen-presenting cells (macrophages) to initiate antigen processing and production of interleukins. The subsequent activation of B- and T cells initiates the production of memory cells. The persistence of the vaccine as an antigen in lymphoid tissue causes the B cells to become antibody-secreting cells that will continue to produce antibody to protect against infection.

The rate and severity of systemic adverse reactions are as follows:

* Significantly greater with DTP compared with DT vaccinated children (Fig. 6.3 and Table 6.15). This suggests that the pertussis component of DTP is the main cause of these reactions. Approximately half of DTP recipients develop fever, usually within 48h of the vaccination. The temperature elevation is usually mild, ranging between 38°C and 39°C and occurs more frequently after the third DTP vaccination. A temperature higher than 39°C is rare (6% in DTP recipients), which may be caused by unusual susceptibility to the vaccine.
* Significantly lower with acellular pertussis vaccine than with the whole cell pertussis vaccine [17].

Fever is a common adverse systemic reaction following vaccination. The timing of onset of fever will vary according to the characteristics of the vaccine received, the age of the recipient and the biological response to that vaccine. For example, fever may start within 48 h of tetanus containing vaccine (DTaP/IPV/HIB vaccines) but occurs 6–11 days after measles containing vaccine, MMR. Children aged 6 months to 4 years have the highest incidence of fever. Fever occurs

* with equal frequency after both DTaP and DT vaccines [18].
* commonly after pneumococcal and meningitis vaccines (10–20%, usually low-grade fever).

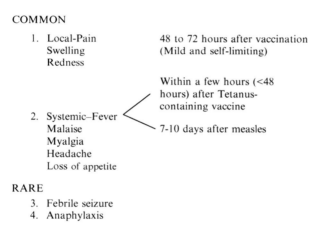

Fig. 6.3 Common and rare complications from scheduled vaccination

	DTP %	DT %
Systemic reactions		
Fever >38°C	46.5	9.3
Fever >39°C	6.1	0.7
Fretfulness	53.4	22.6
Drowsiness	31.5	14.9
Anorexia	20.9	7.0
Vomiting	6.2	2.6
Local reactions		
Redness	37.4	7.6
Swelling	40.7	7.6
Pain	50.9	9.9

Table 6.15 DTP and DT adverse effects following 15,752 and DTP immunization

6

- about a week (range, 6–11 days) following the first dose of MMR vaccine and lasts 2–3 days. This is due to an effective replication of the vaccine virus in the recipient. Fever is less common after a second dose.

Febrile seizures are the most commonly reported neurological event following measles immunization. They occur during the 6–11th day in about 1 in 1,000 children vaccinated with MMR. This rate is similar to that reported in the same period after the single measles vaccine. They do not increase the risk of subsequent epilepsy. Febrile seizures used to occur following DTP (or pertussis) vaccination, with an incidence of 1:1,750 when the third dose of DTP was given after 6 months of age.

Other more serious, but fortunately exceedingly rare, adverse reactions include infantile spasms, hypotonic, hypotensive episodes, or permanent neurological damage. Considerable controversy exists as to whether the pertussis vaccine is actually the cause of these neurological disasters. Neurological complications, such as encephalitis, Reye's syndrome and Guillian-Barre syndrome may occur in one per million vaccinated when compared to one per 1,000 following natural measles. Sub-acute sclerosing panencephalitis has an incidence of approximately one per 2 million vaccinated.

Antipyretics before and after the vaccination can reduce the fever and pain associated with vaccination. Parents should receive information on the possibility of fever and advice for reducing it. The advice should include the information that fever following vaccine is not a contra-indication to further doses. Box 6.2 summarizes the adverse reactions following vaccinations.

6.4.3   Sarcoidosis

Sarcoidosis is a multisystem granulomatous disease of unknown aetiology. The disease most commonly affects the lungs, intrathoracic lymph nodes, eyes the skin. Characteristic histological findings are multiple non-caseating granulomas without necrosis. The lymphocytes

---

Box 6.2 Summary Points of Adverse Reactions Following Vaccinations

> Febrile reaction (fever $\geq 38°C$) is common in children following vaccination.
> Timing of fever is related to the type of vaccine used and the biological response to that vaccine.
> Fever following vaccination is not a contra-indication to further doses.
> Leaflet about common adverse events and their management given to parents at the time of vaccination will help in the management.
> Newer combined vaccines, particularly the acellular component of pertussis vaccine, are less reactogenic and cause less adverse reactions.
> The serious life-threatening events are rare and the fear of these should not deter clinicians in continuing to advise vaccinations to all children.

Table 6.16 Diagnostic criteria and frequent findings in sarcoidosis

Criteria	
• Histology:	Evidence of granulomata and absence of tubercle bacilli
• Microbiology	Negative cultures of sputum and gastric washing
• Radiology	Bilateral hilar adenopathy or pulmonary infiltration
• Skin test	Negative tuberculin test. Positive Kveim test (in 50%)
Frequent findings:	Elevated ACE, hypercalcaemia, hypercalcuria, leukopenia hyperuricaemia, hypergammaglobulinaemia

ACE = angiotensin-converting enzyme

within the granulomas are T- and B cells, with many monocytes and macrophages in various stages of activation.

Children may present with fever, weight loss, arthralgia, erythema nodosum, peripheral lymphadenopathy or loss of vision (due to granulomatous uveitis). Cases are frequently discovered by routine chest X-ray, which classically shows bilateral hilar adenopathy with or without diffuse pulmonary infiltration. Sarcoid granulomas are present in either pulmonary parenchyma or thoracic lymph nodes in 90% of the cases. Diagnostic criteria are shown in the Table 6.16.

Fever has been neglected in studies on sarcoidosis, and some consider fever to be inconsistent with the diagnosis. Studies [19, 20] on fever in sarcoidosis however concluded that:

* the incidence of fever ranges between 2 and 21% of cases, usually low-grade fever.
* it may be the only presenting manifestation, which lasts up to several months as PUO. This is particularly common with hepatic granulomas.

A large study [21] of 75 patients with sarcoidosis found that 41% exhibited fever of significant magnitude and duration, often accompanied by night sweats and chills. Fever reached a peak level of 38.3–39.4°C in 77% of the febrile patients and exceeded 39.4°C in the remaining. The most common type of fever was intermittent, with a daily rise of temperature and subsequent fall to a normal level.

The pathogenesis of fever in sarcoidosis is obscure. Stimulated monocytes from patients with sarcoidosis may produce more IL-1 than normal monocytes do. As there is expansion of the lymphocytes, particularly T-helper cells, these cells spontaneously release IL-2 and INF-γ, which may activate alveolar macrophages to induce fever. The use of prednisolone (1–2 mg kg^{-1}) is the mainstay of therapy. Methotraxate also seems effective.

6.4.4 Familial Mediterranean Fever (see also Chap. 1, Sect. 1.2)

Familial Mediterranean fever (FMF) is a hereditary auto-inflammatory disease characterized by recurrent brief episodes of fever and polyserositis. Persons of Mediterranean ancestry (Armenian and Sephardic Jews) are primarily affected. The disease also occurs among individuals of Arab descent. Inheritance is autosomal recessive. The disease is caused by a mutant MEFV on the short arm of chromosome 16. The defective protein is termed pyrin (from the Greek word for fire and fever), which is present in neutrophils and normally inhibits the pro-inflammatory IL-1β [22]. FMF is confirmed by genetic testing. The onset of clinical manifestations occurs in 20% prior to the age of 5 years, and 80–90% of cases are seen by the age of 20 years.

Diagnostic criteria are:

* Recurring episodes of fever
* Pain in the abdomen (peritonitis), the chest (pleuritis) or the joints (arthritis)

A prodromal period of 4–12 h is usually present and is characterized by loss of appetite and abdominal pain due to peritonitis. About 6–10 h later, fever occurs and rapid recovery ensues within 24–72 h. Many patients undergo at least one abdominal operation for suspected appendicitis before FMF is diagnosed. Recurrent oral aphthae are often present. Pericarditis occurs in less than 1%. Amyloidosis is the principal long-term complication of FMF.

Fever is a constant finding and it may be present before other manifestations. It is characterized by the following:

* A level ranging from 38.5°C to as high as 40°C
* A duration ranging from a few hours up to 3 days (mean, 2 days)
* Recurrences at irregular intervals, sometimes over a course of many months and even years

Cytokines involved in the pathogenesis of FMF include the proinflammatory IL-1β, IL-6, IL-8, TNF-α and INF-γ. Laboratory tests show elevated CRP (or ESR), a mild decrease in serum albumin and increased levels of fibrinogen, haptoglobins and lipoproteins. Proteinuria is the first sign of amyloidosis, and renal or rectal biopsy confirms the diagnosis. Continuous prophylactic colchicine (0.6–1.8 mg daily) is effective in decreasing the frequency of the febrile episodes and preventing the formation of amyloidosis [23].

6.4.5
Hypohidrotic Ectodermal Dysplasia

This genetic condition results from faulty development of the embryonic ectoderm and its derivatives. The two recognized forms are:

* The anhidrotic form (sex-linked) characterized by inability to sweat (anhidrosis), absent or defective teeth (anodontia or hypodontia) and scanty hair (hypotrichosis). Less constant features include depressed nasal bridge, large, deformed ears, wrinkling of the orbital skin, dry skin, lack of body odour, chronic rhinitis, recurrent otitis and hoarseness of voice.
* The hidrotic form (autosomal dominant) showing similar teeth and hair defects but differing by demonstrating normal sweating, dystrophic nails, recurrent paronychia, hperkeratosis of the palms and soles, and nerve deafness. In patients with the hypohidrotic form, sweating is severely diminished or absent owing to a paucity or absence of eccrine glands.

The diagnosis can be confirmed by X-ray of the jaw (looking for the absence of unerupted teeth), skin biopsy (showing absence of eccrine sweat glands) and microscopic study of the finger tips for sweat pores.

The main concerns of children with anhidrotic and hypohidrotic forms are:

* Unexplained "fever" (more correctly hyperthermia), which may be considered as pyrexia of unknown origin as the first clue of the diagnosis before the appearance of other signs. The absence of sweating decreases the normal heat loss by evaporation, resulting in recurrent bouts of hyperthermia as high as 42°C, seizures, brain damage and sometimes death.
* Extreme discomfort in hot weather, and the body temperature increases following physical exertion or whenever the environmental temperature rises. Therefore, the condition is much more serious in a hot climate.

The condition is particularly problematic in infants and young children. Older children and adults experience heat intolerance, but they learn to control their body temperature by drinking cold liquids, wetting their skin and clothes and seeking out cool environments. Heterozygote females experience minor heat intolerance.

Children must be kept in a cool environment with a minimum of clothing. Fans and air conditioning are often required. Activities causing sweating (e.g. sport) should be avoided. An external lubricant may be used regularly if the skin is excessively dry.

6.4.6
Sweet's Syndrome (Acute Febrile Neutrophilic Dermatosis)

Sweet's syndrome, first described in 1964 by Sweet [24] is an acute febrile dermatosis which is rare in children [25]. Most patients are female (around 75%). The widely held view is that the syndrome represents a hypersensitivity reaction. The syndrome is characterized by the following:

* Acute febrile illness (noted in 50% of cases), body temperature 38.5–39.5°C)
* Leukocytosis with neutrophilia
* Raised painful plaques on the upper extremities, face and neck
* Characteristic histological proof of these lesions showing dense polymorphonuclear infiltrates of the dermis, with sparing of the epidermis

The syndrome is commonly associated with neoplastic diseases, such as myelogenous leukaemia and immunodeficiency (e.g. HIV infection). Steroid therapy is effective in treating this usually self-limiting disease (if there is no underlying disease).

6.4.7
Familial Dysautonomia (Riley-Day Syndrome)

This is an autosomal recessive genetic disorder that affects the autonomic, peripheral sensory and motor nerve functions. Ashkenazi Jews are primarily affected. Diagnosis is based on the following:

- Localization of the gene on chromosome 9 (perinatal diagnosis is possible)
- Presence of cardinal features, including decreased pain perception, absence of tears, failure to thrive, increased sweating, swallowing in-coordination (which leads to recurrent aspiration pneumonia), skin blotching, diminished deep tendon and corneal reflexes, mental retardation and hypertension
- Absence of fungiform papillae on the tongue
- Absence of flare after intradermal injection of histamine
- Abnormal vanillylmandelic acid to homovanillic acid ratio in the urine
- Abnormal histological findings of nerve biopsy showing reduced numbers of small myelinated and unmyelinated axons

In a study of 49 neonates, poor sucking was the most frequent clinical neonatal problem, followed by hypotonia and hypothermia [26]. Decreased temperature perception is a cardinal symptom. Defective temperature regulation results in recurrent bouts of hypothermia alternating with periods of hyperthermia. Before the diagnosis is established, children may present as a case of PUO. Aspiration leads to pneumonia and recurrent fevers. Heat stroke with a temperature of 41.6°C has been reported [27]. There is no effective treatment and the prognosis is poor.

6.4.8
Infantile Cortical Hyperostosis (Caffey's Disease)

The symptoms of this rare disease (described by Caffey in 1945) usually appear at the age of 6–8 weeks of life, and are characterized by soft-tissue swelling (particularly facial swelling), cortical thickening, fever and irritability. These symptoms are often mistaken as infection. Although the cause is largely unknown, autosomal dominance inheritance has been suggested for some cases of perinatal onset, which are severe and may be lethal. The condition is otherwise benign, and after several exacerbations and relapses, the affected child undergoes spontaneous regression within the first few years of life.

Fever is usually present in the early stage of the disease. Some affected children may have persistent fever and present as PUO. Temperature is usually low grade, but may occasionally reach 40°C. Prostaglandins may play a role in fever induction. The symptoms, including fever, often respond to corticosteroids and indomethacin. Indomethacin is known to inhibit bone formation.

Laboratory findings include mild increase of CRP, ESR, alkaline phosphatase and leukocytosis. Diagnosis is made by plain X-rays. Biopsy confirms the bone changes.

6.4.9
Fever Associated with Teething

The question as to whether teeth eruption causes further symptoms is controversial:

- In the past, serious diseases were attributed to teething. Hippocrates thought that teething caused itching gums, fever, convulsions and diarrhoea. In 1842, teething was the registered cause of death in 4.8% of all infants who died in London under the age of 1 year and 7.3% of those between the age of 1 and 3 years [28].

* Nowadays, while some still believe that teething produces nothing but teeth [29], others believe, as the majority of mothers do, that it is associated with increased body temperature [30].

There is no strong evidence to support claims of systemic signs, including fever, at the time of teeth eruption. The time of tooth eruption may be associated with increased salivation and irritability in children.

References

Haematology

1. Platt OS, Thorington BD, Brambilla DJ, et al. Pain in sickle cell disease: rates and risk factors. N Engl J Med 1991; 325: 11–16
2. Smith WK, Zhao H, Hodinka RL, et al. Epidemiology of human parvovirus B19 in children with sickle cell anaemia. Blood 2004; 103: 422–7
3. Powars D, Overturf GD, Wilkins J. Commentary in sickle cell and SC disease. J Pediatr 1983; 103: 242–4
4. McIntosh S, Rocks Y, Ritchey K, et al. Fever in young children with sickle cell disease. J Pediatr 1980; 96: 199–204
5. Smith AW, Hendrichse RG, Harrison C, et al. Iron deficiency anaemia and its response to oral iron: report of a study in rural Gambian children treated at home by their mothers. Ann Trop Paediatr 1989; 9: 17–23
6. Gera T, Sachdev HPS. Effects of iron supplementation on incidence of infectious illness in children: systematic review. Br Med J 2002; 325: 1142–4.
7. McKee LC. Fever in megaloblastic anaemia. South Med J 1979; 72: 1423–4
8. Igbal MP. Megaloblastic anaemia in a hospital-based population. Med Sci Res 2000; 28: 45–7
9. Welborn JL, Hersch J. Blood transfusion reactions: which are life-threatening and which are not? Postgrad Med 1991; 90: 125–38

Neoplastic Diseases

10. Sasse EC, Sasse AD, Bandalise SR, et al. Colony-stimulating factors for prevention of myelo-suppressive therapy. Cochrane Libr 2006; no 4.
11. Lobell M, Boggs DR, Wintrope MM. The clinical significance of fever in Hodgkin's disease. Arch Intern Med 1966; 117: 335–42

Rheumatic Diseases

12. Calabro JJ, Marchesano JM. Fever associated with juvenile rheumatoid arthritis. N Engl J Med 1967; 276: 11–18

6

13. Tucker LB et al, Adult- and childhood-onset systemic lupus erythematosus: a comparison of onset, clinical features, serology, and outcome. Rheumatology 1995; 34: 866–872
14. Love LA, Leff RL, Fraser DD, et al. A new approach to the classification of idiopathic inflammatory myopathy: myositis-specific autoantibodies define useful homogeneous patient groups. Medicine (Baltimore) 1991; 70: 360–74
15. Koran G, Lavi S, Rose V, et al. Kawasaki disease: review of risk factors for coronary aneurysms. J Pediatr 1986; 108: 388–92
16. Salo E, Pelkonen P, Pettay O. Outbreak of Kawasaki disease in Finland. Acta Paediatr Scand 1986; 75: 75–80

Fever after vaccination

17. Miller E. Overview of recent clinical trials of acellular pertussis vaccines. Biologicals 1999; 27: 79–86
18. Tozzi AE, Olin P. Common side effects in the Italian and Stockholm I trials. Dev Biol Stand 1997; 89: 105–8

Sarcoidosis

19. Hoffman AL, Millman N, Byq KE. Childhood sarcoidosis in Denmark 1979–1994: incidence, clinical features and laboratory results at presentation in 48 children. Acta Pediatr Int Paediatr 2004; 93: 30–6
20. Pietinalho A, Ohmichi M, Hiraga Y, et al. The mode of presentation of sarcoidosis in Finland and in Hokkaido, Japan. Sarcoidosis Vasc Diffuse Lung Dis 1996; 13: 159–66
21. Nolan JP, Klatskin G. The fever of sarcoidosis. Ann Intern Med 1964; 61: 455–61

Familial Mediterranean Fever

22. McDermott MF. A common pathway in periodic fever syndromes. Trends Immunol 2004; 25: 457–60
23. Zemer D, Pras M, Sohar E, et al. Colchicine in the prevention and treatment of the amyloidosis of FMF. N Engl J Med 1986; 314: 1001–5

Sweet Syndrome

24. Sweet RD. An acute febrile neutrophilic dermatosis. Br J Dermatol 1964; 76: 349–56
25. Boatman BW, Talor RC, Klein LE, et al. Sweet's syndrome in children. South Med J 1994; 87: 193–6

Familial Dysautonomia

26. Axelrod FB, Proges RF, Sein ME. Neonatal recognition of familial dysautonomia. J Pediatr 1987; 110: 946–8

27. Tirosh I, Hoffer V, Finkelstein Y, et al. Heat stroke in familial dysautonomia. Pediatr Neurol 2003; 29: 164–66

Fever associated with teething

28. Guthrie L. Teething. Br Med J 1998; 2: 486
29. Illingworth RS. The Normal Child, 3rd edn. Churchill, London. 1964, pp. 77–80
30. Jaber I, Cohen IJ, Mor A. Fever associated with teething. Arch Dis Child 1992; 67: 233–4

Febrile Seizures

7

Core Messages

> Attacks precipitated by fever can be epileptic or non-epileptic.

> Children with febrile seizures (FSs) are not considered to have epilepsy since their seizure only occurs when the child is febrile (acute symptomatic seizure).

> FSs do not constitute a homogeneous entity.

> The cumulative incidence of FSs in most countries is 2–5%.

> FSs usually occur between 6 months and 3 years. They peak at 18 months and it is rare for their onset to be after 6 years of age.

> FSs are divided into simple and complex. The latter have focal features and/or are prolonged and/or are repeated in the same illness.

> Viral illnesses, particularly human herpes virus 6, precipitate most FSs.

> One third of children who have one FS will have at least one recurrence.

> Recurrent FSs are more likely if the child was young at the time of the first seizure, the fever provoking the first seizure was relatively low, the child suffers from a lot of illness episodes and has a family history of FS.

> The risk of epilepsy following FSs is 7% at 25 years.

> Following one or more FS, risk factors for developing epilepsy are family history of epilepsy, neurodevelopmental problems and complex FS.

> The risk that a child with a FS will have bacterial meningitis is 0–4%.

> Routine brain imaging and EEG is not indicated following a FS.

> Regular prophylactic medication to prevent recurrent FSs is not recommended but rectal diazepam or buccal midazolam may be useful to stop further prolonged FSs.

A.S. El-Radhi et al. (Eds.) *Clinical Manual of Fever in Children.*
Doi: 10.1007/978-3-540-78598-9, © Springer-Verlag Berlin Heidelberg 2009

7

7.1
Introduction and Definitions

The provocation of seizures is one of the best known consequences of fever. Clinical terms include the following:

- The term **'seizure'** implies a paroxysmal event but not a specific mechanism. Seizures can arise as a consequence of cerebral or non-cerebral mechanisms. The latter include cardiac, anoxic and metabolic causes.
- **Convulsions** are paroxysmal events whose clinical manifestations involve prominent muscular activity. Previously the term 'febrile convulsions' was often used synonymously with FS. This is however discouraged as not all FSs are convulsive [27].
- **An epileptic seizure** is a clinical event caused by abnormal electrical activity of neurones in the brain [15]. The principal features of epileptic activity are, compared to normal neuronal activity, excessive and/or hypersynchronous. Epileptic seizures are protean in their manifestations, ranging from subjective feelings or perceptions to states of altered consciousness and convulsions.
- **An epilepsy syndrome** is defined by the non-fortuitous clustering of signs and symptoms (such as seizure type(s), age of onset, EEG and other investigational findings). The concept has proved useful in helping guide individual patient management and determining prognosis. Notwithstanding the assertion that FSs do not constitute a form of epilepsy, it is undoubtedly the case that it has also been useful to consider FSs as constituting an 'epileptic seizure syndrome'. However, the concept that all children with FS have a single, uniformly benign condition is wrong and it is likely that there are a number of FS syndromes.

Fever can be associated with the provocation of seizures at all ages, in those with or without non-FSs and in those with or without other neurological impairments. Moreover, the fever can arise from infectious and non-infectious causes, including infections of the CNS. Previously, the term FS was used loosely to cover all these situations. However, with time it has come to have a much more restricted use. The principal reason for this is that it is far more helpful in terms of guiding management and determining prognosis.

Two definitions of FSs are in widespread use: The US National Institutes of Health [47] defined a FS as follows:

An event in infancy or childhood, usually occurring between 3 months and 5 years of age, associated with fever but without evidence of intracranial infection or defined cause. Seizures with fever in children who have suffered a previous nonfebrile seizure are excluded.

The International League Against Epilepsy (ILAE) [20] defined a FS as follows:

A seizure occurring in childhood after age 1 month, associated with a febrile illness not caused by an infection of the CNS, without previous neonatal seizures or a previous unprovoked seizure, and not meeting criteria for other acute symptomatic seizures.

Bottom line Over the last few decades it has been accepted that FSs, even if recurrent, do not constitute a form of epilepsy, despite the seizures having an epileptic mechanism. The main reason for this is that the seizures only occur when the child is febrile; that is, they are a type of acute symptomatic seizure. In the same way, subjects who have seizures only when intoxicated or withdrawing from alcohol or who have seizures only when hypoglycaemic or during acute electrolyte disturbances are not considered to have epilepsy.

7.2
Epidemiology of Febrile Seizure

A number of large epidemiological studies in Western Europe and America have reported strikingly similar incidence and prevalence rates of FSs. The cumulative incidence or prevalence of FS is as follows:

* 2–5% in Western Europe and USA [61]
* 8.3% in Japan [66]
* 14% in Guam [40, 62]
* 0.5–1.5% in China [76]

Although variations in racial, socioeconomic and child rearing practices are largely unexplained, relevant data concerning the incidence of FS suggest the following:

* If malaria is excluded, there are no clear patterns when one compares developing, including tropical, with developed temperate countries. Rates in some of the former approach those found in the latter.
* Studies in the UK [71] and the Netherlands [49] found no evidence of significant differences between races living in the same country.
* There is evidence of slightly higher rates in Black, compared with Caucasian, children in the USA [48]
* Children of South-Asian (predominantly Pakistani) origin living in Bradford, UK, have significantly higher rates than other children do [3]
* Boys are consistently reported to have a higher incidence of FSs than girls, although this is statistically not significant.
* The incidence of FSs may show seasonal variation, but the patterns are complex and probably quite local, reflecting the epidemiology of childhood infectious diseases [61]
* FSs peak in the early evening.

Bottom Line Febrile seizures are the commonest epileptic seizure disorder affecting children: Between 2 and 5 children in every 100 will be affected.

7

7.3
Mechanisms Underlying Febrile Seizures

7.3.1
Genetic Factors

Why one child with a fever has a FS and another with a similar fever does not remains largely unknown. Genetic factors are clearly important. Proposals include the following:

* Polygenic, autosomal dominant and autosomal recessive models
* Polygenic model in families with probands with a single FS
* Repeated FSs and autosomal dominant model with reduced penetrance fits best [45]
* Linkage studies, showing six genetic loci (FEB 1–6) for FS [1, 43, 45]

Three epilepsies with known gene defects have been described in which FS is an important part of the phenotype:

* **'Generalised epilepsy with febrile seizures plus' (GEFS+)** is characterised by individuals in the same family who have both febrile and non-FSs, in which FSs persist beyond the age of 6 and are associated with generalised or occasionally focal non-FSs. GEFS+ is an autosomal dominant condition in which mutations in four genes have been identified to date. These are the SCN1A, SCN2A, SCN1B genes and the GABARG2 gene. The first three of these code for the $\alpha 1$, $\alpha 2$ and $\beta 1$ subunits of the sodium channel whilst the last codes for the $\gamma 2$ subunit of the $GABA_A$ receptor [31]. Sodium channels play a crucial role in neuronal membrane excitability, and many antiepileptic drugs act at sodium channels. GABA is the principal inhibitory neurotransmitter in the CNS, and GABAergic drugs generally inhibit seizures. To date, no mutations in most GEFS+ genes have been found in populations of FSs not corresponding to the GEFS+ phenotype. An exception is a report on an SCN1A mutation apparently responsible for simple FSs in a family [38].
* **Epilepsy with myoclonic-atonic seizures (Doose syndrome)** is a rare familial type of primary generalised epilepsy, which affects children usually 1–5 years of age without neurological deficits before onset.
* **Dravet syndrome** is an epileptic encephalopathy characterised by the occurrence of FSs, which are often prolonged and focal and associated with relatively low-grade fever. The onset is usually in the second half of the first year of life, followed by a polymorphous epilepsy starting in the second or third year of life. Although initial development is normal, with the onset of the polymorphous epilepsy, stagnation in development and often a true loss of skills occur, leaving the child with severe learning difficulties. The majority of patients have mutations in the SCN1A gene and in atypical cases a significant minority have [19].

7.3.2
Factors Relating to the Immature Brain

During the period when infants are vulnerable to FS, important maturational changes, such as synaptogenesis, are occurring in the brain. Excitatory synaptic neurotransmission mediated by glutamate receptors is central to this. At the same time, important changes are occurring in other neurotransmitter systems, such as the GABA system, and in neuromodulatory peptide systems and in voltage-gated ion channels. It is postulated that these changes confer upon the infants' brain an enhanced excitability and vulnerability to epileptic and FS [32].

7.3.3
Fever-Related Mechanisms

Fever involves the expression and then release of proinflammatory cytokines mainly from monocytic cells which act as endogenous pyrogens. Microglia and astroglia in the CNS can also produce proinflammatory cytokines. Prostaglandins, particularly PGE_2, which is locally produced in the anterior hypothalamus, act as common final mediators for the effect of endogenous pyrogens in controlling the core body temperature set point [30]. A large number of ion channels, including some involved in neuronal excitability, are now known to be highly sensitive to temperature. Proinflammatory cytokines as well as inducing the fever which characterises FS may also directly affect neuronal excitability and hence seizure threshold. They may also do so by other mechanisms. For example, certain neuronal populations, including those in the hippocampus, carry various cytokine receptors.

The Bottom Line The brain of the infant has a lower threshold for epileptic seizures. There may be many reasons for this. We are about to experience an explosion in our understanding of the molecular basis for FSs.

7.4
The Fever and Its Causes

Surprisingly, the standard definitions of FSs do not specify what the temperature must be in order to diagnose a FS. As there are important differences between, say, rectal and axillary measurements, some authorities require a temperature of 38.4 or 38.5°C, while others accept 38.0°C. There is a common belief that the rate of rise of temperature is more important than the ultimate height of the temperature. Evidence to support this is lacking, whereas the evidence implicating the height of the fever is strong. Most FSs occur early in the course of the febrile illness and are sometimes the initial presenting feature.

There is strong evidence that children whose initial FS has occurred with a relatively low fever are at a significantly increased risk of recurrences [13, 23–25, 50]

FSs are precipitated by:

* Viruses, particularly viral upper respiratory tract infections, are the commonest precipitants [42, 69].

    – In Europe and the USA, human herpesvirus (HHV)-6, the cause of exanthem subitum (roseola infantum), is particularly implicated, being responsible for up to a third of initial FS [9, 35] HHV-7 is also linked to a lesser degree to the precipitation of FS.
    – In Asia and in other countries, as well as during epidemics, influenza A virus is a particularly important cause of FS [36, 70]. Other implicated viruses include adenovirus, respiratory syncytial virus and enteroviruses.

7

- Bacterial illnesses are less frequently implicated in the precipitation of FS, and the rate of bacteraemia in children with FSs is less than 2%. FSs are caused by malaria and dysentery due to shigella, but it seems that this is probably related to the height of the fever and electrolyte disturbances rather than the effect of a specific neurotoxin.
- Vaccinations [7]. The risk following MMR is 25–34 per 100,000 children vaccinated, with the seizures occurring 7–14 days after the vaccination co-incident with the post-vaccination fever. The risk following DTP is 6–9 per 100,000, with the seizure occurring on the same day as the vaccination.

It is generally considered that fever caused by non-infectious causes can precipitate FSs in susceptible individuals. However, this appears to be infrequent. Kawasaki disease, which is often associated with high fever, is rarely complicated by FSs [74].

> **Bottom Line** The higher the fever, the more likely the child is to have a FS. HHV-6 is a particularly common precipitant of FSs.

7.5
Clinical Features

7.5.1
Predisposing Factors

Predisposing factors include:

- Age-specific incidence of FS follows a bell-shaped curve, with most occurring between 6 months and 3 years of age. The median age at the first FS is about 18 months. Onset after the age of 6 years is rare.
- Genetic factors are of great importance. A child with at least one parent with a FS has a fourfold increased risk of FSs whilst the risk is increased 3.5 times if a sibling has had a FS [73]. The risk is also slightly increased if a parent has had epilepsy.
- Various pre-, peri- and post-natal factors have been shown to increase the risk of FSs. These include some pre-existing maternal conditions, prematurity, problems in the neonatal period and developmental delay.
- It is important to stress that most children who develop FSs are born after unremarkable pregnancies, have no problems in the newborn period and are developmentally normal.

> **Bottom Line** Most children who have a FS are otherwise normal children in the second year of life.

7.5.2
The Febrile Seizures

FSs are usually convulsive and most are generalised tonic–clonic seizures (GTCS) which are either primarily or secondarily generalised. Unfortunately, many clinicians are prone to diagnose GTCS without obtaining a clear account of the initial tonic phase, characterised by more or less whole body stiffening, followed by the clonic phase of repetitive, rhythmical jerking of the limbs. Hence many more FS are probably diagnosed as GTCS than is actually the case. A significant minority are probably tonic or clonic seizures rather than tonic–clonic in type.

In recent years there have been reports of fever precipitating

* Myoclonic seizures [46, 55]. In some children runs of myoclonic jerks have led to GTCS (as is sometimes seen in juvenile myoclonic epilepsy), strongly suggesting that the myoclonic jerks are epileptic in origin.
* Stonic features. Such children may appear floppy and unresponsive and this may not suggest an epileptic origin to eyewitnesses. The autonomic seizures characterising Panayiotopoulos syndrome often occur in association with fever or are accompanied by fever as an ictal manifestation [28]. This is a relatively common epilepsy syndrome which usually occurs in children of about 4–5 years of age.

Febrile seizures, at least those that are convulsive in type, are usually classified as simple or complex. The terms complicated or atypical are sometimes used in preference to complex. Febrile seizures are complex if they have one or more of the following features:

1. They have focal features (including the occurrence of a post-ictal Todd's paresis).
2. They are repeated in the same illness; some definitions stipulate a recurrence within 24 h of the initial seizure.
3. They are prolonged. Mostly this is defined as lasting 15 min or longer, although some use a cut-off point of 10 min and others of 20 min.

Most authorities suggest that around

* 70% of FSs are simple and
* 30% complex

However, these figures vary depending on how carefully focal features are looked for. It is also worth noting that it is difficult to assess the significance of some relatively subtle 'focal' features, such as eye deviation, which can occur in primarily GTCS. A report (12) indicated that:

* 35% of initial primarily febrile seizures were complex and that in 16.1% this was because of the presence of focal features,
* 13.8% of seizures were multiple
* 13.1% of seizures were prolonged (defined as 10 minutes or more).
* 6.5% of seizures were associated with two complex features (e.g. prolonged and multiple) and 0.7% with three complex features (multiple, prolonged and focal)

Complex FSs are more common in younger children. Children with an initial prolonged FS who have further FSs tend to have prolonged recurrent FSs as well [12].

Although FSs are defined as prolonged if they last 15 min or more, most are considerably shorter than this. Following FSs, the recovery time is usually quite short [53, 54]. A recent study found that full consciousness was regained within a mean of 18 min, compared with more than an hour for seizures of other aetiologies [2].

Bottom Line Remember – not all FSs are tonic–clonic, but if they are, classify them as simple or complex.

7

7.6
Recurrent Febrile Seizures

Population and birth-cohort studies suggest that about one third of children who have had one FS will have at least one recurrence; 15% will have at least two recurrences and 10% will have three or more recurrences [6, 13, 29, 48, 50, 71].
Four main factors have been found to influence the rate or recurrent FS:

* Age at first FS. A young age at first FS is associated with a greatly increased risk of at least one recurrence. The risk of a recurrence in a child whose initial FS occurred at less than 12 months of age is about 40% and falls to about 20% if the initial FS occurred after 18 months of age [10].
* Height of temperature at first FS. El-Radhi et al [25]. found that the risk of a recurrence in those children whose first FS occurred with a fever <40°C was several times higher than in those with a fever >40°C. This finding has subsequently been confirmed by others and it seems that the lower the temperature at the initial FS, the greater the risk of recurrence [13, 23, 24, 50].
* Illness frequency. Several studies have found a strong association between the number of illnesses a child experiences following an initial FS and the risk of recurrent FSs [34, 56, 64, 68]. This is also likely to explain reports that recurrent FSs are more common in those attending day-care facilities. Finally, children who have had a FS and who have a first-degree relative with FSs have a greatly increased risk (possibly a doubling) of recurrent FS [13, 51]. Recurrences usually occur within the first year of the initial FS, with around 90% occurring within 2 years [6, 13, 50, 51].
* Family history of FSs. Other factors that are either not associated with an increased risk of recurrence or else of only a modest increased risk or on which the data are conflicting are sex, family history of epilepsy, type of initial FS (i.e. whether simple or complex), and pre-existing neurodevelopmental abnormalities.

Berg et al [13]. calculated individualised risks for recurrences:

* A child with none of the three factors, namely, young age at onset (<18 months), relatively low temperature (<40°C) and positive family history of FSs had a recurrence risk of 15%.
* A child with one, two and three of the factors had a recurrence risk of 27, 39 and 65% respectively.

Bottom Line One third of children who have one FS will have at least one more. There are well-established risk factors for recurrent FSs.

7.7
Differential Diagnosis (see also Chap. 12, Sect. 17)

There is an important differential diagnosis to consider:

* Epileptic seizure
* Rigors

- Febrile syncope
- Blue breath holding spells and reflex anoxic seizures
- Toxic delirium
- Temper tantrums
- Paroxysmal non-epileptic events resembling seizures, in association with otitis media [63]

In addition, epileptic seizures in infancy and young children may be triggered by minor illness without the child being febrile. It has been suggested that this is a distinct condition [37, 75]

> **Bottom Line** The most important aspect in the differential diagnosis of a child with seizure is the presence of associated fever (that is FS) or its absence (that is an epileptic seizure). Hence it is essential to measure body temperature at the onset at these events as soon as possible.

7.8
Prognosis

7.8.1
Risk of Epilepsy

In determining the risk following FSs the pragmatic definition of epilepsy as being at least two non-FSs is usually used. Only a small minority of children who have had FS will develop epilepsy. Nevertheless, children who have had one or more FSs are at greater risk of developing epilepsy than those who have not.

The following are the main factors that influence whether epilepsy will follow FSs:

- Family history of epilepsy; the type of FS (whether complex or not) and pre-existing neurodevelopmental problems [5, 12, 48, 72]
- The effect of pre-existing neurodevelopmental problems is strong. Annegers et al. [4, 5] found that in children who were neurologically abnormal at birth but later had a FS the risk of epilepsy at age 25 years was 55%, compared with 7% in those who were neurologically normal at birth. Similarly, Verity and Golding [72] reported that children neurologically abnormal from birth who experienced a FS 25% developed unprovoked seizures, compared with 3.4% of neurologically normal children. Following a FS, a child with a family history of epilepsy has a threefold increase in the risk of subsequently developing epilepsy and the risk is more than doubled following complex FSs.

The risk of epilepsy following FSs increases as the number of risk factors increases. If only one of family history of epilepsy, neurodevelopmental abnormalities and complex FSs is present the risk is increased 2- to 3-fold. If two are present the risk is increased 5- to 8-fold and if all three are present, 14-fold [48].

The increased risk of developing epilepsy following FSs persists throughout childhood and into adult life. Hence in previously neurologically normal children who had had a FS [5] the risk of epilepsy is 2% at 5 years, 4.5% at 10 years, 5.5% at 15 years and 7% at 25 years.

7

An alternative way at exploring the association of FS and epilepsy is to look at subjects with epilepsy and antecedent FSs. Studies have shown that the following:

- Overall 13–18% of children with new onset epilepsy have had preceding FSs [14, 16].
- The onset of epilepsy tends to be earlier in those with preceding FSs.
- Both focal and generalised epilepsies are often preceded by FSs.
- Simple FSs are more likely to be followed by idiopathic generalised epilepsies whilst complex FSs are more likely to be followed by focal epilepsies [5, 72].

One of the most important unresolved questions in clinical epileptology is whether FSs cause mesial temporal sclerosis and subsequent temporal lobe epilepsy. There are arguments in favour and against such a causal link:

- Such a sequence has been shown in animal experiments, and retrospective series of adult patients operated upon for temporal lobe epilepsy have found that upwards of 30% of those with mesial temporal sclerosis have had FSs, particularly complex FSs in early childhood [44]. A number of studies have described acute hippocampal abnormalities based on MRI scans following prolonged FSs. In one large prospective study 4 of 44 infants who had had febrile status epilepticus had acute hippocampal abnormalities on MRI. The same study has found evidence that the acute changes are often followed by the hippocampal sclerosis [44].
- In contrast epidemiological studies have not supported a causal link. Recent data has suggested the possibility that pre-existing developmental abnormalities in the hippocampus may predispose to prolonged FSs with the potential for then causing further neurodevelopmental damage (59).

Bottom Line Febrile seizures usually have a good outcome. However, the risk of epilepsy is definitely increased, especially if the FSs were complex.

7.8.2
Neurological, Learning and Behaviour Outcomes

In general, population-based series have been reassuring that FSs (excluding febrile status) are not associated with subsequent new neurological problems or with learning or behavioural problems.

7.9
Febrile Status

Approximately 5% of FSs meet the usual definition of status epilepticus (i.e., a single seizure lasting at least 30 min or a series of seizures lasting at least 30 min without full recovery of consciousness between seizures) and about a quarter of all episodes of convulsive status epilepticus in children are febrile [12, 18].

The outcome after febrile status is controversial:

* Early reports emphasised its high mortality and morbidity. More recently, van Esch et al. [67] reported that of 57 cases, 12 had subsequent new neurological problems, often severe.
* In contrast, Barnard and Wirrell [8] found that febrile aetiology was a predictor of a good outcome after status epilepticus. Shinnar et al. [60] reported the short-term outcome of febrile status in a group of 180 children. Around a third of the episodes were focal. There was a strikingly high number (21%) who had pre-existing neurological abnormalities, but none had developed new neurological problems during the relatively short follow-up period.

Bottom Line If a child has had one episode of febrile status (or prolonged FSs) he or she is at significantly increased risk of another prolonged FS.

7.10
Management

7.10.1
Initial Management

Acute management of FSs includes the management of the child who is still convulsing and management of the child whose FS has stopped. In the former an important priority is to safely and rapidly stop the seizure, best achieved through intravenous route with either diazepam or lorazepam (the latter has significant advantages) as used in the paramedical or hospital setting. In both cases the underlying cause of the fever should be sought and, if appropriate, treated. The appropriate measures for stopping FSs, including febrile status, are no different from those used to stop their non-febrile equivalents and will not be discussed in detail here. Particular attention should be given to:

The history, which explores the illness triggering the febrile seizure, looking in particular for any clues to the likely source of the infection. It is also important to record the details of the attack, both to determine that it was a febrile seizure (remembering that there is a differential diagnosis) and, if it was, whether there were complex features since the presence of these may affect management and will help in discussion with the family on prognosis. Other aspects which should be explored include a search in the child's personal and family history for predisposing factors, such as a family history or a history of adverse perinatal events or developmental problems. It is also important to exclude other possible causes for the seizure, such as drug ingestion, trauma, etc.

The examination, which includes a thorough search for the source of the fever as an essential part of the examination. The clinician will rightly be anxious to exclude meningitis but other possibilities should also be considered. The examination should also look for evidence of raised intracranial pressure and for clues, such as the skin lesions of tuberous sclerosis, which might indicate a susceptibility to epilepsy. Finally, it is important to measure and record the state of consciousness. This is best done using the Glasgow Coma Score.

Laboratory investigation is not always required. Some children, such as older children who are fully recovered and have obvious signs of a viral upper respiratory tract infection, require no investigation except a urinalysis. However, investigations, such as a full blood count, measurement of the CRP and bacteriological and viral studies will be required in most children. Other investigations include the following:

- **Lumbar puncture (LP).** Usually of most importance is the decision as to whether to perform an LP to exclude meningitis. The probability that a child with a FS will have bacterial meningitis is low; a systematic review suggested 0–4% [52]. However, signs of meningism may be absent in young children with meningitis, and meningitis can co-exist with evidence of a septic focus elsewhere. Therefore, most authorities have until recently advocated LP in all children following an initial FS under the age of 12 months and many have advocated routine LP in all below 18 months of age. This approach has been criticised. Carroll and Brookfield [17] advised that 'infants without meningeal signs (irritability, lethargy or bulging fontanelle) who have recovered from their seizure are admitted, and reviewed at 4 h. If no deterioration has occurred and the child appears well, LP is considered unnecessary. Riordan and Cant [58] note that meningitis is very unlikely following simple FS with no symptoms or signs of meningitis and, therefore, LP is not necessary. However, they consider a complex FS an indication for LP. Children usually regain full consciousness quickly after FS. A depressed Glasgow Coma Score 1 h after an apparent FS should be viewed with suspicion. However, LP should not be performed until the child is localizing pain or if there are focal neurological signs or papilloedema. Empirical treatment with antibiotics and antiviral agents to cover bacterial meningitis and herpes encephalitis should be started and LP deferred until clinical and radiological evidence suggests it is safe to do so. It should be noted that LP may be normal in very early meningitis, and therefore, if suspicion remains high it should be repeated 24–48 h later.
- **Routine brain imaging, either by CT or MRI,** is not indicated in children with either simple or complex FSs [22, 65]. However, emergency CT scanning would be appropriate following febrile status or in a child who fails to show the expected rapid recovery following a FS. Neuroimaging would also be indicated if there were persistent neurological signs after a FS and in some children whose family, perinatal or developmental history suggested the possibility of a structural brain abnormality. MRI will be more sensitive but is likely to require sedation or an anaesthetic.
- **EEG** in children who have had a FS is often abnormal [33]. Slow wave activity is common shortly after the seizure and may persist for some days. Subsequently, around a fifth of patients will show paroxysmal epileptiform abnormalities. However, detecting such abnormalities is not helpful in guiding either management or prognosis and therefore EEG is not indicated following either simple or complex FSs [21, 53, 54].

Bottom Line There are no hard and fast rules about which children should have a LP after a FS: Even in those under a year it may not be necessary if the child has no meningeal signs, recovers quickly to full consciousness and can be observed for a few hours. However, the threshold should be lower following a complex FS.

7.10.2
Prevention of Recurrences and Anticonvulsant Therapy

Meta-analysis has shown sodium valproate and phenobarbitone to be effective agents in the prevention of recurrences of FSs, although four children would need to be treated with valproate and eight with phenobarbitone to prevent one FS [57]. Phenytoin and carbamazepine appear to be ineffective. Until the 1990s continuous prophylactic treatment with antiepileptic drugs was the norm in most countries for children who had had one or more FS. Now there is unanimity that such a treatment is not appropriate, except in exceptional circumstances. The following are the reasons for this change:

* The recognition of the benign nature of FSs
* A lack of evidence that such treatment alters the outcome in the relatively small number of children with FSs who subsequently develop epilepsy
* The increased concern regarding the potential adverse effects of the available prophylactic agents

There are numerous reports of the intermittent use of various drugs during febrile episodes to prevent recurrences. Use of phenobarbitone in this way is considered ineffective and the data on which to judge the efficacy of sodium valproate and chloral hydrate are very limited. Most interest has centred on the use of benzodiazepines, particularly diazepam given either orally or rectally. The results have been conflicting, although a meta-analysis found that 11.2% of children treated with diazepam to cover febrile episodes had one or more recurrences, compared with 17.2% treated with placebo [39]. Given the benign nature of FSs, the difficulty in recognising the fever before the seizure and the possible risks of such treatment, most authorities do not recommend this treatment.

Many clinicians prescribe benzodiazepines for the immediate treatment of on-going seizures, whether febrile or afebrile – 'rescue medication'. There is no consensus as to when this should be offered, but most clinicians only use it in selected cases. These include children who have had one prolonged FS, including febrile status, and who are at considerably increased risk of further prolonged FS, including further episodes of febrile status. Medications, which have been used are as follows:

* Rectal administration of diazepam ($0.5\,mg\,kg^{-1}$ per dose) has been widely used. Rectal lorazepam is an alternative. Some advise administration as soon as possible after the seizure has began, while others only for seizures lasting longer than a certain period of time, often 5 min.
* More recently midazolam, which can be given buccally, nasally, rectally and intravenously (the last by paramedics or in hospital), has become popular. The buccal and nasal routes have clear advantages over the rectal route in terms of acceptability. Buccal midazolam, $0.5\,mg\,kg^{-1}$, has been shown to terminate seizures more quickly (median of 8 min) than rectal diazepam, $0.5\,mg\,kg^{-1}$, (median 15 min) and to have a more sustained action [41]. Therapeutic success (seizure cessation within 10 min, no respiratory depression and no recurrence within an hour) was achieved with midazolam in 56% of cases, compared with 27% of cases with diazepam. Families who are given rescue medication to stop seizures must have clear instruction regarding

how and when to administer the medication, how to monitor their child afterwards and when to seek further help.

7.10.3
Antipyretic Measures

Intuitively it should be possible to prevent recurrences of FSs by appropriate use of antipyretic agents such as paracetamol and ibuprofen. In fact studies have failed to show a preventive effect [26]. Parents whose children are febrile are also advised to avoid dressing them in multiple layers. Whether these measures reduce the risk of further FS is unknown. Using an electric fan directly over a febrile child is discouraged since it can paradoxically raise the core temperature by causing peripheral vasoconstriction.

7.10.4
Advice to Parents

The trauma of witnessing your child having any form of epileptic seizure is very considerable. Parents and other witnesses require much reassurance. Fortunately, the fact that the vast majority of children with FSs have an excellent prognosis makes this easier than is the case for many other childhood conditions. Topics that should be covered include the following:

* The nature of FSs – explained in a language appropriate for the understanding of the family
* The risk of the child having suffered damage as a result of the initial seizure (no risk, unless it was febrile status)
* The risk of one or more recurrences
* The risk of subsequent non-FSs, including epilepsy
* The effect on cognition and behaviour
* Prevention of further FSs, including use of rescue medication
* First aid measures
* What to tell others, including nurseries and schools

Although a positive approach is justified, it is a mistake to trivialise the event or to underplay the risk of subsequent epilepsy.

> **The Bottom Line** The most important point of managing children with FSs long-term is to reassure the parents and ensure they know what to do should there be a recurrence.

References

1. Aadenaert D, van Broeckhoven C, De jonghe P (2006) Genes and loci involved with febrile seizures and related epilepsy syndromes. Hum Mutat 27: 291–401
2. Allen JE, Ferrie CD, Livingston JH, Feltbower RG (2006) Recovery of consciousness after epileptic seizures in children. Arch Dis Child 92: 39–42

3. Hamdy A, Ginby D, Feltbower R, Ferrie CD (2007) Ethnic differences in the incidence of seizure disorders in children from Bradford, United Kingdom. Epilepsia 48: 913–916

4. Annegers JF, Hauser WA, Elveback LR, Kurland LT (1979) The risk of epilepsy following febrile convulsions. Neurology 29: 297–303

5. Annegers JF, Hauser WA, Shirts SB, Kurland LT (1987) Factors prognostic of unprovoked seizures after febrile convulsions. N Engl J Med 316: 493–498

6. Annegers JF, Blakley SA, Hauser WA, Kurland LT (1990) Recurrence of febrile convulsions in a population-based cohort. Epilepsy Res 5: 209–216

7. Barlow WE, Davis RL, Glasser JW, et al. (2001) The risk of seizures after receipt of whole-cell pertussis or measles, mumps and rubella vaccine. N Engl J Med 345: 656–661

8. Barnard C, Wirrell E (1999) Does status epilepticus in children cause developmental deterioration and exacerbation of epilepsy? J Child Neurol 14: 787–794

9. Barone SR, Kaplan MH, Krilov LR (1995) Human herpesvirus-6 infection in children with first febrile seizures. J Pediatr 127: 95–97

10. Berg AT (2002) Recurrent febrile seizures. In Baram TZ, Shlomo S (eds) Febrile seizures. Academic Press, San Diego, pp. 37–52

11. Berg AT (1992) Febrile seizures and epilepsy: the contribution of epidemiology. Paediatr Perinat Epidemiol 6: 145–162

12. Berg AT, Shinnar S (1996) Complex febrile seizures. Epilepsia 37: 126–133

13. Berg AT, Shinnar S, Darefsky AS, et al. (1997) Predictors of recurrent febrile seizures: a prospective cohort study. Arch Pediatr Adolesc Med 151: 371–378

14. Berg AT, Shinnar S, Levy SR, Testa FM (1999) Childhood-onset epilepsy with and without preceding febrile seizures. Neurology 53: 1742–1748

15. Blume WT, Luders HO, Mizrahi E, Tassinari C, van Emde Boas W, Engel J Jr (2001) ILAE Commission Report. Glossary of descriptive terminology for ictal semionology: report of the ILAE task force on classification and terminology. Epilepsia 42: 1212–1218

16. Camfield P, Camfield C, Gordon K, Dooley J (1994) What types of epilepsy are preceded by febrile seizure? A population based study of children. Dev Med Child Neurol 36: 887–892

17. Carroll W, Brookfield D (2002) Lumbar puncture following febrile convulsions. Arch Dis Child 87: 238–240

18. Chin RFM, Neville BGR, Peckham C, et al. (2006) Incidence, causes, and short-term outcome of convulsive status epilepticus in childhood: prospective population-based study. Lancet 368: 222–229

19. Claes L, Ceulemans B, Audenaert D, et al. (2003) De novo SCN1A mutations are a major cause of severe myoclonic epilepsy of infancy. Hum Mutat 21: 615–621

20. Commission on Epidemiology and Prognosis. International League Against Epilepsy (1993). Guidelines for epidemiological studies on epilepsy. Epilepsia 34: 592–596

21. Cuestas E (2004) Is routine EEG helpful in the management of complex febrile seizures? Arch Dis Child 89: 290

22. Di Mario FJ Jr (2006) Children presenting with complex febrile seizures do not routinely need computed tomography scanning in the emergency department. Pediatrics 117: 528–530

23. El-Radhi AS (1998) Lower degree of fever at the initial febrile convulsion is associated with increasd risk of subsequent convulsions. Eur J Paediatr Neurol 2: 91–96

24. El-Radhi AS, Banajeh S (1989) Effect of fever on recurrence rate of febrile convulsion. Arch Dis Child 64: 869–870

25. El-Radhi AS, Withana K, Banajeh S (1986) Recurrence rate of febrile convulsion related to the degree of pyrexia during the first attack. Clin Paediatr 25: 311–313

26. El-Radhi A, Barry W (2003) Do antipyretics prevent febrile convulsions? Arch Dis Child 88: 641–642

7

27. Engel J Jr (2001) ILAE Commission Report. Proposed diagnostic scheme for people with epileptic seizures and with epilepsy: report of the ILAE task force on classification and terminology. Epilepsia 41: 796–803
28. Ferrie C, Caraballo R, Covanis A, et al. (2006) Panayiotopoulos syndrome: a consensus view. Dev Med Child Neurol 48: 236–240
29. Forsgren L, Heijbel J, Nystrom L, Sidenvall R (1997) A follow-up of an incident case-referent study of febrile convulsions seven years after the onset. Seizure 6: 21–26
30. Gatti S, Vezzani A, Bartfai T (2002) Mechanisms of fever and febrile seizures: putative role of the interleukin-1 system. In Baram TZ, Shlomo S (eds) Febrile seizures. Academic Press, San Diego, pp. 169–188
31. Ito M, Yamakawa K, Sugawara T, et al. (2006) Phenotypes and genotypes in epilepsy with febrile seizures plus. Epilepsy Res 70S: S199–S205
32. Jensen FE, Sanchez RM (2002) Why does the developing brain demonstrate heightened susceptibility to febrile and other provoked seizures. In Baram TZ, Shlomo S (eds) Febrile seizures. Academic Press, San Diego, pp. 153–168
33. Joshi C, Wawrykow T, Patrich J, Prasad A (2005) Do clinical variables predict an abnormal EEG in patients with complex febrile seizures. Seizure 14: 429–434
34. Knusden FU (1988) Frequent febrile episodes and recurrent febrile convulsions. Acta Neurol Scand 78: 414–417
35. Kondo K, Nagafuji H, Hata A, et al. (1993) Association of human herpesvirus 6 infection of the central nervous system with recurrence of febrile convulsions. J Infect Dis 167: 1197–1200
36. Kwong KL, Lam SY, Que TL, Wong SN (2006) Influenza A and febrile seizures in childhood. Pediatr Neurol 35: 395–399
37. Lee W-L, Ong H-T (2004) Afebrile seizures associated with minor infection: comparison with febrile seizures and unprovoked seizures. Pediatr Neurol 31: 157–164
38. Mantegazza M, Gambardella A, Rosconi R (2005) Identification of a Nav1.1 sodium channel (SCN1A) loss-o function mutation associated with familial simple febrile seizures. Proc Natl Acad Sci U S A 102: 18177–18182
39. Masuko AH, Castro AA, Santos GR, et al. (2003) Intermittent diazepam and continuous phenobarbitone to treat recurrencies of febrile seizures: a systematic review with meta-analysis. Arq Neuropsiquiatr 61: 897–901
40. Mathai KV, Dunn DP, Kurland LT, Reeder FA (1968) Convulsive disorders in the Mariana Islands. Epilepsia 9: 77–85
41. McIntyre J, Robertson S, Norris E, et al. (2005) Safety and efficacy of buccal midazolam versus rectal diazepam for emergency treatment of seizures in children: a randomised controlled trial. Lancet 366: 205–210
42. Millichap JG, Millichap JJ (2006) Role of viral infections in the etiology of febrile seizures. Pediatr Neurol 35: 165–172
43. Minawer M, Hesdorffer D (2004) Turning on the heat: the search for febrile seizure genes. Neurology 63: 1770–1771
44. Mitchell TV, Lewis DV (2002). In Baram TZ, Shlomo S (eds) Febrile seizures. Academic Press, San Diego, pp. 103–125
45. Nakayama J, Arinami T (2006) Molecular genetics of febrile seizures. Epilepsy Res 70S: S190–S198
46. Narula S, Goraya JS (2005) Febrile myoclonua. Neurology 64: 169–170
47. National Institutes of Health (1980). Febrile seizures: consensus development conference summary. Vol 3, No. 2. National Institutes of Health. Bethseda, MD

48. Nelson KB, Ellenberg JH (1976) Predictors of epilepsy in children who have experienced febrile seizures. N Engl J Med 295: 1029–1033
49. Offringa M, Hazebroek-Kampschreur AAJM, Derksen-Lubsen G (1991) Prevalence of febrile seizures in Dutch schoolchildren. Paediatr Perinat Epidemiol 5: 181–188
50. Offringa M, Derksen-Lubsen G, Bossuyt PM, Lubsen J (1992) Seizure recurrence after a first febrile seizure: a multivariate approach. Dev Med Child Neurol 34: 15–24
51. Offringa M, Bossuyt PMM, Lubsden J, et al. (1994) Risk factors for seizure recurrence in children with febrile seizures: a pooled analysis of individual patient data from five studies. J Pediatr 124: 574–584
52. Offringa M, Moyer VA (2001) Evidence based paediatrics: evidence based management of seizures associated with fever. Br Med J 323: 1111–1114
53. Okumura A, Uemura N, Suzuki M, et al. (2004) Unconsciousness and delirious behaviour in children with febrile seizures. Pediatr Neurol 30: 316–319
54. Okumura A, Ishiguro Y, Sofue A, et al. (2004) Treatment and outcome in patients with febrile convulsions associated with epileptiform discharges on electroencephalography. Brain Dev 26: 241–244
55. Rajakumar K, Bodensteiner JB (1996) Febrile myoclonus: a survey of pediatric neurologists. Clin Pediatr 35: 331–336
56. Rantala H, Uhari M, Tuokko H (1990) Viral infections and recurrences of febrile convulsions. J Pediatr 116: 195–199
57. Rantala H, Tarkka R, Uhari M (1997) A meta-analytic review of the preventative treatment of recurrencies of febrile seizures. J Pediatr 131: 922–955
58. Riordan FAI, Cant AJ (2002) When to do a lumbar puncture. Arch Dis Child 87: 235–237
59. Scott RC, King MD, Gadian DG, et al. (2006) Prolonged febrile seizures are associated with hippocampal vasogenic edema and developmental changes. Epilepsia 47: 1493–1498
60. Shinnar S, Pellock JM, Berg AT, et al. (2001) Short term outcomes of children with febrile status epilepticus. Epilepsia 42: 47–53
61. Stafstrom CE (1992). The incidence and prevalence of febrile seizures. In Baram TZ, Shinnar S (eds) Febrile seizures. Academic Press, San Diego, pp. 1–25
62. Stanhope JM, Brody JA, Brink E, Morris CE (1972) Convulsions among the Chamorro people of Guam, Mariana Islands. Am J Epidemiol 95: 299–304
63. Soman TB, Krishnamoorthy KS (2005) Paroxysmal non-epileptic events resembling seizures in children with otitis media. Clin Pediatr 44: 437–441
64. Tarkka R, Rantala H, Uhari M, Pokka T (1998) Risks of recurrence and outcome after the first febrile seizure. Pediatr Neurol 18: 218–220
65. Teng D, Nayan P, Tyler S, et al. (2006) Risks of intracranial pathologic conditions requiring emergency intervention after a first complex febrile seizure episode among children. Pediatrics 117: 304–308
66. Tsuboi T (1984) Epidemiology of febrile and afebrile convulsions in children in Japan. Neurology 34: 175–181
67. van Esch A, Ramla IR, van Steensel-Moll HA, et al. (1996) Outcome after febrile status epilepticus. Dev Med Child Neurol 38: 19–24
68. van Stuijvenberg M, Jansen ME, Steyerberg EW, et al. (1999) Frequency of fever episodes related to febrile seizure recurrence. Acta Paediatr 88: 52–55
69. van Zeijl JH, Mullaart RA, Galama JMD (2002) The pathogenesis of febrile seizures: is there a role for specific infections. Rev Med Virol 12: 93–106
70. van Zejl JH, Mullaart RA, Born GF, Galama JMD (2004) Recurrence of febrile seizures in the respiratory season is associated with influenza A. J Pediatr 145: 800–805

7

71. Verity CM, Butler NR, Goulding J (1985) Febrile convulsions in a national cohort followed up from birth. I. Prevalence and recurrence in the first five years of life. Br Med J 290: 1307–1310
72. Verity CM, Golding J (1991) Risk of epilepsy after febrile convulsions: a national cohort study. Br Med J 303: 1373–1376
73. Wallace SJ (2004) Febrile seizures. In Wallace SJ, Farrell K (eds) Epilepsy in children Arnold, London, pp. 123–130
74. Yoshikawa H, Abe T (2004) Febrile convulsion during the acute phase of Kawasaki disease. Pediatr Int 46: 31–32
75. Zerr DM, Blume HK, Berg AT (2005) Nonfebrile illness seizures: a unique seizure category? Epilepsia 46: 952–955
76. Zhao F, Lavine L, Wang Z, Cheng X, Li S, Emoto S, Bolis CL, Schoenberg BS (1987) Prevalence and incidence of febrile seizures (FBS) in China. Neurology 37 (Suppl 1): 149

Hypothermia

Core Messages

› In pediatrics, most cases of hypothermia occur neonatally, particularly in the immediate period after birth

› At birth, the delivery room should be warm. The baby is dried and placed in direct skin-to-skin contact with the mother to prevent hypothermia and facilitate breast feeding

› Hypothermia in a child who was previously normo-thermic is suggestive of an underlying infection

› Antibiotics should be given to all children with unexplained hypothermia prior to laboratory proof of infection except those with mild early-onset hypothermia

› In older children, drowning is one of the leading causes of death. Determining accurately the body temperature (rectal or tympanic site) has important clinical implications

› Hypothermia has potential therapeutic use as neuroprotective agent in newborn infants with hypoxic ischemic encephalopathy

Hypothermia is defined as a core body temperature (pulmonary, esophageal, rectal, tympanic) of less than 35°C, resulting from increased heat loss or decreased heat production. This temperature is more than two standard deviations below the mean core temperature. In pediatric practice, most cases of hypothermia occur during the neonatal period.

A.S. El-Radhi et al. (Eds.) *Clinical Manual of Fever in Children.*
Doi: 10.1007/978-3-540-78598-9, © Springer-Verlag Berlin Heidelberg 2009

8

8.1
Neonatal Hypothermia

8.1.1
Physiological Considerations

An optimal thermal environment during the first few days of life is associated with an increased survival rate of neonates, particularly among preterm infants. Such an environment is known as "neutral thermal environment" (NTE), defined as a thermal condition in which the metabolic rate of a resting subject (as evidenced by oxygen consumption) is minimal. NTE is also defined as "the ambient temperature at which the rectal temperature of the infant at rest is between 36.7 and 37.3°C." This thermal environment exerts minimal demands on the infant's limited thermoregulatory and metabolic capabilities, so that available energy can be utilized for immune response and growth. Examples of neutral thermal environmental temperatures are shown in Table 8.1.

During gestation, the body temperature of the fetus at about 38°C is on average 0.5°C above the maternal core temperature. In the first few minutes after birth, a fall in body temperature subsequent to heat loss occurs through:

* **Radiation** (heat transfer from the infant's warm skin to cooler surrounding walls).
* **Conduction** (heat transfer to cooler surfaces in contact with the infant's skin).
* **Evaporation** (passive transcutaneous evaporation of water from the infant's skin, which depends primarily on air velocity, environmental temperature, and relative humidity).
* **Convection** (heat loss from the infant's skin to moving air, which depends on air velocity and environmental temperature).

Factors responsible for the increased heat loss are:

Table 8.1 Example of neutral thermal environment temperature ranges in infants weighing <2,500 g (low birth weight) and >2.500

Age (h)	Weight (g)	Temperature range (°C)
0–6	1,500–2,500	32.8–33.8
	>2,500	32.0–33.8
6–12	1,500–2,500	32.2–33.8
	>2,500	31.4–33.8
24–36	1,500–2,500	31.6–33.6
	>2,500	30.7–33.5
36–48	1,500–2,500	31.4–33.5
	>2,500	30.5–33.3
72–96	1,500–2,500	31.1–33.2
	>2,500	29.8–32.8
>96	1,500–2,500	31.0–33.2
	>2,500	29.5–32.0

* Large surface area in relation to body mass. The body mass of an infant is about 5% of that of an adult, while his or her surface area is about 15% of that of an adult. The infant's heat loss is 3–4 times that of an adult.
* Damp skin of the newly born neonate.
* Low subcutaneous fat. Fat insulates against heat loss because of its low thermal conductivity. Vernix caseosa (the white cheesy material coating the skin of neonates) also offers some protection against heat loss.
* Low ambient temperature. In most delivery rooms, the temperature is 22–25°C, resulting in a continuing fall in body temperature at a rate of 0.1–0.3°C min^{-1} unless measures are taken to prevent it.

Table 8.2 lists the main risk factors predisposing to hypothermia in children.
Means to counteract hypothermia and produce heat are:

* **Nonshivering thermogenesis** is an increase in the metabolic rate without shivering, which begins as early as 15 min after birth. The site of nonshivering thermogenesis is brown adipose tissue, which is found predominately in the interscapular area, axillae, perirenal area, and around the large vessels in the chest. These areas feel warmer to the touch. Gradually, the brown adipose tissue is replaced by white adipose tissue as shivering becomes the predominant mode of heat production. In contrast to white adipose tissue, the brown tissue is rich in blood and nerve supply, with high mitochondrial content and high metabolic activity, consuming 20 times more oxygen than white adipose tissue. During cold stress, there is increased lipolysis, induced by noradrenaline. Most of the released free fatty acids (FFA) are re-esterfied or oxidized and both of these reactions produce heat. Although shivering, as seen in adults, does not occur in the newborn infant, muscular activity and restlessness in response to cold have been reported [1].
* **Postprandial thermogenesis** is an increase in metabolic rate (range 12–26%) after feeding to meet the metabolic demand of ingestion and absorption. Following feeding of neonates with room temperature formula, their body temperatures usually fall, particularly in preterm infants. This fall in body temperature triggers a metabolic response, which is greater when neonates are fed by cold milk bottles.

Table 8.2 Summary of risk factors leading to cold stress

Neonatal	
At birth	Cold delivery room, delay in drying the baby and placing in contact with mother hypnotic-sedatives used for the mother
Weight	Small-for-date
Gestation	Preterm
Condition	Asphyxia, infection, cerebral hemorrhage
Older Children	
Swimming pool	At home and unfenced
Immunity	Compromised, e.g., chemotherapy
Tropical	Malnutrition
Labor findings	Hypoglycemia

8

- The infant's response to cold, though not fully developed, is still active. Although debatable whether a newborn infant, particularly the premature, responds to a cold environment as a temporary poikilotherm (no metabolic increase) or as an inefficient homeotherm (weak metabolic response), studies have confirmed that newborn infants, including large preterms, are potentially homeotherms [2, 3]. They are capable of vaso-constrictive response, which is followed by vasodilatation during rewarming. High ambient temperatures produce sweating. However, smaller premature infants behave as poikilotherms, requiring an intervention to maintain body temperature.

Other factors interfering with normal thermoregulation include infection, hypoxia, hypercarbia, hypotension and the child's nutritional state.

8.1.2
Early-Onset Hypothermia

This hypothermia occurring during the first three days of life is common due to large surface areas and minimal fat layers. Neonates thus have a limited thermogenic response to cool surroundings. Body temperature is usually mildly low (rectal temperature 34–35°C). At particular risk are:

- Neonate who are left unattended at birth even for a few minutes or who have not received adequate warmth during resuscitation.
- Preterm infants, those with asphyxia, CNS hemorrhage or brain malformation or those receiving infusion of cold blood for exchange transfusion. Infection is infrequent cause of early hypothermia.

The prognosis of early-onset hypothermia is generally good because it is primarily caused by exposure to environmental cooling. In developing countries, infection and mortality may occur. In one study, three out of 27 children infants aged 1–3 days (11%) showed evidence of infection and one died [4,5] (Table 8.3).

8.1.3
Late-Onset Hypothermia

Hypothermia in older neonates (four-28 days) is less common than the early-onset hypothermia, mainly because a metabolic response to maintain body temperature becomes effective from the second or third day of life. In many developing countries, late-onset hypothermia, often with classic cold injury, is common enough to be an important cause of neonatal death during winter months in developing countries. Infection and malnutrition, rather than exposure to cold, are the most causes of this late hypothermia. Severe infection can be overwhelming and lead to a breakdown of the normal physiological response to cold. Therefore, hypothermia in a child who had been previously normo-thermic is suggestive of an underlying infection. Common bacterial infections causing hypothermia are shown in Table 8.4. Hypothermia may lead to aspiration because lethargy causes swallowing reflexes to be more impaired than suckling reflexes.

Table 8.3 Details of 138 children with neonatal hypothermia [4]

Age (days)	No		Weight (kg)		Temperature		Mortality
	Boys	Girls	<2.5	>2.5	Mean	Range	
1–3	17	10	15	12	32.4	30.0–34.8	1
4–7	18	11	17	12	31.7	22.0–34.6	8
8–14	21	19	26	14	32.0	22.7–34.7	11
15–21	11	8	10	9	33.3	32.0–34.8	6
22–28	15	8	10	9	30.7	23.0–34.0	9

Table 8.4 The rate of bacterial infections and complication in 138 children with neonatal hypothermia [5]

Site of infection/complication	No	%
Urinary tract infection	30	22
Meningitis	19	14
Septicemia	30	22
Pneumonia	64	46
Osteomyelitis	2	1
Pneumothorax	16	12
Total No with infection/complication	83	60

Physical signs to detect infections are unreliable and therefore the following investigations should be carried out:

* A chest X-ray to demonstrate the pneumonia
* LP is required to confirm or exclude meningitis
* Serum bilirubin as hypothermia interferes with the ability of albumin to bind bilirubin, thus increasing the risk of kernicterus
* Blood and urine cultures

Table 8.5 lists the main symptoms and signs in hypothermic children. Hypoglycemia is common and may occur in about half of affected children.

Because of the high incidence of infection and its unreliable symptoms and signs of infection, appropriate antibiotics should be initiated at the outset to all these children with late-onset hypothermia, without waiting for laboratory proof of infection. The overall mortality rate in infants in developing countries is high. Death may occur subsequent to massive pulmonary hemorrhage due to coagulopathy or cardiac arrhythmia.

8.1.4
Cold Injury

The syndrome is characterized by hypothermia in association with the symptoms listed in Table 8.5. Cold injury was first described in 1889 by Henoch as a case of "edema in

Table 8.5 Symptoms and signs of neonatal hypothermia and cold injury

Neonatal hypothermia	
General	Refusal to feed, lethargy
Pulmonary	Shallow and slow respiration, grunting, crepitations on auscultation
Body temperature	<35°C
Skin	Feels cold to touch
Neonatal Cold injury	
General	Refusal to feed, marked lethargy, feeble or no cry
Pulmonary	As above, in addition pulmonary hemorrhage
Body temperature	Usually <32°C
Skin	Red face, hands, and feet giving a false impression of well-being, swelling of the soft tissue, pitting edema, localized hardening (sclerema)
Intestinal	Vomiting, diarrhea
Renal	Oliguria
CNS	Seizures
Blood	Hemorrhagic diathesis
Laboratory findings	Hypoglycemia, coagulopathy, thrombocytopenia, hyperkalaemia, high creatinine

the newborn." In 1957, Mann and Elliot described the full clinical picture of classic cold injury in 14 cases [6]. Body temperature ranged between 27 and 32°C, and hypoglycemia was often present. The most important causative factor reported from developed countries has been cold stress (rather than infection) caused by low environmental temperature during cold winter months. Repeated and lengthy exposures to cold were usually required to produce the syndrome. Neonates were predominately affected. The prognosis of children with cold injury is generally worse than that in children with similar body temperature but without cold injury. Mortality used to be high, ranging between 25 and 60%. Eight out of the 14 children described in this study died. Postmortem findings include pulmonary hemorrhage and pneumonia.

8.1.5
Management of Neonatal Hypothermia

Prevention

Hypothermia can be prevented by:

* Ensuring that the delivery room is warm: 25–28°C (77–82°F)
* Drying and wrapping the baby immediately after birth, using a warm blanket or synthetic insulating material, such as an aluminized polyester sheath. Simple drying and wrapping the baby reduce the post-delivery heat loss by more than 50%

- Placing the baby in direct skin-to-skin contact with the mother (as an alternative to wrapping) and covering the baby and mother together. This is particularly important in developing countries where supervision by nursing staff and temperature in the delivery room are often inadequate
- Putting a warm cap on the baby's head
- Facilitating breast feeding, which prevents hypothermia because of the close body contact with the mother

For babies who are at particular risk of hypothermia (sick or preterm infants), additional measures include:

- Placing the baby in an incubator at a thermo-neutral temperature. Plastic heat shields, double-walled incubators, and adequate humidity (around 65%) reduce water loss in low-birth-weight infants. Servo-controlled incubators maintain the surface temperature of neonates at a predetermined level by varying the input of a radiant heat. For naked infants, this is achieved by adjusting incubator heating to maintain an abdominal skin temperature of approximately 36.5°C.
- The main risk of the servo-controlled device is hyperthermia, which may occur if the probe becomes detached from the infant's skin. They can also mask hypothermia or fever.
- The use of radiant warmers is required if resuscitation or anesthetic procedure is anticipated. A plastic blanket placed over the baby further reduces evaporative heat loss.
- Routine nursing procedures (temperature measurement, nappy change, changing the probe sites, heel pricking) should be minimized. Whenever possible these should be performed through the portholes of the incubator.

In many developing countries, incubators may not be available. Measures to prevent hypothermia may be achieved in simpler ways by:

- Using electric heaters to produce an environmental temperature of 29°C and even higher for the smallest babies
- Maintaining close physical contact with the mother
- Warming the cot by radiant heat or hot-water bottles, day and night
- Remembering that lethargy and poor feeding in a baby who feels cold on touch are the earliest manifestations of hypothermia. Mothers should be alerted to these signals and taught to seek medical help early.

Treatment

Treatment is focused on the following three measures:

1. *Rewarming*, either gradually over an extended period, starting with an ambient temperature of about 20°C and increasing by 1°C every 3 h for infants with chronic cold exposure, or rapidly over a few hours, at a rate of 1–2°C h^{-1}. Rapid rewarming is associated with fewer complications and higher survival rates. Rewarming can be accomplished in an incubator (using the maximum air temperature setting), under a radiant heat source in a warm cubicle or using a heated water-filled mattress. The latter two heat sources

help hypothermic neonates achieve normo-thermia more rapidly than those treated in incubator.

Neonates should be monitored by measuring oxygen saturation, blood gases, blood glucose, clotting factors, and body temperature.

2. *Feeding by nasogastric tube* to avoid the risk of aspiration pneumonia. Milk, preferably breast milk, should be warmed to body temperature of about 36°C. An i.v. fluid containing 10% glucose is indicated not only to correct but also to prevent hypoglycemia, which is arising from an increase in metabolic demand during the rewarming.
3. *Treatment with antibiotics.* An infection should be suspected in any child with unexplained hypothermia. Those with mild early-onset hypothermia do not usually require antibiotic treatment.

8.2
Hypothermia in Older Children

In contrast to newborn infants, who rely on nonshivering thermogenesis to produce heat, older children utilize both metabolic activity and shivering to generate sufficient heat to maintain body temperature. The body temperature can be viewed as a core surrounded by skeletal muscles. At rest, the muscles provide relatively little heat, but when the core temperature falls below 36°C, shivering generates considerable heat energy. Skeletal muscles are surrounded by thermoreceptors; these serve as an important regulator of heat exchange. Figure 8.1 shows the basic mechanisms of heat production in response to cold. Table 8.6 lists the main causes of hypothermia in this age group.

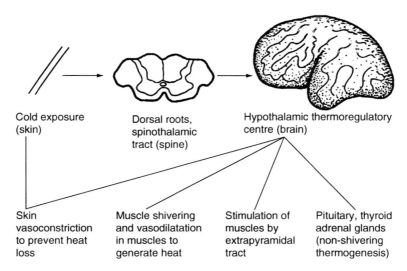

Cold exposure (skin)	Dorsal roots, spinothalamic tract (spine)	Hypothalamic thermoregulatory centre (brain)	
Skin vasoconstriction to prevent heat loss	Muscle shivering and vasodilatation in muscles to generate heat	Stimulation of muscles by extrapyramidal tract	Pituitary, thyroid adrenal glands (non-shivering thermogenesis)

Fig. 8.1 Basic mechanisms of heat production in response to cold

• Accidental
Cold water immersion   Environmental exposure
• Spontaneous
Spontaneous periodic hypothermia   Shapiro's syndrome
• Infection
• Metabolic
• Drug-induced
• CNS-lesions
• Malnutrition
• Therapeutic use

• Induced-hypothermia for surgery
  • Treatment of hypermetabolic state
  • Hypoxic-ischemic encephalopathy

Table 8.6 Main causes and uses of hypothermia

8.2.1
Accidental Hypothermia

Accidental hypothermia is defined as a decrease in core temperature usually in a cold environment, causing an acute clinical problem, which is not caused by failure of the hypothalamic thermoregulatory centre. The most common cause of accidental hypothermia in children is immersion.

Immersion or drowning. Drowning is defined as death by suffocation after immersion in a liquid. In near-drowning the individual survives, at least temporarily. In the USA, where there are 8,000 deaths per year, drowning is the second most common cause of accidental death (after road traffic accidents) and the third leading cause (after road traffic accidents and cancer) of all deaths in children aged 1–14 years (8.4% of all deaths). In Britain, with 700 deaths per year from immersion, drowning is the third leading cause of death (after road traffic accidents and cancer) in children.7

In children, inhalation following immersion is less common than in adults, hence there is a higher survival rate in children than in adults. The lesser degree of inhalation is due to the effect of the diving reflex, which inhibits water aspiration when the face is stimulated by cold water. Immersion causes the following complications:

- **Inhalation of fresh water**, owing to its hypotonicity, causes hemodilution (from absorption of water into the intravascular space), hemolysis and hyponatremia. In contrast, inhalation of salt water, which has an osmolality more than three times that of body fluid, causes withdrawal of water from capillaries and results in hemoconcentration and hypernatremia but no hemolysis.
- **Aspiration** causes pulmonary edema, pneumonia, and pneumothorax.
- **Hypothermia** occurs more rapidly in a child than in an adult because of the child's relatively large surface area to body mass ratio and decreased insulation by fat. Hypothermia causes

Table 8.7 Clinical signs of hypothermic victims in relation to body temperature

Core temperature	Physiology	Signs
35–32	BMR increase	Lethargy, shivering, tachycardia
	Vasoconstriction	Cyanosis, slow respiration
	ADH increase	Diuresis
32–30	BMR decrease	Absent shivering
	Cerebral blood flow decrease	Impaired consciousness, confusion, delirium
	Acidosis or alkalosis	Muscle tone increase, rigidity
30–27	BMR decreases to 50%	Respiration: slow and shallow, skin erythema, edema
	Loss of thermo-regulation	cardiac arrhymia
	Vasodilatation	Loss of consciousness, arrhythmia & conduction defects
<27	Cessation of cardiac functions	Apnoea, asystole, imminent death, from ventricular fibrillation

BMR basal metabolic rate, *ADH* antidiuretic hormone

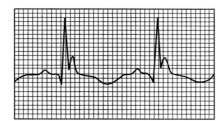

Fig. 8.2 ECG sign in Hypothermia

a decrease in oxygen consumption and metabolic rate. Metabolic processes decrease by about 6% for each 1°C reduction in body temperature, leading to lower oxygen demand. This contributes to the relatively high survival rate of victims.

Table 8.7 lists the main manifestations seen in hypothermic patients in relation to the fall in body temperature. At a core temperature of:

- 35–30°C, compensatory mechanisms are initiated to restore homeostasis.
- <30°C, thermoregulation begins to fail. Unconsciousness and cardiac arrhythmias usually occur. Therefore if a child is conscious he or she is unlikely to have severe hypothermia. ECG abnormalities include bradycardia, prolonged P-R and QT intervals and widening QRS complex with characteristic dome configuration (Osborn waves) at the R-ST junction (Fig 8.2). Atrial and ventricular fibrillations are common.
- <27°C, many hypothermic victims appear dead with asystole and ventricular fibrillation. Other complications include cold diuresis, due to increased antidiuretic hormone

(ADH) activity, acute tubular necrosis, hypotension (after an initial rise in blood pressure), sepsis, rhabdomyolysis, thrombocytopenia, and cerebral edema. Metabolic acidosis and pancreatitis may accompany the severe hypothermic state. Hypoglycemia is a common finding; hyperglycemia may also occur.

Hypothermia victims may respond to resuscitative measures despite the presence of asystole and other complications. Survival and normal cerebral function may occur even with hypoxia for up to 60 min or longer at a body temperature 20°C.

Table 8.8 lists the main investigations for near-drowning victims with moderate to severe hypothermia. The prognosis is related to the duration and the degree of hypothermia. Treatment of hypothermia is discussed at the end of the chapter.

8.2.2
Spontaneous Hypothermia

Spontaneous hypothermia is very rare in children. It is characterized by episodes of hypothermia in individuals who are otherwise well. Shivering may occur at a body temperature of 33.0°C (shivering usually commences in normal people at a body temperature of 36.0°C). Prodromal sweating is found in most cases. No cause has been identified and CT-scan does not usually detect any CNS abnormalities.

Spontaneous hypothermia can occur periodically. Several cases of spontaneous hypothermia have been associated with agenesis of the corpus callosum (Shapiro's syndrome), which generally has a benign, nonprogressive clinical course. There are no associated hypothalamic or CNS lesions [8].

The prognosis of spontaneous hypothermia is good. Management includes adequate insulation to prevent heat loss, particularly during cold exposure.

Table 8.8 Suggested laboratory investigations for patients with moderate to severe hypothermia

Blood investigations	Other investigations
Full blood count	Chest X-ray
Calcium	Abdomen X-ray
Liver function test	Continuous monitoring of ECG
Prothrombin time, fibrinogen	Pulse oximetry[a]

Monitoring of
  Glucose
  Creatinine and urea
  Amylase
  Electrolytes
  Arterial blood gases[b]	

[a] Measurement of oxygen saturation may be inaccurate due to poor perfusion

[b] Arterial blood gases must be corrected for patient's temperature

8

8.2.3
Infection

Exposure to cold adversely affects host defense by suppressing the immune response against the infection. In vitro studies have demonstrated decreased WBC motility, diminished phago-cytosis, and decreased antibody formation at reduced temperature. Animals rendered hypothermic by exposure to cold had decreased survival after challenge with *Salmonella typhimurium* and *Staphylococcus aureus* [9]. Although hypothermia depresses the growth of most pathogenic bacteria, suggesting an apparent beneficial effect during infection, such an effect is usually insignificant compared to the detrimental effect of hypothermia on host defense mechanisms. The rate of mortality due to infection is significantly higher in patients with hypothermia than in febrile or euthermic patients: 71% vs. 37%, respectively, in one study [10].

Infection is a frequent cause of hypothermia in older children and adults, accounting for around 40% of cases in one study [11]. Acute and severe infection, such as pneumonia, septicemia, or meningitis, can cause thermoregulatory failure. Therefore, if a child presents with unexplained hypothermia, investigation should always include a blood culture and a chest X-ray to exclude septicemia or pneumonia. Immunosuppression and malnutrition are significant risk factors for hypothermia during infection.

8.2.4
Drug-Induced Hypothermia

Drugs, principally sedative-hypnotics, may induce hypothermia by counteracting the mechanisms responsible for maintaining the body temperature. Possible actions of these drugs include the following:

- Impairment of the metabolic response needed for non-shivering thermogenesis of the newborn infant
- Depression of the hypothalamic thermoregulatory center
- Interference with the mechanisms for shivering and vasoconstriction. Ethanol predis-poses to hypothermia by being a vasodilator, CNS depressant, a cause of hypoglycemia (see Metabolic causes below), and by increasing the risk of accidents

Drugs capable of causing hypothermia include the following:

- Diazepam administered to mothers in labor may cause apnoeic spells, hypotonia, low Apgar scores, and impaired metabolic response to cold in the newborn infants. A total maternal dose in excess of 30 mg in the 15 h before delivery is capable of producing these adverse effects.
- Chemotherapy for Hodgkin's disease may occasionally cause hypothermia, particularly in patients who were febrile prior to chemotherapy.
- Salicylates or paracetamol administered concomitantly with chemotherapy may increase the risk of hypothermia. The antipyretic ibuprofen has been reported to cause hypothermia in therapeutic doses.
- Other drugs that produce hypothermia include chlorpromazine, hexamethonium, and barbiturate.

8.2.5
CNS Lesions

Occasionally, lesions in the vicinity of the hypothalamus, such as tumor, hemorrhage, or sarcoidosis, may interfere with thermoregulatory mechanisms and produce hypothermia. The occurrence of hypothermia in cases of tumor and hemorrhage is usually terminal.

8.2.6
Metabolic Causes

Patients with hypothyroidism are at increased risk of hypothermia due to decreased metabolic rate. Hypothermia may be the sole manifestation of myxoedema coma. Rarely, hypoglycemia may present as hypothermia as the only manifestation [12]. Correction of the hypoglycemia often increases body temperature. Other metabolic causes include hypopituitarism and hypoadrenalism.

8.2.7
Hypothermia in Malnourished Children (Tropical Hypothermia)

Hypothermia may occur as early as a few weeks of age secondary to malnutrition. Typically the child fails to regain the weight lost during the first few days of life (physiological weight loss). Brown adipose tissue is found to be depleted, which explains why these children show a poor response to cold. Hypothermia is more frequent in marasmus than in kwashiorkor, possibly because of the insulating properties of edema, which may protect against hypothermia. The condition is mainly seen in developing countries

Hypothermia has also been reported in older malnourished children in the tropics. Hypoglycemia and serum electrolyte abnormalities were common and pancreatic necrosis was found in nine out of 19 children examined at autopsy [13]. Reduced subcutaneous fat, which normally serves as an insulating layer against heat loss, is the main predisposing factor to hypothermia.

8.2.8
Management of Hypothermia

Management varies with the nature and severity of hypothermia. Because specific therapy depends upon accurate measurement of core temperature, low-recording thermometers should be available in any emergency setting dealing with hypothermic victims. Management consists primarily of urgent rewarming of the body core. Rewarming may be withheld if supportive measures are unavailable (for example, during transport) to maintain the hypothermic protection. Methods used for rewarming of patients with mild, moderate, and severe hypothermia are summarized in the Table 8.9.

Table 8.9 Methods used for re-warming in patients with mild (using passive re-warming) to severe hypothermia (using in addition active external and core temperature re-warming)

Passive	Warm room, dry blanket, drinking warm fluids, vigorous passive, and active muscle movement
Active external	Warmed blanket, pads, radiant warmer, immersion in hot bath, hot, humidified oxygen at 35–40°C
Core	Warm IV fluids, heated and humidified oxygen, warmed gastric and colonic lavage

- For patients with mild hypothermia (body temperature 33–35°C), simple measures to raise body temperature are sufficient, including transport of the victim to a warm place, removal of wet clothes, covering with a blanket or sleeping bag, drinking warm fluids, and passive as well as active exercise. For the apnoeic immersion victim, once taken from the water, immediate resuscitative measures include clearing water and debris from the airway and application of cardio-pulmonary resuscitation (CPR). Postural drainage of inhaled water is only useful for seawater immersion. With freshwater immersion, the water has moved rapidly from the lung into the vascular system.
- For patients with moderate hypothermia (body temperature 30–33°C), active external warming procedures are required, (in addition to the measures used for mild hypothermia), such as immersion of the trunk in a warm bath at an initial temperature of 30°C and increasing to around 40°C over the next few minutes. If available, inhaled, moisturized air or oxygen warmed at 35–40°C may also be used. Any near-drowning victim with moderate degree hypothermia should be observed in a hospital for a minimum of 1 day because late-onset pulmonary edema may occur as late as 12 h after the accident.
- For children with severe hypothermia (body temperature <30°C), rewarming the core temperature is indicated. One of the best methods for internal rewarming is to make the patient breathe hot, moist air or oxygen. Alternatively, or simultaneously with the above method, submersion in a warm bath aimed at increasing the body temperature slowly (e.g., 0.5–1.0°C h^{-1}) may be used. Additional measures that are essential for survival include the following:

  - Oxygen therapy, 100%, (with or without ventilation). The oxygen flow should be warmed to 35–40°C.
  - Mechanical ventilation as indicated by a rising pCO_2 or a falling pO_2.
  - Fluid and electrolytes therapy aimed at correcting the electrolyte abnormalities, the metabolic acidosis (resulting from carbon dioxide retention and lactic acid accumulation), and associated hypotension. Many victims have hypovolemia, and volume expansion (0.9% sodium chloride, warmed to about 40°C) is essential. Correction of metabolic acidosis with sodium bicarbonate may not be necessary because alkalosis often ensues during rewarming.
  - Intravenous mannitol infusion (1 g kg^{-1} per dose as 20% solution over 30–60 min) for cerebral and pulmonary edema. Overhydration should be avoided. Diuretics and dexamethasone may be helpful.

- Antibiotics are indicated if there is evidence of infection. Infection is unlikely if the hypothermia is due to immersion in clean water.
- Treatment of cardiac arrhythmias according to the nature of the ECG abnormalities. Most, including atrial flutter and fibrillation, disappear spontaneously as the temperature rises. Serious cardiac arrhythmia, such as ventricular fibrillation, requires electrical defibrillation and additional CPR. Although CPR may precipitate ventricular fibrillation (VF), CPR is indicated if the patients have asystole and/or an ECG showing absent QRS-activity. The pulse of a patient with severe hypothermia may not be felt, simulating cardiac arrest and thereby falsely indicating cardiac arrest and the need for external compression. ECG monitoring is therefore vital.

Severe hypothermia may precipitate ventricular fibrillation, which is the most common cause of death. Minimal handling is important to avoid such a risk. Vigorous rewarming also carries the risk of ventricular fibrillation as well as rewarming shock secondary to circulatory insufficiency, which existed during hypothermia, and the additional metabolic burden of rewarming.

8.3
Therapeutic Use of Hypothermia

Perinatal asphyxia or **hypoxic ischemic encephalopathy** (HIE) is responsible for significant disability and death worldwide. Of the 4 million annual worldwide neonatal deaths, 23% are caused by HIE [14]. In the UK, HIE causes death and severe neurodisability in 1–2 per 1,000 term infants [15]. The current management for infants with HIE is supportive, with oxygenation, stabilization of physiologic parameters, and treatment of seizures.

Animal studies and clinical trials have demonstrated that a reduction in temperature of about 3°C (whole body or selective head cooling) applied soon after the onset of HIE was neuroprotective and reduced death and disability rates [16]. Protection was seen largely in infants with a less severe insult. There were no clinically important complications associated with cooling. A recent review analyzing trials of therapeutic cooling for infants with HIE suggested that further data are still needed before cooling becomes the standard treatment for babies with HIE [17].

The exact mechanism of such neuroprotection is still unclear. Table 8.10 lists the likely effects of therapeutic hypothermia following cerebral insult. Hypothermia is associated with a decrease in oxygen demand and an increase in arterial oxygen content, allowing the brain to tolerate circulatory arrest for about 10 min without sustaining damage. The increase in arterial oxygen content is due to a shift of the hemoglobin dissociation curve to the left.

Therapeutic hypothermia obviously contradicts the principles of supportive care for any asphyxiated newborn infant, which include maintaining body temperature at 36.7–37.3°C and the provision of warm humidified oxygen. Prompt and vigorous resuscitation (e.g., intratracheal intubation and ventilation) is presently the most effective method of treating

Table 8.10 Main effects of mild therapeutic hypothermia of about 33°C in HIE

Reduction	Increase
Excitatory neurotransmitters	IL-10 (anti-inflammatory cytokine)
Blood-brain barrier damage	Blood pressure
Cerebral metabolism (O_2 and glucose)	Heart rate
Loss of high energy phosphates	
Secondary cerebral energy failure	
Apoptosis	
Cardiac output	
Platelet function	

HIE-Hypoxic ischaemic encephalopathy

a severely asphyxiated child. However, the application of the therapeutic hypothermia should proceed while other supportive measures are simultaneously given.

Hypothermia has also been proposed as a **treatment for critically ill**, highly febrile patients who have a body temperature >40.0°C. In a study examining this idea by lowering the body temperature to a level of 35–36°C, three of the 13 patients survived, whereas there were no survivors among control group [18]. In another report, cooling was apparently successfully used in the treatment of a child with meningococcal meningitis who was otherwise expected to die [19].

Surgery remains the main indication for therapeutic hypothermia. In cardiac surgery, induction of moderate hypothermia (about 28°C) enables operations (e.g., atrial septal defect) to be carried out on the heart with circulation safely arrested for up to 19 min. At a temperature of 18°C, circulation can be safely arrested for 45 min to repair more complex heart lesions, such as a total anomalous pulmonary venous connection in neonates. In vascular surgery it is used for resection of aneurysms (aortic aneurysm). Neurosurgery also utilizes hypothermia to deal with some intracranial vascular catastrophes, such as a ruptured aneurysm. Unfortunately, cardiac surgery is associated with considerable post-operative morbidity and mortality, including seizures, choreoathetosis, neurodisability, and acute renal failure

Hypothermia has been used to treat patients with cancer. The first attempt to treat malignant tumors by hypothermia was undertaken in 1849 [20]. Systemic or local cooling was applied during 1936–1940 in Philadelphia for therapeutic purposes. The basic observation that stimulated the use of hypothermia to treat patients with cancer was that segments of the body (e.g., extremities) with a relatively low surface temperature of 34.4°C rarely harbor metastasis.

Methods used for induction of cooling include packing the body in ice, use of a refrigerating machine, immersion in cold water, or directing a steam of cold air over the body surface, all aimed at reducing the body temperature to 31–32°C. Lowering the body temperature by drugs (artificial hibernation) also has been achieved by slow intravenous administration of a mixture containing chlorpromazine, promethazine, and meperidine (1:1:2).

References

Neonatal Hypothermia

1. Berg K, Celander O. Circulatory adaptation in the thermoregulation of fullterms and premature newborn infants. Acta Pediatr Scand 1971; 60: 278–84
2. Hill JR, Rahimtulla KA. Heat balance and the metabolic rate of newborn babies in relation to environmental temperature and the effect of age and of weight on basal metabolic rate. J Physiol 1965; 180: 239–65
3. Bell EF, Gray GC, Weinstein MR, et al. The effects of thermal environment on heat balance and insensible water loss in low-birth infants. J Pediatr 1980; 96: 452–9
4. El-Radhi AS, Jawad MH, Mansor N, et al. Sepsis and hypothermia in the newborn infant: value of gastric aspirate examination. J Pediatr 1983; 103: 300–2
5. Radhi AS, Jawad MH, Mansor N, et al. Infection in neonatal hypothermia. Arch Dis Child 1983; 58: 143–5
6. Mann TP, Elliot RI. Neonatal cold injury due to accidental exposure to cold. Lancet 1957; 1: 229–33

Hypothermia in Older Children

7. Immersion and drowning in children. Br Med J 1977; 3: 146–7
8. Slotki IN, Oelbaum MH. Recurrent spontaneous hypothermia. Postgrad Med J 1980; 56: 656–7
9. Previte JJ, Berry LJ. The effect of environmental temperature on the host-parasite relationship in mice. J Infect Dis 1962; 110: 201–9
10. Dorothy NE, Fung P, Lefkowitz M, et al. Hypothermia and sepsis (Letter). Ann Intern Med 1985; 103: 308
11. Lewin S, Brettman LR, Holzman RS. Infections in hypothermic patients. Arch Intern Med 1981; 141: 920–5
12. Kedes LH, Field JB. Hypothermia: a clue to hypoglycaemia. N Engl J Med 1964; 271: 785–7
13. Sadikali F, Owor R. Hypothermia in the tropics: a review of 24 cases. Trop Geogr Med 1974; 26: 265–70

Therapeutic Use of Hypothermia

14. Lawn JE, Cousens S, Zupan J. 4 million neonatal deaths: when?, where?, why?, Lancet 2005; 365: 891–900
15. Levene MI, Evans DJ, Mason S, et al. An international network for evaluating neuroprotective therapy after severe birth asphyxia. Semin Perinatol 1999; 23: 226–33
16. Gluckman PD, Wyatt JS, Azzopardi DV, et al. Selective head cooling with mild systemic hypothermia after neonatal encephalopathy: multicentre randomised trial. Lancet 2005; 365: 663–70
17. Edwards AD, Azzopardi DV. Therapeutic hypothermia following prenatal asphyxia. Arch Dis Child Fetal Neonatal Ed 2006; 91: F127–131

18. Reeves MM, Lewis FJ. Total body cooling in critically febrile patients. Surgery 1958; 44: 84–90
19. Robinson A, Buckler JMH. Emergency hypothermia in meningococcal meningitis. Lancet 1965; 1: 81–3
20. Zingg W. Historical use of hypothermia for cancer. Can J Surg 1983; 26: 97–8

Is Fever Beneficial?

9

Core Messages

› Fever has a long evolutionary history, which by itself supports the hypothesis that fever is an adaptive host response to infection.
› There is considerable evidence that fever promotes host defense against infection.
› Complications and mortality associated with high fever >40°C are closely related to the severity of the underlying disease, not to the level of fever.
› Fever is effectively controlled by the hypothalamic centre and therefore does not climb up relentlessly. Temperatures >42°C are often caused by hyperthermia, not by fever.
› If the febrile child is comfortable, there is little reason to support the practice of routine use of antipyretic medication.
› Parental education is critical in the management of the febrile child.
› Antipyretics do not prevent febrile seizures.
› There is a conflict between research evidence supporting a positive role of fever and the demands of current practice that fever be abolished.

9.1
Evolutionary Arguments for Fever Being Beneficial

9.1.1
Evolutionary History of Fever

One argument that has been used to support the notion that fever is adaptive is that it has a long evolutionary history [1]. Animals such as lizards, turtles, frogs, fish, crickets, scorpions, and beetles develop fever when infected with bacteria, bacterial products, or other "fever-producing" agents (e.g., prostaglandins or bacterial products such as endotoxin).

A.S. El-Radhi et al. (Eds.) *Clinical Manual of Fever in Children.*
Doi: 10.1007/978-3-540-78598-9, © Springer-Verlag Berlin Heidelberg 2009

How can a "cold-blooded" animal such as a lizard develop a fever? Since a fever is due to an elevation in the thermoregulatory "set-point," the "febrile" lizard seeks out a warmer microclimate, thus raising its core body temperature. The same happens to febrile fish, frogs, beetles, or other cold-blooded animals. Even febrile people rely to a large extent on behavioral means to raise body temperature during the rising phase of fever. A variety of behaviors to raise body temperature, which include curling into a fetal position to conserve heat, crawling under a blanket, or drinking hot liquids.

9.1.2
Metabolic Cost of Fever

Why would the metabolic cost of fever be relevant to supporting the argument that fever is adaptive or beneficial? In endotherms, such as birds and mammals, the maintenance of a body temperature of 2 or 3°C above the afebrile level often results in a rise in energy consumption of 20% or more above baseline. This is the result of the Q_{10} effect of increased temperature on various biochemical reactions. If fever did not have some beneficial role, it is highly unlikely that it would have evolved in the first place, since it is so energetically expensive. And, having evolved, it is highly improbable that it would have persisted throughout the animal kingdom.

9.1.3
Might Fever be a Vestige?

Of course, it is always possible that fever is the "appendix" of host responses to infection; that is a vestigial trait. How commonly does this occur? Are there examples of common responses to infection that are truly vestigial in nature (that is has no function)? As indicated through this book, the rise in body temperature during fever is the result of a highly coordinated series of physiological and behavioral responses (e.g., shivering, peripheral vasoconstriction, drinking warm liquids, wearing warm clothing). This rise in body temperature has a metabolic cost, which is associated ultimately with wasting (unless the individual compensates by taking in additional calories, i.e., eats more). It appears the probability that fever is truly a "neutral" trait (or a vestige) is low.

9.2
Arguments for Fever Being Beneficial (Table 9.1)

9.2.1
Effects of Elevated Temperature on Microorganisms

* Animal studies have demonstrated that the bacterial growth rate in experimental pneumococcal meningitis was significantly reduced at elevated temperatures. Gram-negative bacteria, such as Salmonella typhi, were shown to be increasingly susceptible to the bac-

Table 9.1 Summary of arguments for believing fever to be beneficial

Summary
• Fever has a long evolutionary history and is found throughout the Animal Kingdom.
• Fever is energetically expensive, and probably would not be maintained throughout evolution had it no protective or adaptive value.
• There are numerous studies demonstrating a beneficial role of fever.
• Fevers are self-limiting and rarely reach levels that are dangerous.
• The evidence that antipyretic drugs protects against "febrile seizures" is poor.
• Antipyretic drugs, which reduce fever, may counteract the protective effects of fever.
• The principal beneficial effects of antipyretic drugs are their effects on providing comfort to the febrile child (via their "analgesic" or pain-reducing properties).

tericidal effects of normal serum when cultivated at a temperature greater than $37°C$[2]. The growth of viruses was impaired with increased temperatures. Most viruses ceased to replicate at a temperature between 40 and $42°C$. The replication rate of poliovirus at $37°C$ was 250 times than that at $40°C$ [3].

- Human studies: Ancient physicians such as Hippocrates and Rufus of Ephesus used fever to treat various ailments. Fever was the principal form of treatment for syphilis and gonorrhea for centuries. Insufflation of humidified air at $43°C$ (three 30 min sessions at 2–3 h intervals) into the nasal passages of patients suffering from coryza resulted in the suppression of symptoms in 78% of patients [4]. Fever may also be beneficial in patients with meningitis: the presence of fever greater than $40°C$ did not indicate a poor prognosis, but all children presenting with hypothermia died [5]. A study of 102 children with salmonella gastroenteritis from Finland [6] demonstrated a significant negative correlation between the degree of fever and the duration of excretion of organisms. A fever of greater than $40°C$ had the shortest and those without fever the longest duration of bacterial excretion. Fever has therefore a favorable prognostic influence on the length of bacterial excretion. It is, however, not clear whether the above studies are the result of the direct effect of temperature on the growth of the microorganisms or the effect of elevated temperature on host defense responses.

9.2.2
Effects of Elevated Temperature on Defense Mechanisms

- The mobility, phagocytosis, and killing of bacteria by polymorphonuclear leukocytes are significantly greater at temperatures above $40°C$ [7]. Elevated temperatures of $38–39°C$ have a direct positive effect on lymphocyte transformation, the generation of cytolytic cells, B-cell activity, and immunoglobulin synthesis.
- Interleukin-1 is more active at febrile temperature than at an afebrile temperature [8, 9]. Interferon (INF), a potent antiviral agent, has enhanced antiviral activity above $40°C$ [10, 11]. T-cell proliferative response to interleukin-2 and interleukin-1 was greatly increased at $39°C$ compared to $37°C$.

- Fever may act synergistically with antibiotics. Penicillin was found to have a progressive increase of its bactericidal activity as the temperature was raised from 35 to 41.5°C [12].
- There is evidence that elevated body temperatures in the range of 41–42°C can effect the growth of certain tumors. Occasional remissions of Hodgkin's disease occurred after an attack of measles. The metabolism of many types of cancer cell is selectively damaged at temperatures of 42–43°C [13]. Lysosomal enzymes, IL-2, and INF have increased activity at such temperatures, and contribute to tumor cell destruction.

9.2.3
Effects of Suppression of Fever on Underlying Disease

If fever is beneficial, it might be expected that suppression of fever can have a harmful effect. There is some evidence to support this.

- Probably the earliest demonstration of the protective effect of fever was shown in a study of lizards, *Dipsosaurus dorsalis*, infected with a natural pathogen, *Aeromonas hydrophila* [14]. In that study infected lizards were kept in incubators so as to maintain them at their febrile body temperature of 42°C (high fever), 40°C (moderate fever), at their nonfebrile temperature of 38°C, or maintained at body temperatures below normal (36°C or 34°C). The results were striking. The febrile lizards had survival rates of 75% (those at 42°C), 67% (those at 40°C), and 25% (those at 38°C). The lizards kept at below normal body temperatures had even lower survival rates. In a follow-up study, the antipyretic drug sodium salicylate was administered to bacterially infected lizards. This led to an increase in their mortality only when the antipyretic drugs lowered body temperature. All feverish lizards survived, whereas the nonfeverish lizards died [15].
- In human volunteers infected with rhinovirus, the use of antipyretics was associated with suppression of serum antibody response, increased symptoms and signs, and a trend towards longer duration of viral shedding [16]. In a study of children with chickenpox, half of whom received paracetamol four times a day and half received a placebo; the time to total scabbing was slightly shorter in the placebo group (5.6 days) than in the paracetamol group (6.7 days) [17]. Another study from Japan [18] found that the frequent administration of antipyretics to children with bacterial diseases led to a worsening of their illness.
- Many studies have found that hypothermia may impair various defense mechanisms, including delayed and often depressed activity of leukocytes, decreased phagocytosis, and antibody formation as well as increased susceptibility to viral infection. All animals infected with pneumococci, which were rendered hypothermic (body temperature between 30 and 34°C), died, whereas only five of the 31 control animals infected with the same bacteria at normal-to-low febrile levels died [19]. More influenza virus was shed in the nasal washes of ferrets whose febrile response was suppressed by shaving or by treatment with sodium salicylate compared to untreated ones [20]. In a series of children presenting with severe infection, such as pneumonia or septicaemia, it was found that the lower the body temperature, the higher the mortality [21].

9.2.4
The Hygiene Theory

The prevalence of asthma and allergies as well as cancer has increased worldwide for many years and the hygiene theory has been offered to explain the rise [22, 23]. The theory proposes that early exposure to fevers caused by infections (in particular, infection of the upper airways, hepatitis A, and Helicobacter pylori) might protect children against allergic diseases and cancer in later life. It postulates that atopy, or allergy, is Th-2-driven, which is primarily associated with IL-4, IL-5, IL-10, and IL-13 production, whereas infection is Th-1-driven, which is dominated by production of INF-gamma and IL-12. In association with reduced exposure to infections, Th-2 immunity dominates through critical childhood periods, resulting in higher incidence of atopy.

In support of this theory are the following findings:

* The prevalence of atopy is lower among children of large families or those attending day-care nurseries than among children of small families or those not in nurseries.
* Children with older siblings are less likely to develop allergies than children with younger siblings or none at all.
* Children who experienced several febrile episodes during the first year of life have lower incidence of allergy than those with only one or no febrile episode.
* Children exposed to high levels of endotoxin (a major product from Gram-negative bacteria) show reduced prevalence of atopy.
* The use of antibiotics administered during the first year of life is associated with asthma, hay fever, and eczema later on in life. Antibiotics could destroy the beneficial bacteria (probiotics) in the digestive tract.
* Atopic diseases are rare in countries with parasitic infestation.
* A study from Switzerland [24] showed a significant association between febrile infectious childhood diseases and the risk of developing cancer in adulthood.

Thus, we conclude from these intriguing data that exposure to infectious diseases in early childhood, particularly those that may be associated with modest fevers, may protect the child against a wide array of future diseases.

These arguments in favor of fever being protective are facing arguments against fever being beneficial. The next section will review many of those.

9.3
Arguments for Fever Being Harmful (Table 9.2)

9.3.1
Parents' Attitude and Expectation

As fever frequently accompanies childhood illness, it is commonly perceived by parents and physicians as a harmful part of the illness requiring intervention. Part of the reason for this is that fever is often seen as the direct cause of the illness, rather than as a "host defense" response to the illness. Fever is easy to measure, and furthermore even easier to

Table 9.2 Summary of arguments for believing fever to be harmful

Prevailing concepts, arguments largely untrue
  • Parents' attitude and expectation
  • Wide-spread belief among physicians
  • Associated discomfort
  • Risk of febrile seizure
Situation where fever is likely to be harmful
  • Acute stroke
  • Severe sepsis
  • Limited energy supply or increased metabolic rate
  • Bronchiolitis

"treat." Parents worry when their child is feverish and feel that fever may spiral upwards with a possible fatal outcome. Parents often have unfounded anxiety about the possible risks of fever and little or no information about its beneficial role in diseases, and as a result they are convinced that antipyretic measures must be used to lower fever.

Fever phobia, an exaggerated fear of fever in their children, is common among parents of all socio-economic classes. In one study [25], parents began antipyretic medication when their child's temperature was equal or even less than 37.8°C. One of the reasons that parents probably give their children antipyretic medication is not so much because it lowers body temperature (which, of course, it does), but because these drugs are also analgesics. So by giving their children the "antipyretic" medication the child soon feels better. The parent is then relieved that the lowered fever is the cause of the improvement in her/his child. But, this is most likely simply due to the reduction in pain and discomfort caused by the medication.

9.3.2
Prevailing Concepts Among Physicians

Most pediatricians agree that treatment of a febrile child with antipyretics is mostly for the relief of the symptoms of fever. However, many tend to prescribe antipyretics for any child with fever on the basis that antipyretics could prevent its complications. In a study [26] exploring the beliefs and practices of pediatricians in Massachusetts, USA, the majority (65%) of respondent believed that fever itself could be dangerous to a child, with seizures, death, and brain damage being the most serious complications of fever if the temperature is 40°C or greater. Pediatricians may be contributing to fever phobia by prescribing antipyretics for children who are only mildly febrile. As we will describe in a later section (9.4.3) this belief is unfounded.

9.3.3
Associated Discomfort

Children with fever often experience discomfort, headaches and myalgia as a result of cytokine-mediated production of prostaglandins. These symptoms occur during the phase of rising fever, causing reduced activity to the children and thus cause anxiety to their parents. As mentioned above, antipyretics, by also being analgesics, lead to an improvement in the children's level of activity and alertness. When children feel better, an assumption usually emerges that the severity of the disease has been reduced. The elimination of these symptoms (discomfort, pain and aches) is perhaps the main reason why antipyretics have maintained their popularity among parents and have continued in use for over a century.

9.3.4
Risk of Febrile Seizure

In a study [26] from the USA, 49% of pediatricians considered convulsions to be a principal danger of fever and 22% believed that brain damage could result from typical febrile seizure (FS). Early literature [27] reported a mortality rate of 11% in children with FS.

As fever is generally considered to be an essential precursor of a febrile seizure, medical professionals have concluded that antipyretic measures should prevent febrile seizures. Antipyretics continue to be among the most commonly prescribed medications, especially for children at risk of such seizures. Parents are usually advised that the administration of antipyretics to child at risk may reduce the risk of further convulsions. However, as reviewed by Rosman [28], antipyretic therapy has never been shown to prevent febrile seizures. There is now abundant evidence indicating that antipyretics have no effect on preventing further FS. Children with high risk of recurrences of FS (see Chap. 7) develop recurrences in 70–80% while those without these risk factors rarely develop recurrences. Antipyretics are used for both groups of children, suggesting that it is the risk factors, and not the antipyretics, which are responsible for the seizure recurrences. Several randomized, placebo-controlled trials on children at risk of FS found no evidence that the antipyretic paracetamol or ibuprofen, with or without diazepam, was effective in preventing FS during subsequent febrile episodes [29–33]. Furthermore, numerous studies show that a temperature >40°C is associated with decreased incidence of recurrence [34–36]. Thus, a high temperature at the onset of FS is a useful predictor of nonrecurrence.

9.3.5
Views Against the Argument that Fever is Harmful

* Well-planned educational interventions about fever may change parental perceptions and reduce excessive use of health services. This information is best delivered during routine health checks, as parents' anxiety may interfere with their understanding of facts presented when their child is sick.
* About 20% of children seen in the accident and emergency department have a temperature over 40°C and they usually make a full recovery. Fever per se is self-limiting and rarely serious, provided the cause is known and fluid loss is replaced. Fever is most commonly caused by a viral infection of the upper respiratory tract. With fever, unlike hyperthermia, body temperature is well regulated by a hypothalamic set-point that balances heat production and heat loss so effectively that the temperature will not climb up relentlessly and does not exceed an upper limit of 42°C. Within this upper range of 40–42°C, there is no evidence that fever is injurious to tissue. If there is morbidity or mortality, it is due to the underlying disease. The associated fever may well be protective. Although it has been

difficult to define a critical threshold of tissue damage in man (defined as the temperature above which tissue damage occurs), a temperature above 42°C is likely to cause the damage. However, high temperatures are generally caused by hyperthermia, not by fever.

A reduction of symptoms of infection by antipyretics/analgesic drugs is often difficult to contest. It may be considered unkind to withhold these drugs whilst we have a simple and effective remedy to make children feel better. But, what if the use of this medication makes the infection worse? Furthermore, it is not unusual to see a febrile child with mild or no symptoms. In such circumstances there is little evidence to support the practice of routine antipyretic medication. Mild discomfort and myalgia may theoretically be beneficial by minimizing activity during the febrile illness so that available energy is channeled into useful biochemical reactions such as antibody formation.

9.3.6
When Might Fever Truly be Harmful?

Situations whereby fever clearly worsens the prognosis of disease include the following:

* *Acute stroke.* A study [37] showed that high temperature was an independent predictor of poor outcome. Numerous other studies seem to support this observation. For example, Kammersgaard et al. [38] have shown that stroke patients admitted with febrile body temperatures have a worse prognosis than do patients admitted with low or normal body temperature. Some companies are starting to manufacture helmets or other devices to allow the physician to selectively cool the brains of stroke patients
* *Severe sepsis.* In a recent paper, Pollheimer et al. [39] put forth an intriguing hypothesis. Septic patients show a marked muscle depletion of glutamine, which is associated with poor survival. Pollheimer et al. [40] showed that monocytes cultured at "febrile" temperatures in the presence of low glutamine (to simulate severe sepsis) had decreased viability. Thus, these cells that are critically important in fighting infection were severely impeded at febrile temperatures, but only in a low glutamine environment. They hypothesize that when glutamine is restored to the severely septic patient the "benefits of fever would be restored. However, clinical studies are needed to confirm or refute this."
* *Children with bronchiolitis.* A study has shown that the presence of fever did not benefit children admitted with bronchiolitis [41]
* *In situation associated with limited energy supply or increased metabolic rate* (e.g., burn, cardiovascular, and pulmonary diseases, prolonged febrile illness, young children, undernourishment, postoperative state). Fever can increase the metabolic rate and could exert a harmful effect on the disease
* Diseases are associated with high fever (>40°C) for the following reasons:
  - Children with this high degree of fever are likely to be symptomatic
  - With the exception of a few diseases such as Salmonella gastroenteritis and febrile seizures mentioned above, there has been no scientific evidence that high fever is beneficial
  - The prevailing view among physicians and parents is that high fever in particular is harmful and omission of antipyretics seems unethical

9.4
Summary

9.4.1
Lesson from History

- Many scholars of ancient civilizations, particularly the Greeks, believed in the beneficial effects of fever in disease. Hippocratic writings, for example, contain evidence that fever was thought to be beneficial to the infected host. Rufus of Ephesus in the second century AD strongly advocated the beneficial role of fever. He recommended the use of "fever therapy" (such as by malaria) to treat various diseases, including epilepsy. Fever therapy was the principal form of treatment, not only for syphilis and gonorrhea, but also for patients with rheumatoid arthritis and asthma. This belief, held for about 2,000 years, should not be ignored. Virtually all cultures use some form of "fever therapy" in the form of "saunas," or "sweat lodges," or "steam baths," or other ways to raise body temperature artificially. This probably dates back to the Hippocratic era and is based on the "humoral" theory of disease, where one of the forms of therapy was to "cook" the bad "humor."
- Events in the history are known to repeat themselves, and so are medical practice and concepts. It is possible that treatment with fever or hyperthermia could make a comeback and fever could play an important role (or as an adjunct to other therapeutic measures) to treat various diseases when modern medicine may not be capable to do so.

9.4.2
Lesson from Recent Research

- Accumulated data from extensive research into the subject of fever and its role in disease suggest that fever has a protective role in promoting host defense against infection, rather than being a passive by-product.
- Fever exerts an overall adverse effect on the growth of bacteria and some tumors, as well as on replication of viruses. It also enhances immunological processes, including activity of IL-1, T-helper cells, cytolytic T-cells, B-cell, and immunoglobulin synthesis.

Studies on the role of fever in disease in human, particularly in children conclude the following:

- Moderate fever has beneficial effects on a healthy child or adults.
- The effects of a high degree of fever (40–42°C) on pediatric diseases have rarely been studied. Performing clinical studies on child has its own risk, and so it will be difficult to gather such data.
- Our knowledge is extrapolated from studies using animal models or in vitro studies using human tissues.
- There are medical conditions (see below) that do not benefit from associated fever even at lower degree of body temperatures and these have to be treated vigorously with antipyretics.

9.4.3
Authors' Opinion

Fever is one of the oldest known signs of disease. Its description dates back as far as civilization itself, some 5,000 years. Fever is a very common clinical problem, which usually alarms parents. Despite intensive research, few issues in medicine have been more controversial than the biological role of the febrile response, that is, whether fever is beneficial or harmful. There is often a wide perception among doctors and parents that fever is dangerous. Parents have poor understanding of fever and their temperature measurement techniques are inaccurate.

Pediatricians who work with children in hospitals have come to terms that antipyretics (paracetamol without or alternating with ibuprofen) are very often automatically prescribed on the treatment sheet for the single indication, that is, the presence of fever (usually above 38.0°C, sometimes lower). Both, a child who is playful on the ward and another with a significant discomfort due to fever, receive antipyretics. This is the current practice, which is widely accepted. When we focus upon "treating" the fever, we are giving the impression to parents and health professionals that fever is harmful and that antipyresis is beneficial. Scientific evidence does not support this practice. It is the underlying disease not the fever that we should be concerned about. The presence of fever could well be of benefit to the infected host through activation of the immune system.

It is well-established that:

*   The reduction of fever by the use of antipyretics does not usually have a positive role on the underlying disease, nor does it reduce the time of infection.
*   The principal benefit of the antipyretic drug is to make children more comfortable, and that is because the antipyretic drug also has analgesic property.

Research indicates that we are at crossroads, divided between strong research evidence accumulated during the past few decades supporting a positive role of fever (with the exceptions noted earlier in this chapter) and the continued pressures of current practice to lower body temperature (i.e., "treat the fever" as though the fever were the disease). As clinicians, we need to educate our patients and health professionals that:

*   There is accumulating evidence that supports the notion that fever evolved as a host defense mechanism.
*   We should use antipyretic drugs sparingly in our clinical practice.

This may initially cause some dismay among parents because of their perception that their sick and needy children are not being treated. But, if we are to play a leadership role in our fields, we should help to educate the public about the results of research that have been coming forward over the past several decades. To continue the current practice of liberal use of antipyretics may mean that we are ignoring important messages from research.

Although this chapter of the book has stressed the beneficial effects of fever, the author does recognize that the issue as to whether fever is beneficial or not is still controversial, and there are scholars who maintain the view that the function of fever is still uncertain. Although it is difficult to isolate fever as a single parameter in a disease to investigate its function, more effort should be exerted to determine this function in every febrile disease. In particular, we need to know which diseases are likely to benefit from the presence of fever, so that minimal interference during their courses may be considered. On the other hand, we should investigate in which diseases the associated fever may be harmful so that steps are taken to treat it. Also it should be determined what degree of fever is harmful and thus ought to be reduced. Until these types of studies are conducted for a wide assortment of infections, the question of whether most fevers should be left alone or treated in the pediatric or adult patient will remain unanswered.

References

1. Kluger MJ, Kozak W, Mayfield KP. Fever and Immunity, in *Psychoneuroimmunology*, Third Edition, Vol. 1, Academic Press, San Diego. 2001, pp. 687–702
2. Osawa E, Muschel LH. Studies relating to the serum resistance of certain Gram-negative bacteria. J Exp Med 1964; 119: 41–51
3. Lwoff A. Factors influencing the evolution of viral diseases of the cellular level and in the organism. Bacteriol Rev 1959; 23: 109–24
4. Yerushalmi A, Lwoff A. Traitment du coryza infectieux et des rhinitis persistantes allergiques par la thermotherapie. Comp Rendus Seances. Acad Sci (Ser D) 1980; 291: 957–9
5. Wong VK, Hitchcock W, Mason WH. Meningococcal infections in children: a review of 100 cases. Pediatr Infect Dis J 1989; 8: 224–7
6. El-Radhi AS, Rostila T, Vesikari T. Association of high fever and short bacterial excretion after salmonellosis. Arch Dis Child 1992; 67: 531–2
7. Nahas GG, Tannieres ML, Lennon JF. Direct measurement of leukocyte motility: effects of pH and temperature. Proc Soc Exp Biol Med 1971; 138: 350–2
8. Duff GW, Durum SK. Fever and immunoregulation: hyperthermia, interleukin 1 and 2, and T-cell proliferation. Yale J Biol Med 1982; 55: 437–42
9. Murphy PA, Hanson DF, Guo YN, et al. The effects of variations in pH and temperature on the activation of mouse thymocytes by both forms of rabbit interleukin-1. Yale J Biol Med 1985; 58: 115–23
10. Dinarello CA, Bernstein HA, Duff GW, et al. Mechanisms of fever induced by recombinant human interferon. J Clin Invest 1984; 74: 906–13
11. Heron I, Berg K, Cantel K. Regulatory effect of interferon on T cell in vitro. J Immunol 1976; 17: 1370–3
12. Mackowiak PA, Marling-Cason M, Cohen RL. Effects of temperature on antimicrobial susceptibility of bacteria. J Infect Dis 1982; 145: 550–53
13. Donato V, Zurlo A, Nappa M, et al. Multicentre experience with combined hyperthermia and radiation therapy in the treatment of superficially located non-Hodgkin's lymphomas. J Exp Clin Cancer Res. 1997; 16: 87–90
14. Kluger MJ, Ringler DH, Anver MR. Fever and survival. Science 1975; 188, 166–8
15. Bernheim HA, Kluger MJ. Fever: of drug-induced antipyresis on survival. Science 1976; 193: 237–9
16. Graham NH, Burrell CJ, Douglas RM, et al. Adverse effects of aspirin, acetaminophen, and ibuprofen on immune function, viral shedding and clinical status in rhinovirus-infected volunteers. Infect Dis 1990; 162: 1277–82
17. Doran TF, Angelis CD, Baumgarder RA, et al. Acetaminophen: more harm than good in chickenpox? Pediatr 1989; 114: 1045–8

9

18. Sugimura T, Fujimoto T, Motoyama T, et al. Risks of antipyretics in young children with fever due to infectious diseases. Acta Paediatr Jpn 1994; 36: 375–8

19. Muschenheim C, Duerscher DR, Hardy JD, et al. Hypothermia in experimental infections. Infect Dis 1943; 72: 187–96

20. Husseini RH, Sweet C, Collie MH, et al. Elevation of nasal viral levels by suppression of fever in ferrets infected with influenza viruses of differing virulence. Infect Dis 1982; 145: 520–4

21. El-Radhi AS, Jawad MJ, Mansor N, et al. Infection in neonatal hypothermia. Arch Dis Child 1983; 58: 143–5

22. Williams LK, Peterson EL, Ownby DR, et al. The relationship between early fever and allergic sensitization at age 6 to 7 years. J Allergy Clin Immunol 2004; 113: 291–6

23. Custovic A. The hygiene hypothesis revisited: pros and cons. Asthma and immunology 60th anniversary meeting, Denver, Colorado, March 7–12, 2003

24. Albonico HU, Braker HU, Husler J. Febrile infectious childhood disease in the history of cancer patients and matched control. Med Hypotheses 1998; 51: 315–20

25. Schmitt BD. Fever phobia. Am J Dis Child 1980; 134: 176–81

26. May A, Bauchner H. Fever phobia: the pediatrician's contribution. Pediatrics 1992; 90: 851–4

27. Ekholm E, Niemineva K. On convulsions in early childhood and their prognosis. Acta Paediatr 1950; 39: 481–501

28. Rosman NP. Febrile Convulsions, in Fever: Basic Mechanisms and Management, Second Edition, edited by P.A. Mackowiak. Lippincot, Philadelphia. 1997, pp. 267–77

29. Kramer MS, Naimark L, Leduc DG, et al. Risks and benefits of paracetamol antipyresis in young children with fever of presumed viral origin. Lancet 1991; 337: 591–4

30. El-Radhi AS, Barry W. Do antipyretics prevent febrile convulsions? Arch Dis Child 2003; 88: 641–2

31. Schnaiderman D, Lahat E, Sheefer T, et al. Antipyretic effectiveness of acetaminophen in febrile seizures: ongoing prophylaxis versus sporadic usage. Eur J Pediatr 1993; 152: 747–9

32. Van Stuijvenberg M, Derksen-Lubsen G, Steyerberg EW, et al. Randomized, controlled trial of ibuprofen syrup administered during febrile illnesses to prevent febrile recurrences. Pediatrics 1998; 102: 1–7

33. Van Esch A, Steyerberg EW, Moll HA, et al. A study of the efficacy of antipyretic drugs in the prevention of febrile seizure recurrence. Ambul Child Health 2000; 6: 19–26

34. Meremikwu M, Oyo-Ita A. Paracetamol for treating fever in children. Cochrane Database Syst Rev 2002; 4

35. El-Radhi AS. Lower degree of fever is associated with increased risk of subsequent convulsions. Eur J Paediatr Neuro 1998; 2: 91–6

36. Offringa M, Derksen-Lubsen G, Bossuyt P. Seizure recurrence after a first febrile seizure: a multivariate approach. Dev Med Child Neurol 1992; 34: 15–24

37. Azzimondi G, Bassein L, Nonino F, et al. Fever in acute stroke worsens prognosis. Stroke 1995; 26:2040–43

38. Kammersgaard LP, Jorgensen HS, et al. Stroke 2002, 33: 1759–62

39. Pollheimer J, Zellner M, Eliasen MM, et al. Increased susceptibility of glutamine-depleted monocytes to fever-range hyperthermia: the role of 70-kDa heat shock protein. Ann Surg 2005; 241: 349–55

40. Novak F, Heyland DK, Avenell A, et al. Glutamine supplementation in serious illness: a systematic review of the evidence. Crit Care Med 2002; 30: 2022–9

41. El-Radhi AS, Barry W, Patel S. Association of fever and severe clinical course in bronchiolitis. Arch Dis Child 1999; 81: 231–4

Management of Fever (Antipyretics)

10

Core Messages

> Fever in children is a frequent reason for consultation to pediatricians and GPs, estimated to be 30% of the total visits.
> The principal indication for the use of antipyretics is not to reduce body temperature but to make the child comfortable.
> Antipyretics are ineffective in preventing febrile seizures.
> Currently, paracetamol is a first-line choice for fever and pain management.
> Combining two antipyretics has no scientific basis and does not achieve a greater antipyretic/analgesic effect than using either agent alone.
> In therapeutic dose, antipyretics rarely cause adverse events.
> The use of tepid sponging for febrile children is unnecessary because of the availability of antipyretic drugs, which are simpler to use, more effective in reducing body temperature, and produce less discomfort to children.
> One of the most important duties of pediatricians is to differentiate between an ill child (who may need prompt attention, including hospitalization) and a well child who can be sent home. This is learned by experience.
> Fever phobia is common among parents and doctors. This excessive fear of fever is unfounded. It is not the fever that is harmful but the underlying disease. The associated fever may be protective.

10.1
Historical Background of Antipyretics

Ancient Egyptian scholars and the Indians of North America knew the therapeutic benefit of willow tree bark, which contains salicylates. Hippocrates recommended chewing willow leaves as childbirth analgesia. In the mid-eighteenth century, Reverend Edmund Stone in England described the benefit of willow bark "in the cure fever" [1].

A.S. El-Radhi et al. (Eds.) *Clinical Manual of Fever in Children.*
Doi: 10.1007/978-3-540-78598-9, © Springer-Verlag Berlin Heidelberg 2009

In the 1880s, the German synthetic dye industry accidentally discovered acetanilide and antipyrine (1883). These early antipyretics, along with phenacetin (discovered in 1887) and aminopyrine (discovered in 1896) were later withdrawn because of toxicity. Aspirin was synthesized in 1853 and introduced into clinical practice in 1899 by the German drug company, Bayer, which gave it its name. By 1914, aspirin was the world's most widely used drug, not only as an antipyretic and analgesic, but also against hay fever and diabetes mellitus. In 1988, aspirin was removed from the World Health Organization's list of essential drugs following reports linking aspirin and Reye's syndrome (encephalopathy associated with liver necrosis). Paracetamol (in USA – Acetaminophen) was introduced in 1893.

10.2
Mechanisms of Action of Antipyretics

* Antipyretics act centrally by lowering the thermoregulatory set point of the hypothalamic center. This is achieved through inhibition of cyclooxygenase (COX), the enzyme responsible for the conversion of arachidonic acid to prostaglandins (PG) and leukotrienes. Although several prostaglandins can induce fever, PGE2 is the most important mediator. The lowering of the hypothalamic set point leads to a series of physiological responses, including decreased heat production, increased blood flow to the skin, and increased heat loss through the skin by radiation, convection, and evaporation, resulting in a reduction in body temperature.

* Most antipyretics inhibit PG effects on pain receptors, capillary permeability and circulation and leukocyte migration, thereby reducing the classical signs of inflammation. Prostaglandins also produce bronchodilatation and have an important effect on the gastrointestinal tract and renal medulla. Therefore, the expected side effects of these drugs include bronchospasm, gastrointestinal hemorrhage, and renal impairment.

* Antipyretics do not reduce fever to a normal level, reduce the duration of febrile episodes, or interfere with the normal body temperature. They also do not directly interfere with pyrogen formation or with mechanisms of heat loss, such as sweating. Their effectiveness in reducing fever depends on the level of fever (the higher the fever, the more the reduction), the absorption rate, and the dose of the antipyretic.

Table 10.1 Characteristics of an ideal antipyretic

An ideal antipyretic should:
• Give rapid result and be effective in reducing fever by at least 1°C (1.8°F)
• Be available in liquid and suppository form
• Have low rate of side effects in therapeutic doses and low toxicity when taken in overdose
• Have low incidence of interaction with other medications and rarely contraindication in pediatric doses
• Be safe
• Be cost effective

10.3
Choosing an Antipyretic

An ideal antipyretic is expected to have the characteristics shown in Table 10.1.

The choice of antipyretics has been narrowed to paracetamol and ibuprofen following the recommendation against aspirin use. Before that, aspirin had the advantage over paracetamol because of its low cost and its anti-inflammatory effect. Ibuprofen is more expensive and has more side effects than paracetamol (see later).

10.4
Indications for Antipyretics

The main indication for prescribing an antipyretic is not to reduce body temperature but to relieve the child's discomfort and thereby the parent's anxiety. There is little evidence to suggest that reduction of body temperature in itself is beneficial. Current pediatric practice for a febrile child includes the use of antipyretics when the temperature is greater than 38.5 or 39°C. With the reduction of fever, the activity and alertness of children may improve, while the improvement in mood or appetite is less pronounced.

10.5
How Beneficial are the Antipyretics?

Antipyretics are among the most commonly used medications in children. Fever is the leading cause for seeking a physician's attention (30% of consultations), and antipyretics are prescribed almost routinely to reduce it. The answer to the important question as to whether antipyretics should be used to lower body temperature depends on whether fever is deleterious or beneficial to children. Table 10.2 summarizes arguments for and against the use of antipyretics.

Table 10.2 Summary of arguments for and against the use of antipyretics

In favor of antipyretic use	Against antipyretic use
Prevailing concept that fever is harmful	Fever per se is self-limited and rarely serious
Fever if untreated may rise to a dangerous level, causing CNS damage	Fever, unlike hyperthermia, is regulated by an effective thermoregulatory center. It does not climb up relentlessly
Relieving parental anxiety	Educating parents can reduce their fear
Risk of fever seizures (FS)	No scientific evidence that they prevent FS
	Fever has a protective role against infection
	Antipyretic drugs have adverse effects and occasional fatalities

10

Arguments for the Use of Antipyretics

* Parents' attitude and expectation

Antipyretics are often prescribed because parents are worried when their child is feverish and feel that fever may spiral upward with a possible fatal outcome. Parents often have unfounded anxiety about the possible risks of fever and no information about its beneficial role in diseases. Practically all parents remain convinced that antipyretic measures must be used to lower fever.

* Prevailing concepts among physicians

Most pediatricians agree that treatment of a febrile child with antipyretics is for the relief of the symptoms of fever. However, many tend to prescribe antipyretics for a child with any degree of fever. In a study [2] exploring the beliefs and practices of pediatricians in Massachusetts, USA, the majority (65%) of respondents believed that fever itself could be dangerous to a child, with seizures, death, and brain damage being the most serious complications if the temperature was 40°C or greater. Pediatricians may be contributing to parental fever phobia by prescribing antipyretics for children with mild fever.

* The risk of febrile seizures (FS)

Fever can cause a brief benign convulsion in 3–4% of all children. In a study from the USA, 49% of pediatricians considered convulsions to be a principal danger of fever and 22% believed that brain damage could result from FS [3]. As the essential precursor of a FS is fever, physicians have concluded that antipyretic measures should prevent FS. Parents with children at risk of FS are usually advised that the administration of antipyretics can prevent further FS.

There is now abundant evidence against the previously assumed risks of FS. It is now well established that antipyretics are ineffective in the prevention of FS. Two large population-based studies [4, 5] found no deaths or persistent motor deficits directly attributed to FS. A temperature >40°C with the first seizure was associated with a decreased incidence of recurrence of FS [6,7]. An evidence-based search [8] concluded that antipyretic drugs are ineffective in preventing FS and should not be recommended for preventing further FS.

* Associated discomfort

Febrile children often experience discomfort, headaches, and myalgia resulting in reduced activity and causing anxiety to the parents. Antipyretics by being analgesics lead to an improvement in the children's level of activity and alertness. The elimination of these symptoms (discomfort, pain, and aches) is the mean reason why antipyretics have maintained their popularity among parents.

This point, a reduction of symptoms of fever by antipyretics, is difficult to contest. It is unkind to withhold antipyretics while we have a simple and effective remedy to make children feel better. However, it is not unusual to see a febrile child with mild or no symptoms. In such circumstances if parents have received an explanation about the nature of their child's illness, there is little evidence to support the practice of routine antipyretic administration.

Arguments Against the Use of Antipyretics

- Fever is self-limiting and well controlled.

Fever per se is self-limiting and rarely serious provided that the cause is known and fluid loss is replaced. Fever is commonly caused by a viral infection of the upper respiratory tract. Antipyretics have no influence on the clinical course of the disease or on the number of subsequent febrile days. With fever, unlike hyperthermia, body temperature is well regulated by a hypothalamic set point that balances heat production and loss so effectively that the temperature will not climb up relentlessly and does not exceed an upper limit of 42°C. Within this upper range of 40–42°C, fever is not injurious to tissue. About 20% of children seen in the emergency room have temperatures over 40°C and they usually make a full recovery. If there is morbidity or mortality, it is due to the underlying disease. The associated fever may well be protective.

- The effects of fever on microorganisms and defense mechanisms.

Studies have demonstrated that the bacterial growth rate in experimental pneumococcal meningitis is significantly reduced at elevated temperatures [9]. Gram-negative bacteria, such as *salmonella typhi*, were shown to be increasingly susceptible to the antibacterial effects of serum when cultivated at a temperature >37°C [10]. There was a significant inverse correlation between the degree of fever and the duration of excretion of organisms. A fever of greater than 40°C had the shortest and those without fever the longest duration of bacterial excretion [11].

If fever is considered beneficial, antipyretics may have harmful effects. In one study, the administration of the antipyretic sodium salicylate to lizards with bacterial infection increased their mortality. All febrile lizards survived, whereas all afebrile lizards died [12]. A study from Japan [13] found that the frequent administration of antipyretics to children with bacterial diseases led to a worsening of their illness.

Fever enhances immunological processes, including mobility of polymorphonuclear cells, activity of interleukin-1, T helper cells, and cytolytic T cells, as well as B cell activity and possibly immunoglobulin synthesis [14].

- Side effects and fatalities.

Antipyretics are known to cause adverse reactions and some fatalities. In the UK, paracetamol has been one of the most popular choices for suicide attempts in adolescents and adults, causing 100–150 deaths annually. In the USA, paracetamol-associated overdoses account for 56,000 emergency visits, and 26,000 hospitalizations, with approximately 450 deaths each year. About 100 of these deaths are unintentional [15].

10.6
Antipyretics (See Table 10.3 for summary points)

Antipyretics are among the world's most used medications. As a group, these drugs differ chemically but have in common mechanisms of action, including antipyresis, analgesia, anti-inflammatory effect, and platelet inhibition (paracetamol does not possess the latter two activities). A brief classification of antipyretics is shown in Table 10.4.

Table 10.3 Summary points of antipyretics

• The current practice considers the liberal use of antipyretics a necessity and demands measures to abolish it, often at low degree of fever. Fever phobia is widespread among parents and physicians. More education is needed to alleviate this excessive fear of parents about fever.

• Antipyretic drugs, by being analgesics, reduce not only the fever but also the pain. Children feel better and we assume that when we reduce fever we reduce the severity of the disease. The elimination of these symptoms (discomfort, pain, and aches) is perhaps the main reason why antipyretics have maintained their popularity among parents and have continued in use for over a century.

• There is no evidence that fever, in contrast to hyperthermia is injurious to tissue. If there is morbidity or mortality, it is due to the underlying disease. The associated fever may well be protective.

• Until properly controlled studies have assessed the risk of combining the two antipyretics, paracetamol and ibuprofen, practitioners and parents may be advised to use paracetamol alone in the treatment of febrile children.

• Antipyretics have no influence on the clinical course of the disease and do not reduce the mean number of days of subsequent fever.

• Drastic measures to lower body temperature have no scientific basis, are distressful to patients, and are counterproductive.

• Physical measures (fan, tepid sponging) for fever are unnecessary and unpleasant for the child; their use is discouraged. Instead, offering extra fluids, keeping the room cool, and dressing the child in light clothing are encouraged.

Table 10.4 Medications/measures known to lower body temperature

Para-aminophenols
  Paracetamol
	Endogenous antipyretics
	  Arginine vasopressin
	  Alpha-melanocyte stimulating hormone

Propionic acid derivatives
  Ibuprofen
  Naproxen
	Physical measures
	  Bed rest
	  Tepid sponging

Salicylates Aspirin	

Other NSAIDs
  Nimesulide
  Diclofenac	

10.6.1
Paracetamol (Acetaminophen)

Effects and Dose
Paracetamol is an active metabolite of acetanilide and phenacetin. Currently, paracetamol is the most commonly used antipyretic and analgesic drug in pediatric practice. Table 10.5 shows some clinical data on the available preparations of paracetamol.

Table 10.5 Recommended doses of some paracetamol preparations, their advantages, and disadvantages

	Oral	Rectal	Intravenous
Available	Tab: Panadol (500 mg) Liquid: Calpol (120 mg/5 ml; or 250 mg/5 ml)	Paracetamol 60, 125, or 500 mg	Paracetamol infusion 10 mg ml^{-1}
Dose	10–15 mg/kg^{-1} at 4–6 h or 60–75 mg/kg^{-1} per day for children; 4 g/day for adults	Same as oral	15 mg/kg^{-1}
Neonate	20 mg/kg^{-1} start, then 10–15 mg/kg^{-1} every 8–12 h	20 mg/kg^{-1} start, then 15 mg/kg^{-1} BD	
Advantage	Well tolerated, good absorption	Used if the oral route is unsuitable or impractical, e.g., vomiting, drowsiness, coma	Penetrates readily in CSF, rapid central analgesia, bypassing the delayed absorption of enteral route
Disadvantage	May cause vomiting, abdominal pain. A high carbohydrate meal may reduce absorption and interfere with fever reduction	Absorption is slower and more variable than the oral form	Few indications, e.g., intraoperative or post-operative analgesia, not as an antipyretic

Dose	Expected temperature reduction (°C)
5 mg/kg^{-1}	0.3–0.4
10–15 mg/kg^{-1}	1.2–1.4
20 mg/kg^{-1}	1.4–1.6

Table 10.6 Antipyretic effect of commonly used paracetamol doses 2–3 h after administration (initial body temperature 39.5°C)

A dose of 5 mg kg^{-1} body weight paracetamol achieves an insignificant temperature reduction (Table 10.6). Following administration of a therapeutic dose, fever begins to fall in about 30 min, a nadir is reached in about 2 h, and recurrence of fever is observed in 3–4 h. A peak plasma level is reached in about 30 min. Clearance is reduced in neonates; a dose at 8–12 h intervals is recommended.

Side Effects

Paracetamol has remarkably few and mild side effects when administered in ordinary doses. It does not cause gastrointestinal bleeding, analgesic nephropathy, or coagulopathy.

Table 10.7 Adverse reactions of paracetamol

Gastrointestinal	Vomiting, abdominal pain
Dermatological	urticaria, erythema multiforme, purpura
Respiratory	bronchospasms
CNS	Dizziness, irritability, blurred vision, hypothermia
Other	May prolong viral shedding in some infections, e.g., varicella, causing no alleviation of symptoms and may prolong the illness

Table 10.7 shows the main reported side effects, all of which are rare in clinical practice, except perhaps abdominal pain and vomiting (incidence around 1%). Reported cases of bronchospasms must be unusual because paracetamol is recommended as a substitute for aspirin in asthma patients. Paracetamol may rarely interfere with glucose homeostasis in the liver, causing hypoglycemia.

Drugs reported to interact with paracetamol include warfarin, metoclopromide, beta-adrenergic blockers, and chlorpromazine.

Overdose

Toxicity of paracetamol is infrequent in children, and fatalities below the age of 13 years are almost unknown. It has a wide therapeutic margin, and only a much higher dose ($>15\,g$ in adult and $150\,mg\,kg^{-1}$ in a child) is associated with significant hepatotoxic effects. It has been suggested that the sulfate (the predominant metabolite of paracetamol found in children below the age of 12 years), in contrast to the glucuronide (the predominate metabolite found in adults), protect children from liver toxicity. As paracetamol is minimally bound to plasma protein (10%, while salicylate is 70–90% bound), elimination from the body is rapid. Therefore, chronic toxicity from accumulation, seen commonly with salicylates, is unknown.

Major complications from paracetamol toxicity include the following:

- Liver necrosis: Paracetamol and its two major metabolites, sulfate and glucuronide, are not toxic. Instead, a minor intermediate (N-acetyl-p-benzoquinonimine) is highly reactive with hepatocytes, causing necrosis. The ingestion of a toxic dose or a blood level higher than $300\,mg\,dl^{-1}$ at $4\,h$ after intake is likely to produce liver necrosis.
- Other complications: These include acute tubular necrosis, hypophosphatemia, renal failure, thrombocytopenia, hypothermia, encephalopathy, cardiomyopathy, hyperglycemia, hypoglycemia, metabolic acidosis, and coagulation defects.

Management of paracetamol toxicity includes the following:

- Plasma paracetamol measurement should be performed $4\,h$ after ingestion.
- Activated charcoal is administered to minimize the drug absorption.
- The specific antidote is N-acetylcysteine, which acts mainly by enhancing glutathione stores and providing a glutathione substitute. A standard dose consists of $300\,mg\,kg^{-1}$ administered intravenously over a $20\,h$ period. This treatment prevents most complications, including deaths. Hepatic toxicity rarely occurs when N-acetylcysteine is begun within $10\,h$ of ingestion (see Fig. 10.1).

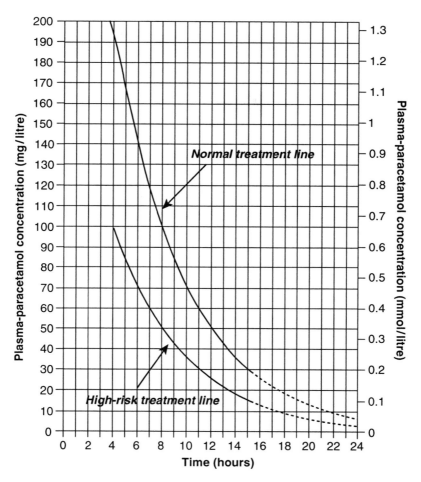

Fig. 10.1 Treatment of paracetamol poisoning according to its concentration and time of its intake

Criteria associated with poor outcome include arterial pH <7.30 after the first day of overdose, prolonged prothrombin time, high serum creatinine, and the presence of encephalopathy.

10.6.2
Ibuprofen

This drug (propionic acid derivative) became the only nonsteroidal anti-inflammatory drug (NSAID), approved as an antipyretic in the USA since 1984 and in the UK since 1990.

10

The drug is well absorbed from the gastrointestinal tract, reaching a peak serum concentration in about 1 h. A suspension is available for children who are at least few months of age. Its anti-inflammatory and analgesic properties provide additional therapeutic advantages over paracetamol in the treatment of various febrile infectious diseases. Rectal ibuprofen is available, e.g., for perioperative pain control. Ibuprofen is used as follows:

• Antipyretic: The maximal effective level of antipyresis can be achieved with a dose of 5 mg kg^{-1} for at least 3–4 h. A dose of 10 mg kg^{-1} is more potent and has longer lasting fever suppression than paracetamol. The onset of antipyresis tends to be earlier, and the effect greater in infants than in older children.
• Antipyretic, analgesic, and anti-inflammatory effects in juvenile idiopathic arthritis (JIA): A dose of 20–40 mg kg^{-1} per day has a greater therapeutic effect and fewer side effects compared with aspirin in a dose of 60–80 mg kg^{-1} per day.
• Anti-inflammatory agent, which has been shown to retard the progression of lung disease in cystic fibrosis [16].
• Prostaglandin inhibitor: Intravenous ibuprofen is effective in closing a patent ductus arteriosus in premature infants (comparable with indomethacin) with minimal effect on renal function.

Toxicity

Ibuprofen has favorable therapeutic benefits with few adverse effects compared with its widespread use. Drug-related adverse reactions (Table 10.8) are mostly dose related and occur more often than those associated with paracetamol. On the other hand, adverse

Table 10.8 Dose-related adverse reactions to ibuprofen

Organ	Antipyretic dose	Anti-inflammatory dose	Overdose
GI system	Vomiting, nausea, abdominal pain, diarrhea	Vomiting, nausea, abdominal pain, diarrhea, blood	Vomiting, nausea, abdominal pain, diarrhea, blood
CNS	Irritability, headache, agitation aseptic meningitis*	Irritability, headache, agitation aseptic meningitis*	Confusion, blurred vision, nystagmus, seizure, coma
Skin	Rash	Rash	Rash
Renal		Edema, Na retention, proteinuria, hemorrhage, increased creatinine	Renal failure
Liver		Increased enzymes	Increased enzyme
Hematology		Agranulocytosis, hemolytic anemia	
Other		Hyperthermia, hearing loss, teratogenic (gastroschisis)	

*Ocurring particularly in patients with systemic lupus erythematosus (SLE)

reactions from ibuprofen are less than those associated with aspirin. In a metaanalysis involving 46,000 patients, the incidence of digestive events was 5%, with 0.02% upper gastrointestinal bleeds [17].

Children after an ingestion of 100 mg kg^{-1} are unlikely to present symptoms. Even doses of 300 mg kg^{-1} are often asymptomatic. Management of a case with toxicity includes activated charcoal and general supportive care. There is no specific antidote against ibuprofen toxicity.

10.6.3
Aspirin

Until 1980, aspirin was the most widely used antipyretic and analgesic in pediatric practice. Aspirin had about 70% share of the USA market, with paracetamol taking the remaining 30% market. In the UK, the trend was approximately the opposite. Trials comparing equal doses of aspirin and paracetamol demonstrated an identical antipyretic effectiveness, with aspirin being more effective for analgesia. Following reports linking Reye's syndrome and aspirin, the Committee on Infectious diseases of the American Academy of Pediatrics concluded in a report in 1982 that aspirin should not be given to any child with varicella or with possible influenza.

Aspirin is used as an:

* Antipyretic/analgesic: Although aspirin is no longer recommended for such an indication, it is still frequently used. As the half life of salicylate blood level is 3–4 h, 4–6 times daily in a dose of 10–15 mg kg^{-1} is appropriate.
* Anti-inflammatory in rheumatic diseases, such as JIA and rheumatic fever: An initial dose of 80 mg kg^{-1} in 3–4 divided doses is followed by a dose adjusted to maintain a serum salicylate level of 20–30 mg dl^{-1}. As Reye's syndrome has been reported in patients with JIA treated with aspirin, the drug has lost popularity in recent years to treat connective tissue diseases.
* Antithrombotic agent for its antiplatelet and fibrinolytic activity: This is recommended in children with Kawasaki disease, congenital heart diseases and in adults with coronary heart disease.

Reported adverse effects are shown in Table 10.9. Adverse effects occurring with a salicylate serum level of less than 20 mg/100 ml are generally considered side effects, while those occurring at a higher level are considered poisoning. Features of adverse effects and poisoning often overlap.

Groups who are at high risk of developing adverse effects include:

* Children with viral infections, particularly with upper respiratory tract infection or varicella (see later Reye's syndrome).
* Pregnant women who are generally advised to avoid aspirin because of the increased risk of the following:
   – Perinatal hemorrhage for both mother and offspring if aspirin is ingested within 5 days of delivery

Table 10.9 Reported adverse reactions to aspirin

Organ	Manifestation
General	Elevated body temperature, sweating, dehydration
Respiratory	Hyperventilation
Gastrointestinal	Vomiting, abdominal pain, gastric ulcer, hemorrhage
Liver	Increased liver enzymes, abdominal pain, hepatitis, Reye's syndrome (RS)
CNS	Headaches, dizziness, irritability, confusion, tinnitus
Skin	Rash, often urticarial, angioedema
Kidney	Interstitial nephritis, papillary necrosis
Platelets	Hemorrhage, diminished coagulation

- Closure of ductus arteriosus in utero, which can contribute to persistent fetal circulation postnatally
- Interference with uterine contractility
- Possible stillbirth
- Possible (but unconfirmed) fetal malformation. Teratogenicity includes increased risk of certain cardiac defects, such as aortic stenosis, coarctation of the aorta, hypoplastic left ventricular syndrome, and transposition of the great vessels

- Glucose-6-phosphate dehydrogenase (G6PD) deficiency: Aspirin is considered to be an hemolytic agent in individuals with G6PD deficiency, and children with this disorder are advised against its use.
- Asthma: Aspirin-induced sensitivity includes wheezing, urticaria, rhinorrhea, and angiedema. Aspirin inhibits the synthesis of prostaglandin, which exerts a bronchodilatatory effect.
- Patients with bleeding tendency or undergoing surgical procedure because of irreversible inhibition of platelet function.

Poisoning may result from the following:

- Accidental or therapeutic salicylate ingestion: The latter is more encountered in paediatric practice.
- Ingestion of oil of wintergreen (methyl salicylate): This can cause severe salicylate poisoning and death (one teaspoon may be lethal).

Table 10.10 summarizes the pathophysiological abnormalities leading to the main features of aspirin intoxication.

Whereas in older children and adults respiratory alkalosis predominates the clinical picture, in young children the phase of respiratory alkalosis is brief, and by the time the child reaches the hospital, metabolic acidosis mixed with respiratory alkalosis is usually established. In infancy or in severe salicylate poisoning, marked disruption of the acid–base status may occur, manifesting as low blood pH. The presence of only respiratory alkalosis may signify either mild or early poisoning. Table 10.11 lists the clinical findings of aspirin poisoning according to the degree of severity.

Table 10.10 Pathophysiological mechanisms and the resulting clinical findings in aspirin overdose

Pathophysiological findings	Leading to
Direct stimulation of respiratory center in the CNS	Hyper- and tachypnea, low pCO_2, increased pH, alkaluria
Inhibition of Krebs cycle enzymes	Acidosis (pH < 7.32) due mainly to accumulation of pyruvate and lactic acid
Increased metabolism of lipids	Vomiting, acidosis, accumulation of ketone bodies, and ketonuria
Stimulation of hepatic glucogenesis and failure of tissue to utilize glucose	Glucose↑, or↓ (the latter is often a feature of chronic intoxication)
Increased metabolism, osmotic diuresis, increased excretion of bicarbonate, starvation	Dehydration, loss of salt and water, accumulation of ketone bodies, hypokalemia, hyponatremia

Table 10.11 Signs of salicylate poisoning according to the amount of ingested salicylate and salicylate blood levels

Degree	Intake (mg kg^{-1})	Serum level (mg dl^{-1})	Expected findings
Mild	100–150	20–40	Hyperpnea, vomiting, tinnitus, lethargy, mild dehydration
Moderate	150–300	40–60	As above, but more severe, plus disorientation, fever
Severe	300–500	60–100	Coma, seizure
Potentially fatal	>500	>100	

Investigation should include the following:

- Blood for FBC, salicylate level, glucose, liver function tests, prothrombin time, gas analysis, bicarbonate, electrolytes and urea, ketone bodies, and osmolality.
- Urine pH: The ferric chloride test is useful. When positive, the urine color turns violet or purple indicating the presence of salicylate.
- ECG monitoring.

Management (see Table 10.12)

Reye's Syndrome (RS)

This syndrome was first described as a clinical entity by Reye in Australia in 1963. It affects children of any age, but most patients are in the age group of 6–8 years.

10

Table 10.12 Management of aspirin poisoning and RS

- Admission to an intensive care facility, with monitoring of vital signs, water and electrolyte balance, blood gas analysis, and pH of the urine. There is no specific antidote.
- Activated charcoal
- Correction of fluid, electrolyte, and blood gas imbalance. Large amount of fluid in the first hours of admission are often needed to correct dehydration
- Forced alkaline diuresis may be beneficial to increase salicylate elimination. Bicarbonate ($1-2$ mEq kg^{-1}) may be required to correct acidosis, but vigorous alkali therapy may be dangerous.
- Coagulation defects are treated with vitamin K derivative.
- In cases of RS, prompt blood exchange transfusion and early diagnosis can significantly reduce case fatality.
- High body temperature is treated with tepid sponging.
- In severe poisoning not responding to the above measures or if symptoms worsen, hemodialysis should be considered. Respiratory failure necessities artificial ventilation.

RS is defined as an acute noninflammatory encephalopathy associated with fatty metamorphosis of the liver. Diagnostic criteria are:

- Alteration in the level of consciousness
- Threefold or greater rise in levels of alanine and aspartate transaminases (normal <40 U l^{-1}), ammonia (>100 μmol l^{-1}), hypoglycemia (<2.4 mmol l^{-1} (40 mg/100 ml), prolonged PT (>4 s))
- Normal CSF
- No other explanation for the hepatic or cerebral abnormalities
- Histological findings (not essential for the diagnosis), which include small droplets of fat infiltration without inflammatory changes under the light microscope and electron microscopy showing abnormal hepatocyte mitochondria with varying degree of enlargement, decrease in matrix density, and loss of mitochondrial dense bodies

The definite cause of RS remains unclear, but appears to be the result of interactions between viruses (influenza A and B, adenoviruses, varicella) and medications. It is possible that aspirin enhances virulence of certain viruses by blocking the antiviral effect of interferon. Other factors such as toxins (aflatoxins) and genetic predisposition have also been suggested to cause RS.

The following factors support the association between aspirin and RS:

- A statistically significant correlation between the development of RS and administration of aspirin during a viral infection.
- A similarity between salicylate toxicity and RS: Both conditions may show vomiting, hyperventilation and confusion, acid–base abnormalities and most significantly similar hepatic histological findings with fatty infiltration and preservation of lobular structure.
- The occurrence of RS in children taking salicylate for connective tissue diseases.
- A progressive decline in the incidence of RS with the drastic reduction in the use of aspirin since 1988.

Clinical features are characterized by a mild prodromal viral illness (such as URI or varicella) followed abruptly by the following:

* Vomiting followed by alternation of consciousness (lethargy, delirium, coma) and often convulsions
* Varying degrees of hypertonicity, continuing convulsions, and decerebrate rigidity, indicating a poor prognosis
* Liver enlargement
* An EEG with generalized slow wave activity

For management of aspirin poisoning and RS, see Table 10.12.

10.6.4
Other Antipyretics

* **Naproxen**, also anti-inflammatory and analgesic, has a long plasma half-life of about 14 h. Therefore, twice-daily administration is appropriate. It is effective in patients with cancer.
* **Indomethacin** is not used as an antipyretic in children because of the availability of other antipyretics with less adverse reactions. Its complications include gastrointestinal (vomiting, bleeding, ulcers) and CNS symptoms (headache, dizziness, confusion). The drug is effective in the treatment of fever in cancer.
* **Dipyrone** is another pyrazolone derivative but unlike paracetamol it has a high rate of toxicity, particularly agranulocytosis, which led to its withdrawal from the USA market in 1977. It is still used in many parts of the world (dose: 15 mg kg⁻¹). The drug is no longer recommended for use in children.
* **Salicylamide** is rarely used nowadays as an antipyretic. It is less effective than paracetamol or aspirin in reducing fever.
* **Antipyrine** was widely used as an antipyretic throughout the world but has been withdrawn because of toxicity, particularly agranulocytosis.
* **Nimesulide** is an NSAID with antipyretic, anti-inflammatory, and analgesic activities. A dose of 5 mg kg⁻¹ per day three times daily has a prompt antipyretic effect. Adverse reactions include abdominal symptoms, gastrointestinal bleeds, hypothermia, and elevated liver enzymes (to be avoided in liver disease).
* **Chlorpromazine** is an antipyretic through both a central hypothalamic and a peripheral vasodilatory effect. Surface cooling potentiates the effect of chlorpromazine and may result in hypothermia and postural hypotension.

10.6.5
Steroid Antipyresis

Steroids have an antipyretic effect, and patients receiving long-term steroids may have either no fever or a reduced fever in response to infection. Usually, fever suppression lasts about 3 days following withdrawal of steroids. The effect is due to reduced production of interleukin-1 (IL-1) by macrophage, causing the following:

* Blunted acute-phase responses with ongoing infections
* Suppression of lymphocyte activity and local inflammatory response
* Inhibition of prostaglandin release

10.7
Combining Antipyretics

In recent years, it has become a common practice to combine the two antipyretics paracetamol and ibuprofen to treat febrile children in hospital and at home. This practice is discouraged (Table 10.13) [18].

10.8
Physical Treatment

Physical methods used to lower body temperature include:

* **Bed rest:** Intense physical activity can increase body temperature in febrile and afebrile individuals. However, the movement of a febrile child during normal activity is usually not intense enough to do that. It is the general impression of many pediatricians that febrile children who are not resting in bed recover as quickly as children who rest in bed. Therefore, enforcing bed rest in febrile children is not only ineffective but may be undesirable and psychologically harmful. In one controlled study of 1,082 febrile children, bed rest was not found to have a significant effect on temperature reduction [19].
* **Alcohol sponging** using either 70% ethyl alcohol or 70% isopropyl alcohol in water is an effective method for reducing fever, and may be superior to sponging with tepid water. Alcohol inhalation during sponging can induce hypoglycemia and coma. This method is contraindicated.
* **Tepid sponging:** Tepid is the only recommended water temperature for sponging. The use of tepid sponging for febrile children is unnecessary because of the availability of antipyretic drugs, which are simpler to use, more effective in reducing body temperature, and cause less discomfort to children. Furthermore, in treating fever vigorously by

Table 10.13 Combining antipyretics: key points

Paracetamol is frequently used in an alternating manner with ibuprofen for the treatment of febrile children. This practice is not recommended because of the following:
• There is presently no scientific evidence in support of this practice.
• There is no evidence that a greater antipyretic effect influences the underlying disease or duration of fever.
• It may suggest to the parents that fever is a grave situation.

combining an antipyretic drug with physical methods, parents may be given the impression that fever is harmful and antipyresis is beneficial. The scientific evidence does not support this practice. When doctors and parents feel that sponging is necessary (e.g., high body temperature >40°C, which is not responding to antipyretic medications), it is important to use it after administering antipyretic medication to ensure lowering of the hypothalamic set point.

• Using cool or cold sponging is contraindicated. This opposes the physiologically raised set point of the thermoregulatory center of the hypothalamus, which causes shivering leading to a rise of body temperature. Cold sponging causes vasoconstriction, which raises body temperature. Furthermore, the cold sponging is uncomfortable to the child.

• Total body surface cooling: Several methods have been used for total body surface cooling, including cooling blanket, ice packs, air conditioner, and circulating ultrasonic humidifier. These methods are primarily indicated to treat patients with hyperthermia (Chap. 2).

10.9
Management of Fever in Hospital

10.9.1
Assessing a Febrile Child

A febrile child may present either with localized signs of infection (fever with a source), fever without localizing signs (found in 20% of all febrile children), or rarely with fever of unknown origin. This classification is clinically useful since each has common causes. For example, an upper respiratory tract infection is the most common cause of fever with localized signs while urinary tract infection is the most common bacterial cause in febrile children without localizing signs (see for details Chap. 1).

Management should include taking history, performing physical examination and laboratory investigation:

• History, focusing on:

  - Onset, duration, and the degree of fever recorded at home
  - Presence of similar symptoms in other family members
  - Pattern of feeding, degree of activity, playfulness at home
  - Preexisting disease
  - Previous administration of antibiotics

• Physical examination, which is performed in two parts:

  - Observation of items to predict serious bacterial infection (Table 10.14). These items, combined with a history and physical examination, can identify most serious diseases in children.
  - Physical examination, looking particularly for a focus to explain the fever.

Table 10.14 Observation scale to differentiate between febrile ill and well children

Observation item	Signs not suggestive of a serious illness (e.g., viral illness)	Signs suggestive of a serious illness (e.g., serious bacterial infections)
Cry:	Strong	Weak and moaning
Stimulation:	Content	Continual cry, hardly respond
Alertness:	Alert, slightly drowsy	Falls asleep, difficult to arouse
Color:	Pink	Pale, mottled, ashen
Breathing:	Normal	Tachypnea, grunting
Response:	Smile	No smile, face dull or anxious
Playfulness:	Play	No
Feeding:	Well	Not interested
Eye contact:	Present	Absent

- Investigation, taking into consideration that:
  - In a child with localized signs of infection, investigation should be minimal and focus on a diagnostic test most likely to provide a diagnosis.
  - Screening tests include full blood cell count (FBC), looking particularly at the WBC count, CRP, and urine dipsticks.
  - In small children, chest auscultation is unreliable and chest X-ray is usually necessary to diagnose pneumonia.
  - Blood culture is essential in an ill child without a focus of infection.
  - Pulse oximetry is a mandatory test for any ill child.

The ultimate goal of assessing a febrile child is to identify the child with serious bacterial infection so that appropriate antibiotics may commence to treat the infection (see later).

10.9.2
Measurement of Body Temperature

Measurement of temperature (see also Chap. 4) is an essential part of the routine examination for all patients attending the A & E department and GP surgery. Disagreement still exists as to the best thermometer and anatomical site for temperature measurement.

An ideal thermometer should have the following characteristics:

1. Accuracy, i.e., a reliable thermometer for predicting fever and reflecting core body temperature, in various age groups
2. Easy and convenient usage by patient and practitioner
3. Short duration of temperature measurement
4. Comfort and avoidance of embarrassment
5. No cross infection
6. Not influenced by ambient temperature
7. High safety factor
8. Low cost and cost effectiveness

Most hospitals and GP surgeries use the electronic thermometer, which has replaced mercury in glass thermometer. The major advantages of these electronic devices are their rapid response and the ease in reading the digital measurement. One question that still exists is the choice of anatomical site for the temperature measurement by the electronic thermometer: axillary (AT), rectal (RT), or sublingual = oral temperature (OT).

* There is universal agreement that AT is inaccurate and insensitive when compared with any core temperature (that is from the pulmonary artery, esophagus, or bladder) with the exception of afebrile neonates in neonatal units where the environmental temperature and humidity are maintained at optimum levels. A systematic review of 20 studies comprising 3,201 children confirmed the inaccuracy of AT [20].
* RT measurement is more accurate than axillary measurement. However, the procedure is frightening for small children and may be psychologically harmful for older children. In addition, it is time-consuming, requiring often a private room, undressing, and the attendance of a nurse. It may rarely cause rectal perforation. RT is reliable only if the body is in thermal balance and reacts slowly to changes in temperature. RT is contraindicated in certain children, such as neutropenic oncology or HIV-infected patients.
* The OT is not used in children less than 5 years of age and this is the group with the highest incidence of fever.
* There are many potential benefits to infrared ear thermometry (IRET). The technique is fast and easy to use without risk of cross-infection and is not influenced by environmental temperature. A reduction in the numbers involved in a nosocomial outbreak of vancomycin-resistant enterococcus and *clostridium difficile* infection has been achieved by replacing rectal and oral thermometers with tympanic membrane thermometers [21]. The use of tympanic thermometers saves nursing time and is therefore cost effective. In recent years, tympanic thermometers have become very popular both with health professionals and at home. In the USA, 65% of pediatricians and 64% of family practice physicians regularly use IRET [22].

In conclusion, an ideal thermometer involves a combination of the best instrument and most appropriate site. Tympanic thermometry appears to offer such a combination as it provides an accurate assessment of core body temperature in about 2 s. In addition, this technique is clean, safe, and cost effective.

10.9.3
When Should a Febrile Child be Admitted to Hospital?

Febrile children should be considered for hospital admission if:

* They are neonates (less than 28 days).
* They appear toxic or ill looking (irritability, inconsolable crying, lethargy).
* There is a history of PUO or prolonged fever.
* Serious bacterial infection (SBI) is suspected or present.
* They present with bloody diarrhea, increased abdominal tenderness, or drowsiness.
* There are associated skin petechiae.

- An infant has fever $>40°C$, particularly $>40°C$ without a focus.
- The child has his/her first febrile seizure (FS).
- There is tachypnea, grunting, rash, headaches, or vomiting.
- Parents appear unreliable and follow-up is not assured.
- They have significant risk factors such as immunodeficiency or SCA.
- They have abnormal laboratory results such as WBC $>20,000$, or high CRP.
- The patient is a young child with urinalysis suggestive of UTI.

Febrile children may be sent home provided that:

- They appear well and playful.
- A urine sample has been sent for culture or urine dipsticks are negative for nitrate and WBC.
- A follow-up appointment is arranged within 24–48 h if fever persists.
- Parents are informed that children should return if condition worsens.

Children with fever usually do not require antibiotics. Children with suspected or confirmed SBI, or with abnormally high WBC or CRP and who appear well, can be managed with IV or IM Ceftriaxone. A follow-up in 24 h should be arranged.

10.9.4
When to Use Antipyretics?

Antipyretics may be indicated as a matter of routine in the following conditions:

- Symptomatic fever with pain, discomfort, delirium, excessive lethargy. Antipyretics serve here to improve the child's well-being, allowing the child to take fluid and reduce parental anxiety.
- Children with bronchiolitis: A study has shown that the presence of fever did not benefit children admitted with bronchiolitis [23].
- In situations associated with limited energy supply or increased metabolic rate (e.g., burn, cardiovascular and pulmonary diseases, prolonged febrile illness, young children, undernourishment, and postoperative state): Fever can increase the metabolic rate and could exert a harmful effect on the disease.
- High fever ($>40°C$) for the following reasons:

  - Children with this high degree of fever are likely to be symptomatic.
  - With the exception of a few diseases such as Salmonella gastroenteritis and febrile seizures mentioned earlier, there has been no scientific evidence that high fever is beneficial.
  - The overwhelming and prevailing view among physicians and parents is that high fever in particular is harmful and omission of antipyretics therefore seems unethical.

When not to use antipyretics:

- A child who does not have one of the aforementioned conditions, that is a child who is well with minimal symptoms despite the fever. This constitutes a substantial proportion group of febrile children.

- Physical measures such as a fan or tepid sponging are discouraged. These are unnecessary and unpleasant for the child. Rather keep the room cool and open the window.

10.9.5
Proposed Guidelines for the Use of Antibiotics

Antibiotics are indicated for febrile children in the following indications:

- All children with a focus of infection suggestive of a bacterial disease.
- All neonates and ill-looking children (see the observation scale in Table 10.14).
- Children with high fever >40°C and less than 36 months of age who have no focus of infection may receive Ceftriaxone while waiting for culture results.
- Children without focus of infection whose screening tests (FBC, CRP, urine dipsticks) are abnormal.

10.10
Management of Fever at Home

10.10.1
Temperature Measurement

Parents use body temperature to determine their child's state of health. When their child is ill they like to know their temperature and use touch and thermometers to determine fever [24]. Although parents take temperatures regularly many are unable to either accurately take a temperature or read a thermometer (30–46%) [25–27]. Despite this, parents initiate activities to reduce fever based on incorrect readings and sometimes normal temperature [28]. Parents judge how their child must feel by how they themselves feel when they have a similar temperature. This is inaccurate as children have higher body temperatures than adults; body temperature does not stabilize to adult levels until puberty [29].

It is unnecessary to monitor frequently the child's temperature, and parents must be advised against this. Daily temperature checking, preferably in the morning, is sufficient to determine continuation of fever [30]. However, when children feel very hot or are miserable, it is advisable to take temperatures more frequently. An incorrectly high temperature measurement leads to unnecessary antipyretic use. Another unfortunate aspect of depending on temperature assessment is that parents might not seek medical assistance for a lethargic, toxic child with a low-temperature reading.

Parents must be informed about circadian influences on body temperature and to not be overly concerned by a slight rise in temperature late afternoon and early evening, which can be as high as 1°C [31–33]. Health professionals must provide accurate, consistent advice about temperature taking and assist parents to accurately take their child's temperature with the thermometer they use at home.

10

10.10.2
Assessing a Febrile Child

Parents are alerted to the possibility that their child may be febrile by the following:

- Changes in the child's normal behavior: Over time, parents learn to recognize their own child's fever-specific behavior and will touch the child to see if they are *hot*; if so, most parents take the child's temperature.
- The child being often flushed, refusing food and fluids, and not sleeping well.

Guidelines for parents' assessment of their child have been developed by the National Collaborating Centre for Women's and Children's Health [34] and include the child's:

- Skin color: does the child have normal color of the skin, lips, and tongue; or does the child look pale or is the child's skin mottled or ashen?
- Activity levels: are they normal and is the child responding normally to social cues, staying awake, or able to be wakened easily; does the child have a strong normal cry; or is the child not responding normally to social cues, needing prolonged stimulation to awaken the child, listless and lethargic with reduced activity levels?
- Respiratory rate: are there signs of nasal flaring, tachypnea; is the respiratory rate normal for the child; is there evidence of grunting; can they see moderate or severe drawing in of the chest?
- Hydration: do the child's skin, eyes, and moist mucous membranes appear normal or do the mucous membranes look dry; in infants, are they feeding normally or poorly; is there a reduction in urine output or skin turgor; or is there bile-stained vomiting?
- Fever: have they had a fever for more than 5 days; are they younger than 3 months and have a temperature of 38.0°C or greater; or are they between 3 and 6 months and have a temperature of 39.0°C or greater?
- Joints: is there swelling of a limb or joint; is the child not weight-bearing on a limb or not using an extremity; or is there a new lump?
- Other signs: does the child have a nonblanching rash, bulging fontanel, neck stiffness, fits; or does the child have any focal neurological signs?

10.10.3
Antipyretic Measures

The administration of the common medications used as antipyretic and analgesic, paracetamol and ibuprofen, leads to a reduction in discomfort and temperature in a febrile child. This can cause confusion about the role of analgesics/antipyretics and support beliefs that reduction of fever may reduce the severity of the illness [35–37]. Although professionals may report positive attitudes about the benefits of fever, continuing education in fever management is needed to change the uninform practice of antipyretic overuse [38, 39].

Antipyretics are parents' preferred method of managing fever, and there has been an increase in this preference over the past two decades from 67% to more than 90% (91–95%) [40, 41]. Of concern for health professionals is that similar to temperature-taking parents' antipyretic administration is often incorrect both in dose or frequency [42, 43]. Underdosing increases health service usage and encourages alternating antipyretics to maintain normal temperature. Overdosing is potentially harmful.

Many parents expect antipyretics to normalize fever and prevent its recurrence. As antipyretics does nor normalize body temperature or prevent recurrences of fever, parents' concerns increase leading to increased antipyretic use, including alternating antipyretics, and increased health service use. Alternating antipyretics is an increasingly common practice with parents. Reports suggest that this practice has risen from 27% in 2001 to between 52 and 67% in 2007 [44]. Parents alternate the drugs in order to prevent overdosing or unwanted side effects from one antipyretic; some considered this safer than monotherapy. On the other hand, despite relying on antipyretics to reduce fever, many parents (73%) believe that antipyretics can cause harm such as liver and kidney damage, unconsciousness or death and stomach irritation [41]. The continued use of antipyretics even though parents believe that they may be harmful highlights parental concern about fever and the need to control it.

Many health professionals recommend that parents alternate antipyretics although:

* There is lack of evidence of the safety of this practice.
* The practice can increase parents' fever phobia.
* It also increases the risk of incorrect dosing, which is more likely with ibuprofen than paracetamol.
* It increases parental preoccupation with the height of the fever and the need to control it to prevent adverse events. It increases their fears, which in turn increase antipyretic and health service use.

Recognition of the need for caution in advising parents to alternate antipyretic is readily available [33]. This practice should only be considered on an individual basis following advice from a health professional who provides parents with written instructions indicating antipyretic preparations, doses, and frequency of administration. Alternating is not recommended as routine practice [45, 46].

Parents need to understand that all drugs, including antipyretics, have potentially noxious side effects. Those reporting adverse events following ibuprofen administration are fewer as it is a newer drug [47–49]. However, ibuprofen has been reported to be associated with more adverse drug reactions than paracetamol (10:6); it is not recommended as a first-line treatment [50]. There is an urgent need for parents to realize the need for accuracy and caution with the use of these drugs despite their ready availability in many stores. The use of antipyretics and advice about their use should always be directed by competent health professionals [51, 52].

10.10.4
When to Contact the GP?

Fever remains a common factor influencing parents to seek medical advice. The overuse of health services for self-limiting viral infections has been the impetus for early fever-management education interventions [53–55]. To ensure that parents seek medical advice it is important that physicians educate them about the following:

10

- Beneficial effects of fever
- Thermoregulation, in particular that fever is well controlled, does not climb up relent-lessly and does not damage the brain
- Benign nature of febrile seizures and that antipyretics can not prevent them
- Rational use of antipyretics and that they are not always needed for fever
- Higher rate of febrile episodes in children compared with adults

Parents should seek medical advice immediately when the child is:

- Younger than 3 months, unless following DPT immunization
- Fever is 40.5°C (105°F) or higher
- Crying inconsolably or whimpering
- Difficult to waken
- Cries when touched
- Has a stiff neck
- Suffers from severe headache, neck stiffness, or light hurts their eyes
- Purple spots are present on the skin
- Having trouble in breathing, even after the nose is cleared
- Unable to swallow, and drooling saliva
- Looks or acts very sick
- Looks *sick*, pale, lethargic, or weak

Call the doctor in the next 24 h if your child:

- Has fever in the range 40–40.5°C (104°–105°F) especially if the child is younger than 2 years
- Complaints of burning or pain on urination
- Has had a fever for more than 24 h without an obvious source or location of infection
- Refuses to drink
- Persistently vomits
- Has pain
- Shows no improvement in 48 h
- Continues with fever and is under 6 months of age
- Shows signs of drowsiness

Call the doctor during office hours if the child:

- Has been febrile for more than 72 h
- Had a fever that went away for 24 h or more and has returned
- Has a history of febrile convulsions
- You have any other concerns or questions

10.11
Fever Phobia and Its Management

Fever, a common occurrence in childhood, is a frightening experience for parents. They believe that fever is harmful and brings about febrile convulsions, brain damage, death, dehy-dration, and discomfort and therefore must be controlled. Concerns have changed over time:

- In the 1980s, parents were more concerned about brain damage (38–46%) than febrile seizures (FS) (15–39%) [56].
- Twenty years later, although still concerned about brain damage (21–53%), parents are more concerned about FS (32–70%) [57].
- More parents awaken a sleeping febrile child for administration of antipyretics (66–92% vs. 48–53%, respectively, in 1980) [58, 59].

These concerns reflect parents' fever phobia. Some health professionals contribute to parents' fever phobia through the following:

- Continuing reports of febrile convulsions and brain damage [2, 36]
- Recommendation of regular antipyretics, even alternating antipyretics, despite evidence that fever is not harmful and antipyretics do not prevent febrile convulsions [8, 60–63]
- Unnecessarily advising to reduce fever [64]
- Distributing conflicting information from doctors about illness severity and their proposed management, which increases parents' uncertainty about how to care best for their febrile child [65]

To address parents' fever phobia, health professionals must update their own knowledge about fever and consistently advise parents to do the following:

- Manage fever in an evidence-based manner
- Manage their febrile children at home including careful observation of the child's interaction with the environment and response to fever
- Prevent dehydration by encouraging fluids, i.e., small, frequent drinks of clear liquid, e.g., water or diluted juice
- Reduce distressing symptoms such as pain and discomfort with recommended doses of analgesics [66, 67]
- Observe the child closely, focusing on the child's well-being rather than temperature
- Maintain an awareness that mild to moderate fever is beneficial and supports the immune system
- Make the child comfortable, dressing them in light clothing, not overdressing
- Provide a light blanket for children who are cold or shivering
- Selectively reduce fever with medications when fever is:

  - Greater than 39.0°C and associated with discomfort
  - 40°C or higher, and
  - In all children who are irritable, miserable, or appear to be in pain

- Accurately medicate their child as follows for children up to 6 years:

  - Paracetamol: 15 mg kg^{-1} every 4 h up to four times a day.
  - Ibuprofen, always administered with food or milk: check labeling as dosage is age-related until 2 years (ibuprofen is not recommended for all children, check the recommendations for your country), then 10 mg kg^{-1} 3–4 times a day.
  - Aspirin should be avoided.

- Do not continue giving regular medication for more than 48 h without having your child assessed by a doctor.

10

References

1. Lekstrom JA, Bell WR. Aspirin in the prevention of thrombosis. Medicine 1991; 70: 161–178
2. May A, Bauchner H. Fever phobia: the pediatrician's contribution. Pediatrics 1992; 90: 851–854
3. Kramer MS, Naimark L, Leduc DG. Parental fever phobia and its correlates. Pediatrics 1985; 75: 1110–1113
4. Nelson KB, Ellenberg JH. Prognosis in children with febrile seizures. Pediatrics 1978; 61: 720–727
5. Verity CM, Golding J. Risk of epilepsy after febrile convulsions: a national cohort study. Br Med J 1991; 303: 1373–1376
6. El-Radhi AS. Lower degree of fever is associated with increased risk of subsequent convulsions. Eur J Paediatr Neurol 1998; 2: 91–96
7. Offringa M, Derksen-Lubsen G, Bossuyt P. Seizure recurrence after a first febrile seizure: a multivariate approach. Dev Med Child Neurol 1992; 34: 15–24
8. El-Radhi AS, Barry W. Do antipyretics prevent febrile convulsions? Arch Dis Child 2003; 88: 641–642
9. Small PM, Taeuber MG, Hackbarth CJ, et al. Influence of body temperature on bacterial growth rates on experimental Streptococcus pneumoniae meningitis in rabbits. Infect Immun 1986; 52: 484–487
10. Osawa E, Muschel LH. Studies relating to the serum resistance of certain gram-negative bacteria. J Exp Med 1964; 119: 41–51
11. El-Radhi AS, Rostila T, Vesikari T. Association of high fever and short bacterial excretion after salmonellosis. Arch Dis Child 1992; 67: 531–532
12. Bernheim HA, Kluger MJ. Fever: effect of drug-induced antipyresis on survival. Science 1976; 193: 237–239
13. Sugimura T, Fujimoto T, Motoyama T, et al. Risks of antipyretics in young children with fever due to infectious diseases. Acta Paediatr Jpn 1994; 36: 375–378
14. Lwoff A. Factors influencing the evolution of viral diseases of the cellular level and in the organism. Bacteriol Rev 1959; 23: 109–124
15. Nourjah P, Ahmad SR, Karwoski C, et al. Estimates of acetaminophen (paracetamol) associated overdoses in the US. Pharmacoepidemiol Drug Saf 2006; 15: 398–405
16. Lands LC, Milner R, Cantin AM, et al. High- dose ibuprofen in cystic fibrosis. Canadian safety and effectiveness trial. J Pediatr 2007; 151: 249–254
17. Moore N, Noblet C, Breemeersch C. Focus on the safety of ibuprofen at the analgesic-antipyretic dose. Therapy 1996; 51: 458–463
18. Mayoral CE, Marino RV, Rosenfeld W, et al. Alternating antipyretics: is this an alternative? Pediatrics 2000; 105: 1009–1012
19. Gibson JP. How much bed rest is necessary for children with fever? J Pediatr 1958; 54: 256–261
20. Craig JV, Lancaster GA, Williamson PR, et al. Temperature measured at the axilla compared with rectum in children and young people: systemic review. Br Med J 2000; 320: 1174–1178
21. Brooks S, Khan A, Stoica D, et al. Reduction of vancomycin-resistant Enterococcus and Clostridium difficile infections following change to tympanic thermometers. Infect Control Hosp Epidem 1998; 19: 333–336
22. Silverman BG, Daley WR, Rubin JD. The use of infrared ear thermometers in pediatric and family practice offices. Public Health Rep 1998; 113: 268–272
23. El-Radhi AS, Barry W, Patel S. Association of fever and severe clinical course in bronchiolitis. Arch Dis Child 1999; 81: 231–234

24. Walsh AM, Edwards HE, Fraser JA. Influences on parents' fever management: beliefs, experiences and information sources. J Clin Nurs 2007; doi: 10.1111/j.1365–2702.2006.01890.x
25. Fischer H, Moore K, Roaman RR. Can mothers of infants read a thermometer? Clin Pediatr 1985; 24: 120
26. Porter RS, Wenger FG. Diagnosis and treatment of pediatric fever by caretakers. J Emerg Med 2000; 19(1): 1–4
27. Taveras EM, Durousseau S, Flores G. Parents' beliefs and practices regarding childhood fever - A study of a multiethnic socioeconomically diverse sample of parents. Pediatr Emerg Care 2004; 20(9): 579–587
28. Crocetti M, Moghbeli N, Serwint J. Fever phobia revisited: have parental misconceptions about fever changed in 20 years? Pediatrics 2001; 107(8): 1241–1246
29. Lorin MI. Pathogenesis of fever and its treatment. In: McMillan JB, DeAngelis C, Feigin RD, Warshaw JB (Eds). Oski's Pediatrics: Principles and Practices. Philadelphia: Lippincott, 1999. pp. 848–850
30. Schmitt BD. Fever in childhood. Pediatrics 1984; 74(Suppl): 929–936
31. Brandon SL, Phyllis CZ. Circadian rhythm sleep disorder. Chest 2006; 130: 1915–1923
32. Samples JF. Circadian rhythm: basis for screening fever. Nurs Res 1985; 34: 377–379
33. Waterhouse J, Drust B, Weinert D, et al. The circadian rhythm of core temperature: origin and some implications for exercise performance. Chronobiol Intern 2005; 22(2): 207–225
34. National Collaborating Centre for Women's and Children's Health. Feverish illness in children. Royal College of Obstetricians and Gynaecologists (RCOG Press), UK, 2007
35. Karwowska A, Nijssen-Jordan C, Johnson D, et al. Parental and health care provider understanding of childhood fever: a Canadian perspective. Can J Emerg Med 2002; 4(6): 394–400
36. Walsh AM, Edwards HE, Courtney MD, et al. Fever management: paediatric nurses' knowledge, attitudes and influencing factors. J Adv Nurs 2005; 49(5): 453–464
37. Lagerlov P, Helseth S, Holager T. Childhood illnesses and the use of paracetamol (acetaminophen): a qualitative study of parents' management of common childhood illnesses. Fam Pract 2003; 20(6): 717–723
38. Isaacs SN, Axelrod PI, Lorber B. Antipyretic orders in a university hospital. Am J Med 1990; 82: 580–586
39. Mackowiak PA. Diagnostic implications and clinical consequences of antipyretic therapy. Clin Infect Dis 2000; 31: S230-S33
40. Schmitt BD. Fever phobia: misconceptions of parents about fevers. Am J Dis Child 1980; 134(2): 176–81
41. Walsh A, Edwards H, Fraser J. Over-the-counter medication use for childhood fever: a cross-sectional study of Australian parents. J Paediatr Child Health 2007; doi:10.1111/j.1440–1754.2007.01161.x
42. Goldman RD, K0 K, Linett LJ, et al. Antipyretic efficacy and safety of ibuprofen and acetaminophen in children. Ann Pharmacother 2004; 38(1): 146–150
43. Li SF, Lacher B, Crain EF. Acetaminophen and ibuprofen dosing by parents. Pediatr Emerg Care 2000; 16(6): 394–397
44. Wright AD, Liebelt EL. Alternating antipyretics for fever reduction in children: an unfounded practice passed down to parents from pediatricians. Clin Pediatr 2007; 46: 146–150
45. Schmitt BD. Concerns over alternating acetaminophen and ibuprofen for fever. Arch Pediatr Adol Med 2006; 160: 197–202
46. Goldman RD. Alternating ibuprofen and acetaminophen may be more effective in the treatment of fever in children. J Pediatr 2006; 149: 140–141

47. Lesko SM, Mitchell AA. An assessment of the safety of pediatric ibuprofen: a practitioner-based randomized clinical trial. J Am Med Assoc 1995; 273(12): 929–133

48. Lesko SM, Mitchell AA. The safety of acetaminophen and ibuprofen among children younger than two years old. Pediatrics 1999; 104: e39

49. Anderson BJ. Comparing the efficacy of NSAIDs and paracetamol in children. Paediatr Anaesth 2004; 14: 201–217

50. Titchen T, Cranswick N, Beggs S. Adverse drug reactions to nonsteroidal anti-inflammatory drugs, COX-2 inhibitors and paracetamol in a paediatric hospital. Br J Clin Pharmacol 2005; 59: 718–723

51. Blatteis CM. Endotoxic fever: new concepts of its regulation suggest new approaches to its management. Pharmacol Therapeut 2006; 111: 194–223

52. Mackowiak PA. Temperature regulation and the pathogenesis of fever. In: Mandell GL, Bennett JE, Dolin R (Eds). Principles and Practices of Infectious Diseases. Philadelphia: Curchill Livingstone, 2000. pp. 604–622

53. Casey R, McMahon F, McCormick MC, et al. Fever therapy: an educational intervention for parents. Pediatrics 1984; 73: 600–605

54. Robinson JS, Schwartz M, Magwene KS, et al. The impact of fever education on clinic utilization. Am J Dis Child 1989; 143: 698–704

55. Walsh AM, Edwards HE. Management of childhood fever by parents: literature review. J Adv Nurs 2006; 54: 217–27

56. Abdullah MA, Ashong EF, Al Habib SA, et al. Fever in children: diagnosis and management by nurses, medical students, doctors and parents. Ann Trop Paediatr 1987; 7: 194–199

57. Al-Eissa YA, Al-Sanie AM, Al-Alola SA, et al. Parental perceptions of fever in children. Ann Saudi Med 2000; 20: 202–205

58. Kramer MS, Naimark LE, Leduc DG. Parental fever phobia and its correlates. Pediatrics 1985; 75: 1110–1113

59. Al-Eissa YA, Al-Zamil FA, Al-Sanie AM, et al. Home management of fever in children: rational or ritual? Intern J Clin Pract 2000; 54: 138–142

60. Vestergaard M, Basso O, Henriksen TB, et al. Risk factors for febrile convulsions. Epidemiology 2002; 13: 282–287

61. Meremikwu M, Oyo-Ita A. Paracetamol for treating fever in children (Review), Report Art. No.: CD003676. DOI: 10.1002/14651858.CD003676 2002

62. Wright AD, Liebelt EL. Alternating antipyretics for fever reduction in children: an unfounded practice passed down to parents from pediatricians. Clin Pediatr 2007; 46: 146–150

63. Pearce C, Curtis N. Fever in children. Aust Fam Pract 2005; 34: 769–771

64. Schmitt BD. Fever in childhood. Pediatrics 1994; 94: 929–936

65. Walsh AM, Edwards H, Fraser J. parents' childhood fever management: a community survey and instrument development. J Advan Nurs 2008; 63: 376–388

66. Connell F. The causes and treatment of fever: a literature review. Nurs Stand 1997; 12: 40–43

67. McCarthy PL (Ed). Fevers and the Evaluation of the Child with who has Fever. Philadelphia: Saunders, 1999. pp. 157–163

Fever and Complimentary Medicine   11

Core Messages

> CAM = Complimentary medicine (practice used in addition to conventional) and alternative medicine (practice used instead of conventional).
> Practically all human cultures have used some form of CAM.
> CAM aims to treat the patient as a whole; treatment attempts to stimulate the self-healing abilities of body.
> While conventional medicine is largely science-based, CAM is largely based on beliefs. Part of the success may be due to placebo effects.
> More research is needed to determine what practice in CAM is superior to the conventional medicine so that it can be advocated for wider use.
> CAM should be evidence-based and procedures scientifically based.
> Consumers of herbal or homeopathic products are advised to take them only if these are officially licensed, and not for prolonged use. Chinese herbal medicines with complex ingredients are best avoided due to reported side effects.
> There has been little research in CAM on the subject of fever or febrile illness. Trials are needed to assess the effect of herbal antipyretic medicine on the treatment of fever.

11.1
Homeopathy

Homeopathy is considered as a holistic system of medicine that uses highly dilute substances in an attempt to stimulate the body's potential for self-healing. It was developed two centuries ago by the German doctor Samuel Hahnemann, who thought that the side effects of the orthodox drugs were unacceptable. He then began to investigate the healing power of natural remedies. His research was published between 1811 and 1821 in six volumes *Materia*

A.S. El-Radhi et al. (Eds.) *Clinical Manual of Fever in Children.*   251
Doi: 10.1007/978-3-540-78598-9, © Springer-Verlag Berlin Heidelberg 2009

11

Medica Pura. The homeopathic practice is based on the principle that if a symptom picture is correctly matched to its compatible remedy then the patient would be swiftly cured.

The following drugs have been used in homeopathy to treat fever:

- **Belladonna**: It is said to be most beneficial in the first few hours of fever. It can cause hallucination and confusion.
- **Aconitum napellus (monkshood)**: It is poisonous in large quantity.
- **Chamomilla (German Chamomile)**: This agent has been advocated for young children with teething and for older children with prolonged fever. Its main therapeutic use is for digestive disturbance. It can be rubbed into the painful area of the gum.
- **Tanacetum parthenium** (feverfew or wild quinine): This herbal preparation is used as a traditional remedy for migraine and fever.

Homeopathy is one of the most controversial methods of complimentary medicine, mainly because of the high dilution of the substances used. The effect of homeopathy is often considered to be no more than a placebo effect. What is the available scientific evidence?

- When all double-blind trials and/or randomized trials and placebo-controlled trials with homeopathy were studied, the results of the metaanalysis showed that the clinical effect of homeopathy is not completely due to placebo. However, homeopathy was not found to be efficacious for any single clinical condition [1].
- In searching placebo-controlled trials of oscillococcinum for treatment of influenza and fever, this homeopathic medicine was found to slightly reduce the duration of the symptoms [2].
- A placebo-controlled trial in children with recurrent upper respiratory tract infections showed a small but insignificant difference in symptom score in favor of the homeopathic medicines [3].
- In a controlled trial, a homeopathic medicine (Viburcol) was compared with acetaminophen (paracetamol). Viburcol was found as effective as the antipyretic and better tolerated [4].

11.2
Herbal Medicine

Herbal treatment of fevers aims to support the cleansing process initiated by body to increase its resistance.

The following plants are known to reduce body temperature:

- **Feverfew** (*Tanacetum parthenium*) is a perennial aromatic herb, which has been used medicinally for a variety of indications, for example, reduction of fever (hence its name), vasodilatation, sedation, and uterine stimulation. It was well known to ancient Egyptian and Greek physicians. Feverfew appears to exert an inhibitory action on prostaglandin production by preventing its production from arachidonic acid. Its extracts inhibit the release of enzymes from polymorphonuclear leukocytes, hence its effectiveness in the management of arthritis. The extracts are effective in treating and preventing migraine. As an antipyretic, feverfew is currently not in use. Feverfew should not be used in children younger than 2 years of age, and it is contraindicated in pregnancy. It also can cause contact dermatitis and mouth ulceration.

* **White willow bark** (*Salix alba*) was used as an anti-inflammatory and analgesic medicine in ancient Mesopotamia, China, and among native Americans. The white willow is a source of salicin, which was isolated in 1820s and eventually led to the synthesis of aspirin. It has been used as an antipyretic and in rheumatic diseases. It is not recommended in children because of the risk of Reye's syndrome.

* **Anise seed** (*Pimpinella anisum*) is a pleasant-tasting plant, initially native to Egypt, but cultivated in many parts of the world. Anise has anti-inflammatory cytotoxic properties (particularly on colon cancer), and it is used to treat fever, bronchitis, and sore throat. Anise seed is contraindicated in pregnancy.

* **Licorice** (*Glycyrrhiza glabra*) has been used for thousands of years as a treatment for inflammatory conditions through its steroid-like actions. Its strong anti-inflammatory action is utilized to treat pain and fever. Although it is related to steroids, it does not cause gastric or intestinal ulcer. It does not suppress the bone marrow. Prolonged or high dose of licorice may produce mineralocorticoid adverse effects.

* **Ginger** (*Zingiber officinale* roscoe) was used in the Middle East for centuries before it moved to Europe. It has been used for numerous ailments, ranging from dyspepsia, fever, cholera, and malaria. It encourages the body to produce sweat and fight inflammation such as certain types of arthritis. It is currently used for nausea and depression.

* **Yarrow** (*Achillea millefolium*) has an anti-inflammatory action and also a cooling effect in fevers by stimulating sweating. A combination of garlic, ginger, and lemon is considered by herbalists as the classic remedy for flu.

* **Elder flowers** (*Sambucus nigra*) are used in the treatment of many febrile respiratory conditions, particularly those associated with phlegm (colds, flu, bronchitis, and sinusitis). Although these flowers are effective against certain pathogens, such as *Salmonella typhi* and *Vibrio cholerae*, the clinical relevance of this effect is uncertain. The stems must not be used, as they contain cyanide.

11.3
Aromatherapy

Aromatherapy, meaning treatment using scent, is a particular branch of herbal medicine. The ancient Egyptians are generally regarded as the founders of aromatherapy, and aromatic oils were described on papyri from 1500 B.C. The Greeks had a penchant for decorating their heads with fragrant flowers, a form of psychoaromatherapy. Hippocrates advocated daily aromatic bath and scented massage to prolong life. Arab physicians harnessed the power of aromatic oil and floral waters (camphor and rose water) to purify the air and protect themselves from disease. The crusading knights brought these *Arab perfumes* to Europe. The word aromatherapy was first used in 1937 by the French chemist Rene-Maurice Gattefosse. His research revealed that volatile extract distilled from certain aromatic plants had a good effect on the skin. He also found that essential oils applied to the skin could be absorbed into the bloodstream where they interact with the body's chemistry.

Essential oils are volatile, odoriferous liquid components of aromatic plants. At least 150 essential oils have been extracted for use in aromatherapy. Although essential oils can be used as steam inhalation, aromatherapists tend to favor massage as the most effective way of therapy. Because the oils are highly concentrated, they must not be swallowed.

11

Table 11.1 Some essential oils known to reduce fevers

Essential oils	Clinical effects
Eucalyptus (*eucalyptus globules*)	Antiseptic, diuretic, and deodorant (should not be used for small children)
Peppermint (*Mentha piperita*)	Remedy for digestive problems; reduces sweating, thus producing cooling effect on body. It has a stimulant effect, hence not to be used at night
Lemon (*citrus limon*)	Stimulates the body defences to fight infection; diuretic, laxative
Lavender (*lavandula angustifolia*)	Relaxing: useful for irritability and low concentration (e.g., for children with ADHD) insomnia
	Analgesic: for headaches, neuralgia, muscular pain, shingles, rheumatism
	Anti-inflammatory: flu, colds

The aromatic plants are antiseptic (notably eucalyptus), possessing antiviral and antibacterial action. The plants have been shown to reduce body temperature (Table 11.1).

11.4
Safety of Homeopathy, Herbal Medicine, and Aromatherapy

The safety of these three forms of alternative medicine remains a concern. Some products are uncontrolled, as many countries do not recognize them as medicines. Although the toxicity of certain herbal medicines is well recognized, the incidence of such toxicity is unknown [5]. Herbal products should be free from toxic ingredients and contamination, such as residues of pesticides. Some Chinese medicines contain complex ingredients, which have been associated with serious adverse reactions, such as liver damage by *Dictamnus dasycarpus*, and renal failure by *Stephania tetrandra* and *Magnolia officinalis* (both used as slimming products). Although homeopathic medicines may appear to be too dilute to cause toxic effects, they may however contain toxic metals such as arsenic, cadmium, and mercury.

Consumers of these products are advised to take them only if these products are officially licensed and as directed, and not for a prolonged use. Chinese herbal medicines with complex ingredients are best avoided.

11.5
Acupuncture

Acupuncture was established as part of Traditional Chinese Medicine (TCM) since prior to third century B.C.E. [6] The celebrated physician Zhang Zhong Jing (150–219 A.D.) with his *Treatise on Febrile Disease* categorized and outlined treatment for different types of fever as the disease progressed through the body. Although primarily an herbal text, his work provided the theoretical framework for the acupuncture treatment of fevers. Since the Song dynasty (960–1279 AD), pediatrics has been a recognized as subspecialty of TCM recognized with techniques specific to the different clinical realities that children present.

Table 11.2 Outcome of evidence-based medicine applied to various medical conditions, which treated by acupuncture[2]

Conclusively positive	Inconclusive	Conclusively negative
Dental pain	Addiction	Weight loss
Low back pain	Asthma	Smoking cessation
Migraine	Stroke	
Nausea and vomiting	Rheumatic diseases	

Acupuncture is increasingly common in medical practice today, and among adults, there is substantial evidence supporting its effectiveness in treating such conditions as chronic pain and nausea and vomiting. In particular, there is empirical support for the efficacy of acupuncture in treating various conditions of chronic pain affecting particularly the musculoskeletal system (see recent review by Tan et al., 2007) [7]. Acupuncture needling releases various transmitters (endorphins, serotonin, norepinephrine), which inhibit the transmission of pain impulses. Application of the rules of evidence-based medicine to acupuncture proves it to be effective for some conditions and ineffective for others [8] (Table 11.2).

In contrast to the large number of trials on acupuncture in adults there have been relatively few studies in pediatric populations, including only a very small number of trials of acupuncture for pain complaints in children (see Tsao and Zeltzer, 2005) [9]. There is a conventional view that children are afraid of needles, and for this reason, clinicians may hesitate to recommend acupuncture because of concerns regarding its acceptability [10]. However, there is also evidence that at least among children in chronic pain acupuncture treatment is highly acceptable [11].

Despite the lack of scientific evidence on the treatment of pediatric fevers with acupuncture, there continues to be a rich tradition and abundant empirical evidence for the treatment of such conditions. This tradition includes the recognition that fevers are caused by *external pernicious influences*, what we now call viruses or bacteria, and the interplay between these influences and the constitution of the patient determines the kind of treatment that is applied [12]. Fever causes marked release of pyrogenic cytokines IL-6 and TNF-alpha (Chap. 3). Although electroacupuncture in rats has demonstrated a reduction of hypothalamic production of proinflammatory cytokines, including prostaglandin-E2, IL-6, IL-1 beta mRNAs levels, acupuncture is not usually used clinically to decrease body temperature.

Acupuncture has proved to be very safe and adverse events are extremely rare [13]. Serious adverse events have been estimated to be 0.05 per 10,000 treatments [14]. The most common serious adverse events are hepatitis B and C and HIV infection. It is advisable to ensure that the practitioner is familiar with the treatment of children and uses disposable needles.

11.6
Reflexology

This is a holistic, noninvasive technique aimed to treat imbalances within the body. It is based on the principle that all parts of the body are interdependent and that the body has to maintain a state of balance for optimum energy flow and health. This balance is achieved by applying pressure on certain points (on the feet, hands, and ears) that correspond to every organ and

11

gland of the body. By exerting pressure on these *reflex points* one can stimulate or sedate the nerve pathways linking these points to the corresponding organs. The treatment is said to stimulate the normal function of the organ involved to secrete hormone or enzyme.

Reflex areas, which may be used to treat fevers are:

- Pituitary gland reflex area (hypothalamic/pituitary point) situated in the centre of the great toe: This area is thought to control the autonomic functions as well as the regulation of body temperature.
- Facial reflex area located in the first three toes of each foot: This area is also recommended for teething troubles accompanied by fever.
- Top of the ear: This area is thought to be ideal for any inflammatory condition or fever. It is said to have a soothing and analgesic effect on the body.

11.7
Massage

For thousands of years, massage has been used to heal and to soothe the sick. Ancient Chinese and Indian texts describe various massage techniques. Greek and Roman physicians used massage as one of the principal means of relieving pain. Hippocrates wrote, "The physician must be experienced in many things, but assuredly in rubbing." Massage was almost forgotten during the Middle Ages, but was revived in the sixteenth century by the French doctor Ambroise Pare, and later at the beginning of the nineteenth century by a Swede Per Henrik Ling (1776–1839).

Massage will not calm a fever. It is not recommended for febrile illness, and it is contraindicated with high fever.

11.8
Shiatsu

Shiatsu means *finger pressure* in Japanese, and it combines massage and acupuncture without the use of needles. It originated in China between 2000 and 3000 B.C. and was later adopted by the Japanese. It is practiced through a layer of clothing, in contrast to most types of massage.

This method is based on traditional Oriental philosophy and medicine, which believes that everything in existence is a manifestation of energy. The universal energy, called Ki, is required to flow around the human body smoothly in order to maintain optimum health and prevent diseases. Shiatsu practitioners believe that that the body has 12 energy channels (or meridians). Pressure on certain points along these meridian channels is to *unlock energy from being impeded*. Certain points are believed to treat fevers, including the following:

- The end of the elbow flexure (also help to treat cough, sore throat)
- Between the seventh cervical and first thoracic vertebra (also help to treat cold, asthma, and headaches)

11.9
Chiropractic

Chiropractic (meaning *done by hand*) was founded in 1895 and is based on the belief that the body has an inherent ability for self-healing if nerve impulses are allowed to travel freely between the brain and the rest of the body. This is usually performed by manipulation of the spine. A variety of physiotherapy exercises are used to help relax muscles before manual adjustment is made.

11.10
Osteopathy

This method of healing teaches and practices the following:

*   The body is a unit that functions as such.
*   The body has its own self-protecting and self-regulating mechanisms.
*   Structure and function are reciprocally interrelated.

Diseases according to osteopathy are chiefly due to loss of structural integrity, which can be restored to harmony or equilibrium by manipulation. Practitioners focus on history, observation, and palpation. The later involves tissue tone, texture, temperature, and moisture. This is followed by manipulation and thrust, such as high-velocity, low-amplitude, and muscle energy techniques, which have been the mainstay of osteopathic treatment. Although diseases affecting the musculoskeletal system are the main reasons to use this form of treatment, symptoms such as fever are also targeted. Osteopathy may include treatment of nutrition, occupational therapy and physiotherapy, psychotherapy, various types of medicines, and spiritual support.

11.11
Spiritual Healing

Spiritual healing is the oldest practiced therapy used in some forms in every culture. It is defined as a purposeful intervention by one or more persons aiming to help others by means of focused intention, touch, religious direction, or intercessory prayer, without the use of conventional physical or chemical therapy. Spiritual healing is not recommended by medical professionals as an alternative to conventional treatment. However, many support its supplemental usage. In many instances, it has been used as a last resort treatment when conventional treatment has had little or no effect.

Practitioners of this method believe that they can penetrate the body through energies that surround the body. Emotional disorders, such as anxiety and depression, often respond to spiritual healing. A literature search to identify studies published between 1999 and 2003 describing the effect of religion on health outcomes showed that religious intervention

11

such as intercessory prayer decreases the duration of fever in patients with sepsis and the length of hospital stay as well as improves the success rate in in-vitro fertilization [15].

References

Homeopathy

1. Linde K, Clausius N, Ramirez G, et al. Are the clinical effects of homeopathy placebo effects? A meta-analysis of placebo-controlled trials. Lancet 1997; 350: 834–43
2. The Cochrane Library 2006; no. 1 (CD001957)
3. de Lange de Klerk ESM, Blommers J, Kuik DJ, et al. Effect of homeopathy on daily burden of symptoms in children with recurrent upper respiratory tract infections. Br Med J 1994; 309: 1329–32
4. Derasse M, Klein P, Weiser M. The effects of a complex homeopathic medicine compared with acetaminophen in the symptomatic treatment of acute febrile infections in children. Explore (NY) 2005; 1: 33–9
5. Choonara I. Safety of herbal medicines in children. Arch Dis Child 2003; 88: 1032–33

Acupuncture

6. Kan-Wen Ma. Acupuncture; its place in the history of Chinese medicine. Acupunct Med 2000; 18: 88–99
7. Tan G, Craine MH, Bair MJ, et al. (2007). Efficacy of complementary and alternative medicine (CAM) interventions for chronic pain. J Rehabil Res Dev 2007; 44: 195–222.
8. Ernst E. An evidence-based approach to acupuncture. Acupunct Med 1999; 17: 59–61
9. Tsao, JCI., Zeltzer, LK. Complementary and alternative medicine approaches for pediatric pain: A review of the state-of-the-science. Evid based Complement Alternat Med 2005; 2: 149–59
10. Kemper KJ, Sarah R, Silver-Highfield E, et al. On pins and needles? Pediatric pain patients' experience with acupuncture. Pediatrics 2000; 105(4, Part 2): 941–7
11. Zeltzer LK, Tsao JCI, Stelling C, et al. A Phase I study on the feasibility of an acupuncture/hypnotherapy intervention for chronic pediatric pain. J Pain Symptom Manage 2002; 24: 437–46
12. Scott J, Barlow T. (1999) Acupuncture in the Treatment of Children, 3rd Edition. Eastland Press, CA
13. Rampes H. (1998). Adverse reactions to acupuncture, in *Medical Acupuncture: A Western Scientific Approach*, Filshie J, White A. Eds., Churchill Livingstone, Oxford, UK, p. 375
14. White A. Acupuncture in medicine. Acupunct Med 2004; 22: 122–33

Spiritual Healing

15. Coruh B, Ayele H, Pugh M, et al. Does religion activity improve health outcomes? A critical review of recent literature. Explore (NY) 2005; 1(3): 186–91

Core Messages

> Establishing a diagnosis from several clinical presentations is a common challenge in paediatrics that needs knowledge and experience to solve. This chapter provides clinicians with a guide to clinical and laboratory means to reach a diagnosis of the most common febrile diseases.

> Infection is the most likely diagnosis in a child with fever, where the fever is usually of short duration and is associated with a focus in about three quarters of cases and without a focus in the majority of the remaining cases.

> Viral infections, affecting mainly the upper respiratory tract (URT), are the cause of fever in about 90-95% of febrile children. It is the physician's primary role to identify the remaining 5-10% of children who have a bacterial infection and who may require antibiotic treatment.

> Nowadays, most cases of tonsillitis, otitis media and pneumonia, during the first years of life, are caused by a viral infection.

> In the tropics, bacterial and parasitic infections are more common than in developed countries and are important causes of mortality of millions of children.

> Pyrexia of unknown origin is considered when fever persists for more than one week: it's cause is unknown despite investigation. In contrast to adults, PUO in children is mostly due to infection followed by collagen and vascular causes.

> The diagnosis of fever of non-infectious origin is considered after excluding an infection. This is done by history, physical examination and laboratory tests.

> Persistent and/or insidious fever of a low degree (< 39.5°C), the absence of chills and diurnal rhythm of fever are suggestive of non-infectious fever.

> An important cause of elevated body temperature is heatstroke, which is due to a combination of heat, high humidity, excessive wrapping and lack of fluids.

A.S. El-Radhi et al. (Eds.) *Clinical Manual of Fever in Children.*
Doi: 10.1007/978-3-540-78598-9, © Springer-Verlag Berlin Heidelberg 2009

12

12.1
Differentiating Fever of Infectious and Noninfectious Origin

Main causes of fever:

- Infections (Bacterial, virus, TB, parasitic, rickettsia) are by far the most common cause of fever in children. Infection remains the likely diagnosis in a febrile child until proven otherwise.
- Noninfectious (collagen/vascular, malignancy, drugs, allergy, recent immunization, periodic fevers).

Diagnosis that fever is caused by an infection is supported by the following:

- Underlying conditions predisposing to infections (e.g., Immunocompromised status, splenectomy, sickle cell anemia, neonates and young infants, intravascular catheters)
- Fever of 40°C or greater, presence of chills, diurnal fluctuation of fever
- A focus for infection (e.g., tonsillitis, pneumonia). In case of fever without a focus, the diagnosis can usually be rapidly established by laboratory means (e.g., UTI, malaria)
- Short duration of fever occuring, for example, in viral infections
- Rapid response to antibiotics in bacterial infections
- Concomitant herpes labialis
- Leukocytosis >20,000 in bacterial and leukopenia <5,000 in viral infections
- High procalcitonin (PCT) levels. PCT is low in viral infections and inflammatory diseases, for example, connective diseases and neoplasma

Diagnosis that fever is not caused by an infection is supported by the following:

- History (e.g., recent vaccination, drug intake)
- Persistent or insidious fever of low degree (<39.5°C)
- Associated pruritic rash, multiple joint involvement
- Negative bacterial cultures in blood, stool, urine, and CSF
- Absence of chills and diurnal rhythm of fever
- Exclusion of an infection by history, physical examination, and laboratory tests
- Fever not responding to antibiotics but responding to steroids
- Absence of leukocytosis and left shift, presence of antinuclear factor (ANF)

12.2
Differentiation Between Viral and Bacterial Infections

Although high and prolonged fever is more often caused by bacterial than by viral infections, affecting mainly the upper respiratory tract (URT), are the causes of fever in about 90–95% of febrile children. It is the physician's primary role to identify the remaining 5–10% of children who have a bacterial infection and who may require antibiotic treatment. Those with viral infection will usually require only symptomatic treatment. With stomatitis, varicella, or other readily identified exanthems, the cause of the fever is apparent, and further diagnostic evaluation may not be required. Patients with impaired immune status (on chemotherapy), sickle cell disease, human immunodeficiency virus infection, or cystic fibrosis should be considered to have a bacterial infection until proved otherwise. Often, however, it is difficult to differentiate viral from bacterial infections. Although high and prolonged fever is more often caused by bacterial than viral infection, such fever may frequently be caused by respiratory virus infections (Table 12.1).

Diagnosis of viral infection can be made using detection of viral antigen with enzyme immunoassay (ELA), fluorescent antibody (FA), or electron microscopy.

Serologic proof requires demonstration of a significant rise in IgG antibody between acute and convalescent sera or demonstration of virus-specific IgM antibody.

Table 12.1 Differential diagnosis between viral and bacterial infections

Features that increase the likelihood of viral infection	Features that increase the likelihood of bacterial infection
Many organs are involved at the same time, mostly affecting the URT	Localized to one organ (ears or tonsils)
Attendance of nursery or being in contact with people with similar symptoms	High fever (>39°C), duration (>3 days), and the presence of rigor, herpes labialis
Well-appearing, playful, and interacts well with his parents	Irritable, lethargic child, who looks ill with a weak cry and who is uninterested in the surroundings
Normal CRP and leukocytes (leukocytosis is rare in viral infections with few exceptions, such EBV and CMV). Leukopenia, lymphocytosis (or lymphocytopenia), and thrombocytopenia. Neutrophilia as an early sign of some infections, for example, chickenpox.	High CRP, ESR, WBC, absolute neutrophil count. In parasitic infections (malaria, leishmania), initial leukocytosis is often followed by leukopenia, monocytosis, thrombocytopenia, and eosinophilia
Reduced cytokines levels except INF-α level. Normal procalcitonin	High procalcitonin (PCT)[a] level >1.2 ng ml^{-1} and a higher level (>5 ng ml^{-1}) in severe bacterial infections

[a] PCT is a precursor of the hormone calcitonin found in small quantities in healthy subjects (<0.10 ng ml^{-1}). It offers higher sensitivity and specificity than CRP and WBC to differentiate between viral and bacterial infection.

12

12.3
Periodic Fever (see also Chap. 1, Sect 1.2)

Periodic fever (PF) is characterized by episodes of fever recurring at regular or irregular intervals. Each episode is followed by one to several days, weeks, or months of normal temperature. Examples are seen in malaria (termed tertian when the febrile spike occurs every third day or quartan when the spike occurs every fourth day) and brucellosis (see Chap. 5). The differential diagnosis of the hereditary causes of periodic syndrome is shown in Table 12.2.

FMF and PFAPA are the most common causes of PF. Fever is a constant finding and it may be present alone before other manifestations. Fever is usually greater than 39°C and may reach 40.5°C. FMF occurs in individuals from Mediterranean ancestry who usually present with loss of appetite and abdominal pain due to apparent peritonitis. About 6–10 h later, fever occurs and rapid recovery ensues within 24–72 h. While patients with FMF usually respond dramatically to colchicine 0.6 mg hourly for four doses, for those with PFAPA, steroid therapy is very effective in controlling fever and other symptoms within 2–4 h. IgD is elevated in the majority of cases of PFAPA.

TRAPS (TNF-receptor associated periodic syndrome) is rare and occurs in many ethnic groups. Fever usually lasts 2–3 weeks, which distinguishes it from FMF. HIDS is very rare and has been described mostly in Western Europe.

FCUS (familial cold urticaria syndrome) and MWS (Muckle-Wells syndrome) are characterized by recurrent episodes of fever, which starts 1–2 h after exposure to cold and lasts <24 h, occurring before the age of 6 months.
The differential diagnosis of this syndrome is the following:

• Acquired cold urticaria – does not present with fever and is unusual so early in life
• FMF – longer duration of episodes, arthritis, and abdominal pain
• Hyper IgD – longer episodes, diarrhea, and increased IgD
• TRAPS – longer episodes of periorbital edema

Table 12.2 Differential diagnosis of hereditary periodic fever syndromes

Disorder	Inheritance	Fever duration	Periodicity	Clinical features	Labor tests/etiology
FMF	AR	1–3 days	3–6 weeks	Polyserositis (abdominal, chest pain) synovitis, myalgia	↑Inflammatory markers, gene mutations MEFV on chromosome 6
Cyclic neutropenia	AD	5–7 days	3 weeks	Pharyngitis, gingivitis, mouth ulcers, lymph-adenopathy, cellulitis	Neutrophils <200, mutations of the gene neutrophils elastase (ELA2): chromosome 19
TRAPS	AD	Weeks	Irregular	Muscle cramps, vomiting and diarrhea, migratory arthralgia, migratory rash, periorbital edema	↑Inflammatory markers
HIDS	AR	4–6	4–8 weeks	Abdominal pain, headache arthralgia, lymph adenopathy, diarrhea	↑IgD, IgA, and mevalonic acid in the urine. TNF and the enzyme MVK are low
PFAPA	sporadic	3–5 days	3–6 weeks	Aphthous stomatitis pharyngitis, lymphadenitis	Inflammatory marker
MWS/FCUS/ NOMID/CINCA	AD	Irregular	Irregular	Urticaria, conjunctivitis progressive deafness, arthritis, chronic meningitis, skin rash	Mutations in CIAS1 gene on chromosome 1q44

FMF Familial Mediterranean fever; *TRAPS* tumor necrosis factor receptor-associated periodic syndrome; *HIDS* Hyperimmunoglobuliaemia D and periodic fever syndrome; *NOMID* neonatal-onset multisystem inflammatory disease; *CINCA* chronic infantile neurologic cutaneous and articular syndrome; *PFAPA* periodic fever, aphthous stomatitis, pharyngitis, and adenitis; *MWS* Muckle-Wells syndrome; *FCUS* Familial cold urticaria syndrome; *AR* autosomal recessive; *AD* autosomal dominant; *GCSF* granulocyte colony stimulating factor; *NSAIDs* nonsteroidal anti-inflammatory drugs

12

12.4
Unexplained Fever (Pyrexia of Unknown Origin, PUO)

Unexplained fever or PUO indicates the presence of fever without a focus due to a single diagnosis which remains obscure after a week of intense investigation. Although the degree of fever, age of the child, and the results of initial screening tests (CRP, WBC) are not in themselves diagnostic, a combination of history, examination, and the results of these tests can provide important clues to the underlying diagnosis. Table 12.3 shows the most common diagnoses of PUO.

Table 12.3 Main causes of PUO

Causes	Pattern of fever	Clues to diagnosis
Infection (60–70%)		
TB	Persistent, low grade fever often lasting for weeks, night sweats	Cough, weight loss, history of contact with an infected person
HIV	Fever occurs in 85% of cases. Unexplained, persistent or intermittent for >1 month is common	Mononucleosis-like symptoms with sore throat, myalgia, arthralgia, rash, lymphadenopathy. Lab findings: low WBC and platelets
Cat-scratch fever	Fever occurs in about 30% with a range of 38–39°C in mild cases; more severe cases present with high and persistent fever	Kitten exposure, papule at the site of inoculation, regional lymph-adenopathy, abdominal pain, splenomegaly
Endocarditis	Insidious, low-grade fever, night sweats	Splenomegaly, tender nodes (Osler's node), subungal (splinter) bleeding, pre-existing CHD, heart murmur, anemia, low platelets
Typhoid fever	Ladder-like increase of fever to reach 40–41°C. If untreated with antibiotics, the temperature remains continuous at 39–40.5°C for 2–3 weeks before abating slowly. RB is typical	Abdominal tenderness, delirium, and hepatosplenomegaly. At the end of the first week, roseate detected in 20–40%, on chest and abdomen. Lab findings: leucopenia, anemia, thrombocytopenia, and increased liver enzymes
Brucellosis	Incidence in 90–100%, either insidiously over several days or sudden with chills, rising sharply to 40.5°C and swinging considerably. Pattern is remittent, and often periodic. RB is common	History of direct contact with infected animals or their discharge, or through consumption of infected milk, or milk products. Arthralgia/arthritis, hepato-splenomegaly. Leukopenia
Q-fever	Sudden onset of high fever up to 40.5°C. There is no typical pattern. Diagnosis should be always considered in children with PUO	Persons at risk of infection are those who work with cattle, sheep, or their products. Flu-like symptoms, headaches, arthralgia, myalgia, hepatitis, pneumonia
Viral (e.g. EBV, CMV)	80% have pharyngeal form with lymphadenopathy, and 20% present with fever alone (typhoidal form). Fever may last 4 days to 2 or 3 weeks peaking on the fifth day of illness. Fever is frequently intermittent, with ranges 38.5–39.5°C, but rarely higher than 40°C	Fatigue, periorbital edema, splenomegaly. Cases with fever alone require blood tests to confirm diagnosis. Leukocytosis with lymphocytosis is often present

(continued)

12

Table 12.3 (continued)

Causes	Pattern of fever	Clues to diagnosis
Noninfection Collagen and vascular (20%)		
Still's disease	The commonest pattern is intermittent, often hectic, with a daily rise in the evening, then falling to normal in the morning. As the fever continues, the pattern may become double quotidian. Other febrile patterns include continuous and periodic	Leukopenia, rash, generalized lymphadenopathy and splenomegaly. Persistent arthritis for >6 weeks
SLE	SLE may present abruptly with fever, simulating an acute infection, or may develop over months with only episodes of fever, malaise, arthralgia, and weight loss. Fever ranges from moderate to high, occurring in 80–85% and accompanying the facial erythematous rash in about 40% of cases	Butterfly facial rash, leukopenia, renal involvement, anemia, thrombocytopenia
Malignancy (5%)		
Lymphoma	Neoplastic fever (usually <39°C that respond to naproxen) should be considered after exclusion of an infection. Some patients present with relapsing Pel-Ebstein fever (high fever for 10 days, regularly alternating with a few days or weeks of normal temperature)	Cervical lymphadenopathy, mediastinal and/or hilar mass. Night sweats, weight loss, pruritis
Miscellaneous (10%)		
For example, FMF	Fever usually last 48–96h, peaking within 1–3 days Fever may be the only feature, presents as PUO	Polyserositis, inherited as AR. Symptom-free Intervals range from days to months, even longer, rash (erysipelas-like) usually anterior leg
Undiagnosed (10%)		

URT upper respiratory tract; *EBV* Ebstein Barr virus; *MCV* cytomegalovirus; *RB* relative bradycardia

12.5
Hyperthermic Conditions

The most important causes of hyperthermia are heatstroke, malignant hyperthermia (MH), neuroleptic malignant syndrome (NMS), serotonin syndrome (SS), drugs, and hemorrhagic shock and encephalopathy (HSE)

Condition	Diagnostic clues
Heatstroke	
	Infants are at high risk
	Causes are extreme heat, high humidity, excessive wrapping, lack of fluids. Infants left unattended in a car. It is the result of exposure to heat and inability to sweat
	Rapid onset and an increase within few minutes of body temperature to 40°C or greater
	Signs: flushed, dry, and hot skin, not sweaty, disorientation, headache
MH	
	Family history may be positive (multi-factorial)
	Event occurs during anesthesia, primarily halogenated inhalation, and succinylcholine anesthesia
	Diagnosis: Exposure of biopsied muscle tissue to caffeine or halothane
NMS	
	Caused almost exclusively by antipsychotics, including all types of neuroleptics
	The disorder typically occurs within 2 weeks of the initial treatment
	First symptom is muscular rigidity, followed by high fever, sweating, unstable BP, tachycardia, confusion, delirium
	Increase of CPK and metabolic acidosis are usual findings
	NMS and SS share similar features but they can be distinguished by the difference shown in Table 12.4. NMS should also be differentiated from the more common adverse drug reaction characterized by the presence of rash (often urticaria), itching, blood eosinophilia, wheezing, and usually no fever.
HSE	A very rare condition, characterized by an acute onset of shock (poor perfusion, low BP), occurring predominately in 3–8 months old infants. HSE resembles heatstroke

Table 12.4 Differential diagnosis of SS and NMS

Feature	SS	NMS
Mechanism	Serotonin excess	Dopamine antagonism
Cause	SSRIs, antidepressants; Drug interaction enhances Serotonin transmission	Typical antipsychotic, haloperidol, and atypical antipsychotic (e.g., clozapam, resperidone)
Onset of symptoms	Minutes to hours	Days to weeks
Fever	Low-grade fever	Higher degree of fever
Neuromuscular	Myoclonus, hyper-reflexia euphoria, rapid eye movement	"lead pipe" rigidity
Gastrointestinal	Diarrhea, vomiting	Diarrhea, vomiting
Metabolic acidosis	Rare	Common
Rhabdomyolysis	Rare	Common
Elevated transaminases	Rare	Common

12

12.6
Unexplained Hypothermia

At rest humans produce 40–60 kilocalories (kcal) of heat per square meter of body surface area through generation of cellular metabolism. The body looses heat through radiation, conduction, convection, and evaporation (see Chap. 8)

* Decreased heat production

    – Hormonal: Hypopituitarism, hypoadrenalism, hypothyroidism. These conditions are considered particularly if patients do not respond to conventional therapy
    – Metabolic: Urea cycle disorders (defects in the nitrogen metabolism), particularly arginosuccinic aciduria (an autosomal disorder of the urea cycle, which is characterized by the triad of hyperammonia, encephalopathy, and respiratory alkalosis)
    – Transfusion/infusion of cold blood or fluids, gastric lavage using cold fluids or for peritoneal dialysis
    – Hypoglycemia
    – Severe and overwhelming infection, such as sepsis or septic shock
    – Severe malnutrition and starvation, such as anorexia nervosa

* Increased heat loss

    – Cold delivery room
    – Drugs causing vasodilatation
    – Spontaneous periodic hypothermia, which may be associated with absent corpus callosum (Shapiro's syndrome). There is an absent shivering and profuse sweating. Episodes usually last hours to days. The condition is usually benign

* Impaired thermoregulation

    – Cerebral bleeding, hypoxic ischemic encephalopathy
    – Menke's kinky hair syndrome, an x-linked inherited disorder of copper metabolism
    – Prader Willi syndrome. The syndrome is associated with disturbance in thermoregulation, causing unexplained hyperthermia or hypothermia. This risk is high in very cold weather or postoperative period
    – Drugs

* Sedative-hypnotics: Benzodiazepines, barbiturates, opiates antidepressants, antipyretics (rare side-effects of antipyretics), and organophosphate poisoning

12.7
Pharyngitis/Tonsillitis

The major cause of bacterial pharyngitis is Group A β-hemolytic streptococcus (GABHS), accounting for 10–20% of cases in children. Most causes of pharyngitis are viral, including EBV, adenovirus, coxsakie A viruses (Table 12.5).

Table 12.5 Differential diagnosis of pharyngitis

Pharyngitis	Features	Diagnosis
GABHS	School age, absence of symptoms of URTI (e.g., coryza, hoarseness), exudates on tonsils, deviation of the uvula, high fever	Rapid antigen test, throat swab culture, ASO titre. High WBC and CRP
Viruses	Preschool age, presence of rhinorrhea, conjunctivitis, and cough. No response to antibiotics, thus longer duration of fever	Diagnosis is usually clinical. Viral study is not necessary
EBV	Older children and adolescents, gray membrane on tonsils, lymphadenopathy, splenomegaly,	Monospot test (sensitive in 90% and 95% specific), IgM for EBV
Herpangina (Coxsakie A virus)	Preschool age, ulcers on whitish-gray base, and a red border on soft palate, high fever	Clinical, diagnostic tests unnecessary
Scarlet fever	Tonsillitis, punctuate, erythematous blanchable exanthem, accentuated on skin folds and creases, tongue is bright red, with white coating (strawberry tongue)	Positive throat swab culture for streptococci, ASO titre rising fourfold
KD	Most affect children <5 years, persistent fever, lymph-adenopathy	(see diagnostic criteria, Chap. 6)
Peritonsillar abscess	High fever (40–41°C), toxic appearance, history of tonsillitis with an afebrile period or continuing fever, asymmetric uvula deviation, torticollis	Clinical diagnosis

URTI upper respiratory tract infection; *EBV* Ebstein Barr virus; *KD* Kawasaki disease

12.8
Differential Diagnosis of Pneumonia and Chest Infiltration

Pneumonia is a primary infection of the parenchyma of the lung, which is much less common than secondary bacterial infection complicating an acute bronchiolitis. The diagnosis of pneumonia can only be established with certainty by a chest X-ray. It is important to note the following:

* A viral URTI often precedes the onset of bacterial pneumonia.
* Pneumococcal pneumonia cannot be differentiated from other bacterial or viral pneumonias with certainty. Therefore, antibiotics are usually administered once a radiological pneumonia is diagnosed.

In the differential diagnosis of pneumonia:

* Salicylate poisoning with features of hyperthermia and tachypnoea
* Any illness causing respiratory distress, for example, bronchiolitis, tuberculosis, congestive cardiac failure, aspiration of a foreign body, atelectasis

Bacterial pneumonia can be diagnosed by the following findings:

* *Pneumococcal pneumonia*

  – Typical age >4 years of age
  – A brief URTI is followed by shaking chills, then fever as high as 41°C, followed by tachypnoea, a dry cough, delirium, and abdominal pain
  – Chest findings include chest retraction, flaring of alae nasi, and fine rales on the affected side. Initially, there may be dullness on the affected side. Classic signs of consolidation are noted on the second and third day of illness producing bronchial breathing
  – Radiological evidence of consolidation
  – Leukocytosis of 20,000 cells mm^{-3} or more
  – Isolation of the organisms from the blood (positive in 10%), or from pleural fluid aspirate or bronchoscopic washing

* *Mycoplasma pneumonia*

  – Onset is insidious with fever, headaches, and abdominal pain, followed by cough.
  – May present with similar clinical and radiological features of other pneumonias. However, children with *M. pneumonia* appear well despite the extent of the X-ray lesions. Chest X-ray often shows peribronchial and perivascular interstitial infiltrates.
  – Diagnosis is made by fourfold rise in antibody titre, a single titre of 128 or more, IgM antibodies, and serum cold-agglutinins.
  – A high CRP or ESR and a normal WBC are fairly characteristic.

* *Staphylococcal pneumonia*

  – Occurs most commonly under 1 year of age, often with a history of staphylococcal skin lesions and URTI

- Abruptly, the infant's condition worsens rapidly with the onset of high fever, cough, and signs of respiratory distress, such as tachypnoea, grunting, sternal and subcostal retraction, and nasal flaring
- Radiological evidence of nonspecific bronchopneumonia early in the illness. The infiltrate soon becomes patchy. Pneumatoceles of varying size are common. Pleural effusion, empyema, and pneumothorax

* *Haemophilus influenza pneumonia* has become very uncommon because of vaccination. Although it may be difficult to distinguish clinically and radiologically from other types of pneumonia, the progression is more insidious and the course is usually prolonged.

Viral pneumonia has the following characteristic findings:

* It is the most common type of pneumonia, particularly in young children most commonly caused RSV.
* It cannot be definitely differentiated clinically and radiologically from other types of pneumonias, particularly mycoplasma pneumonia.
* Most viral pneumonias are preceded by several days of respiratory symptoms, including rhinitis and cough. Onset is usually more gradual than in bacterial pneumonia. Dyspnea with retractions and nasal flaring is more common in young children. Physical examination is often not diagnostic.
* Temperature usually ranges from 38.5 to 40°C.
* Radiological findings may mimic those of bacterial pneumonia. Suggestive of viral etiology is a diffuse infiltrate, especially in the perihilar areas. Several segments of more than one lobe are often involved.
* Leukocytosis is usually under $20,000\,\text{mm}^{-3}$.
* Failure to respond to antibiotics.

Chest infiltrates.

* Diffuse pulmonary infiltrates suggest infection, edema, hemorrhage, interstitial lung disease. Causes can be confirmed using high-resolution CT-scan
* Hilar lymphadenopathy. Bilateral suggest sarcoidosis. Unilateral suggests TB
* Ground-glass opacities (a hazy increase in lung attenuation through which lung vessels are seen). Acute presentation suggests respiratory distress syndrome, pneumonia, pulmonary hemorrhage, or eosinophilic pneumonia

Chest infiltrates may occur in all types of pneumonia, more characteristically in the following:

* *Pneumocystis carinii*, which consists of generalized granular pattern and bilateral pulmonary infiltrates. There is a relative paucity of pulmonary findings for the severity of distress. Cough and fever may be absent.
* *Pulmonary tuberculosis.* In primary TB, mediastinal lymphadenopathy, causing partial or complete obstruction of the bronchus. With complete obstruction there is atelectasis of the distal segment, with dullness on percussion and diminished breath sounds. Rarely is there a classic pulmonary infiltrate with hilar lymphadenopathy. In post-primary TB, the early change shows a well circumscribed, homogenous shadow, commonly in the apices.

12

12.9
Abdominal Pain (AP)

The most common febrile causes of AP include gastroenteritis, GE, appendicitis, mesenteric adenitis, urinary tract infection, UTI, referred pain, pancreatitis, or intussusception.

The differential diagnosis between gastroenteritis, appendicitis, and mesenteric adenitis (Table 12.6), particularly between the latter two, can be difficult. When appendectomy is carried out, 30–40% do not have appendicitis and 20% are found to have mesenteric adenitis. Missed cases of appendicitis occur particularly in young children who may be afebrile (20%) and have often diarrhea.

UTI presentation is usually with high fever without focus, particularly in young children, and with lesser degrees of fever and flank pain in older children. Diagnosis is established by urinalysis.

Intussusception is characterized by paroxysms (every 10–20 min) of colicky AP. The child appears well between these paroxysms. There is usually a palpable mass and a bloody red, currant stools. Pyrexia may occur as a late sign.

Table 12.6 The differential diagnosis between gastroenteritis, appendicitis and mesenteric adenitis

Gastroenteritis	Appendicitis	Mesenteric adenitis
History of diarrhea in other family members	Fever, ranges 38–39°C, is present in 80%	History of an URTI, or the presence of URTI on examination
Crampy AP	Pain, often crampy, starts in the periumbilical region, moves after a few hours to the right iliac fossa. Vomiting and fever follow. Examination shows localized tenderness, guarding and rebound in the RLQA. Moving, jumping, and coughing worsen the pain	AP is more diffuse than in appendicitis. However, the diagnosis is one of exclusion, particularly appendicitis, and it is often made at laparotomy
Diarrhea. Vomiting is usual in Rota-virus GE, rare in salmonella, and unusual in Shigella GE	Pain precedes vomiting. Very young children may have diarrhea, which is usually not pronounced as in gastroenteritis	Vomiting precedes pain
↑WBC and CRP in bacterial and usually normal in viral GE	WBC >15,000, high CRP	WBC <15,000, normal CRP
	High resolution ultrasound scan can differentiate conditions mimicking appendicitis and may suggest the diagnosis	CT image often shows the enlarged mesenteric lymphnodes (5–15 mm), with thickened wall of the terminal ileum

RLQA right lower quadrant of abdomen; *URTI* upper respiratory tract infection; *AP* Abdominal pain

Referred pain either from a viral URTI or pneumonia. It is characterized by:

* AP, which is usually mild to moderate and diffuse
* Physical examination of the respiratory system usually reveals the diagnosis

Crohn's disease. Children usually present with fever, headache, anorexia, oral ulcers, perianal skin tag/fistula, growth failure, vague crampy abdominal pain, often mimicking appendicitis, and erythema nodosum. High CRP, anemia, and thrombocytosis are fairly characteristic.

Enteric fever has the following characteristic clinical course:

* The onset is insidious with fever (without shaking chills), present in almost all patients, associated with headache, cough, and abdominal pain.
* Symptoms gradually increase over 2–3 days, with constipation, nausea, and anorexia.
* The temperature continues to rise in a stepwise fashion to reach 40–41°C. If untreated with antibiotics, the temperature remains continuous at 39–40.5°C for 2–3 weeks before abating slowly. In young children the onset of fever is more often abrupt. Sustained or intermittent fevers are more common than the stepwise pattern of fever. In all ages, fever may continue for many days despite antibiotic therapy, and the child does not become afebrile until the end of the therapy.

Pancreatitis

* Risk factors are intake of the anticonvulsant valproate, hyperlipidemia, biliary tract disorder, or family history of pancreatitis
* Abdominal pain/tenderness (occurs in 80%), which is persistent, radiating to the back
* Vomiting/retching (incidence about 75%)
* Fever/chills (incidence in about 25%)
* Elevated serum lipase and amylase level
* Imaging studies: ultrasonography and CT-scan

Amebic Liver abscess

The common clinical symptoms and signs are abdominal pain (85%), fever and chills (75%), and abdominal tenderness (70%). The location of the abscess is predominantly in the right lobe (75%).

12

12.10
Gastroenteritis

Most diarrheal diseases in children living in developed countries are mild and self-limited, and do not require hospitalization or laboratory evaluation. In a young child who is ill enough to require hospitalization, laboratory investigation of the stool is indicated to determine the cause of the diarrhea and those cases in which antibiotics may be needed.

The three major presentations of diarrhea are shown in Table 12.7. The single most helpful, initial laboratory test is the stool white cell assessment.

Table 12.7 Differential diagnosis in febrile infectious diarrhea

Diarrhea	Fever	Fecal WBC	Likely cause
Watery, no blood, or mucus	Variable	Absent	Toxigenic *E. coli*, traveler's diarrhea, cholera, clostridium
Crampy, blood and mucus, no vomiting	Usually present	Present	Shigella, *E. coli* 017:H57, Yersinia campylobacter, Amoeba (in endemic area)
Watery diarrhea with vomiting	Variable	Variable, mostly monocytes	Rotavirus and Norwalk virus (in winter), adenovirus, salmonella (in summer/fall)

12.11
Jaundice

Jaundice is very common during the neonatal period. It is not discussed here as the causes are almost always afebrile. After the neonatal period, infection remains the most common cause of jaundice worldwide. Hepatitis A (HA) used to be a common infectious disease, but its incidence rate has declined significantly in developed countries. Jaundice should be differentiated from xanthochromia (carotenemia), which is due to carotene deposits in the skin. The sclera remain normal. Table 12.8 facilitates the differential diagnosis of jaundice.

12

Table 12.8 Differential diagnosis of jaundice

Condition	Fever	Distinguishing features	Diagnosis
Acute hepatitis A, B, C, D, E	Common, low grade, appears first; jaundice follows when the fever is normal	80% of cases: asymptomatic. Presentation with malaise, nausea, anorexia, abdominal pain, dark urine, and acholic stools	Abnormal LFT, with high SGPT > SGOT. IgM anti-HA for each virus
Autoimmune hepatitis	Occurs in about 40%	Pallor 100%; jaundice in about 60%	Anemia, positive auto-antibodies
Drug-induced hepatitis	Variable nonspecific pattern of fever	Drugs causing toxicity (e.g., Rifampicin, paracetamol, valproate, INH)	Abnormal LFT, negative IgM for viruses. History of drug intake
Mononucleosis	100% of cases, variable degree	Pharyngitis, lymphadenopathy	Positive EBV-IgM and Monospot
Leptospirosis	High, occurring in almost all cases. Relative bradycardia	Animal exposure, myalgia, subconjuntival bleeding renal involvement adrenal dysfunction, drowsiness	Isolation of organisms and/ or fourfold rise in antibody titre
Malaria	High, intermittent	Jaundice is usually mild, anemia, splenomegaly	Smear for malaria
Typhoid fever	Stepladder rise until the end of the first week, also noted during the day	Jaundice appears at the peak of fever, abdominal symptoms.	Isolation of *S. typhi* from blood, stool, or bone marrow. IgM
Hepatic abscess	High hectic	Right upper quadrant pain and tenderness	Ultrasound scan
Reye syndrome	Mild and infrequent	History of aspirin intake and a flu-like symptoms; decreasing consciousness	See Chap. 10 for diagnostic criteria
Yellow fever (YF)	Sudden and high for 2–3 days, then remits, followed by another spike, relative bradycardia	In contrast to the gradual onset of hepatitis, jaundice in YF appears 3–5 days of high fever	Isolation of virus or IGM enzyme immunoassay

12.12
Coma

Children have a reduced conscious level if they score less than 15 on the modified Glasgow coma score (GCS) or if they are alert (A), responsive to voice (V), to pain (P) or are unresponsive (U) on the AVPU scale.

The main causes are the following:

Intracranial Infections (The Paediatric Accident and Emergency Research Group, 2005)

Bacterial Meningitis

Children with reduced conscious level but no neck stiffness should be suspected if they have fever and two of the following:

* Rash
* Irritability
* Bulging fontanelle; neck stiffness in older children

Herpes simplex encephalitis (HSE)

HSE should be suspected clinically in a child with reduced conscious level if one or more of the following four are present:

* Focal neurological signs
* Fluctuating conscious level for 6 h or more
* Contact with herpetic lesions
* No obvious clinical signs pointing towards the cause

The clinical suspicion of HSE is strengthened by the following:

* MRI scan with nonspecific features of HSE
* Abnormal EEG with nonspecific features of HSE
* CSF positive for herpes simplex virus DNA in PCR

Intracranial Abscess

Should be suspected in a child with a reduced conscious level with the following:

* Focal neurological signs +/− clinical signs of sepsis
* Signs of increased ICP

Diagnosis is confirmed by imaging.

TB Meningitis

Should be suspected in a child with a reduced conscious level and the following:

* Clinical signs of meningitis (see typical CSF findings Chap. 6)
* Insidous, low grade fever
* Cranial nerve palsy, particularly the sixth nerve
* Contact with a case of pulmonary TB

Diagnosis is established from a CSF sample by a positive PCR for TB DNA.

Shock
Circulatory shock is diagnosed if one or more of the following signs are present:

* CRT >2 s
* Mottled cool extremities
* Diminished peripheral pulses
* Systolic BP is less than 5% for age
* Decreased urine output <1 ml kg^{-1}h^{-1}

If shock is present, look for signs of the following:
Sepsis, trauma (blood loss, tension pneumothorax, cardiac tamponade), anaphylaxis (urticarial rash, wheeze, stridor, swollen lips/tongue), or heart failure (enlarged liver, peripheral edema, distended neck veins, heart murmur)

Sepsis
Defined as the systemic response to infection, sepsis is suspected if two or more of the following four are present:

* A body temperature of >38°C or <35.5°C, or history of fever at home
* Tachycardia
* Tachypnoea
* A rise in WBC of 15,000 mm^3 or a fall of 5,000 mm^3, or if there is non-blanching petechial or purpuric skin rash [please check]

Investigations: chest X-ray, throat swab, urine culture if urinalysis is positive for leukocytes and/or nitrate, LP, PCR from blood for meningococci and pneumococcus, coagulation studies (activated partial thromboplastin time), PT, fibrinogen, fibrinogen degradation products, skin swab if areas of inflammation are present, joint aspiration if signs of septic arthritis are present, a thick and thin smear for malarial parasites if foreign travel to endemic area, intracranial imaging, if no other source of infection determined

Afebrile conditions with reduced conscious level: Trauma, metabolic illness (hyperglycemia, hypoglycemia, hyperammonaemia, nonhyperglycemic ketoacidosis, drug-related)

12.13
Fever in Diseases Mainly Occurring in Tropics

The list of tropical diseases causing febrile diseases is very large and beyond the scope of this book. The most common causes of febrile diseases in the tropics are those occurring worldwide, for example, URTI, LRTI (pneumonia), diarrhea, UTI. Table 12.9 shows the main tropical diseases, their geographical distribution and tests to diagnose them. Risk factors, which may lead to various tropical diseases are shown in Table 12.10.

Table 12.9 Main tropical diseases, their endemic geographical areas and tests to diagnose them

Agents	Endemic geographical area	Diagnosis
• Parasitic diseases		
• Malaria	P. vivax: India, C. America P. falciparum: Africa. P. vivax & falciparum: SE Asia	Giemsa-stain: Thick Thin blood smear
• Leishmaniasis	India, Africa, Mediterranean area, S. America	Identification of L. splenic or BM asp.
• Schistosomiasis	Africa, Middle East, South America (S. Mansoni)	Findigof Schistosome eggs in urine or stool
• Bacterial diseases		
• Enteric Fever	Middle East, India, and S. America	Isolation of bacteria in blood, stool, urine. PCR In blood
• Brucellosis	Mediterranean area, India, parts of S. America	Isolation of the bacteria in blood, BM. Serum agglutination test
• Leptospirosis	World-wide	Isolation of bacteria, serologic testing
• TB	World-wide, particularly Africa, Asia	FAB identification by culture or ZN-stain
• Amoebiasis	Throughout the tropics	Stool culture, Anti-amoebic antibody test
• Viral diseases		
• Yellow fever	Central and West Africa, South America	virus isolation, IgM enzyme immune assay
• HIV	World-wide, particularly Africa, India, China	HIV p24 antigen, IgA & IgG antibody, HIV DNA or RNA by PCR
• Dengue fever	South East Asia, W. Africa	IgM, IgG in paired sera (≥4-fold rise)
• Lassa fever	Nigeria, Sierra Leone, Liberia	Virus isolation, IgG in paired sera (≥4-fold rise)
• Hepatitis	Africa, Asia	IgM antibody
• Haemorrhagic fever	Depending on the type of disease (e.g. Omsk Haemorrhagic Fever in Romania and Russia)	Virus isolation from throat washing, IgG (≥4-fold rise in paired sera)
• Rickettsial diseases		
• Q fever	World-wide	Serology: 4-fold rise of paired fluorescent antibody titre
• Epidemic typhus	Africa, South America	Fluorescent antibody Assay, PCR

Table 12.10 Risk factors, which could lead to various tropical diseases

Risk of infection is increased	Disease
Ingestion of unpasteurized milk	Brucellosis, enteric fever, Bovine TB, *Salmonella enteritis*
Exposure to mosquitoes	Malaria, dengue fever, filariasis, yellow fever
Ingestion of uncooked meet	Toxoplasmosis
Exposure to area with ticks	Lyme disease, relapsing fever, tick typhus, Q Fever
Direct contact with animals, or contaminated soil or urine	Leptospirosis

12.14
A Febrile Child with a Non-Blanching Rash

Petechial rash is characterized by extravasation of blood from capillaries, venules, or arterioles, which persists after pressure, for example, by a glass slide or drinking glass. The majority of cases (90%) are nonbacterial and nonlife threatening. About 10% of cases have septicemia, which requires immediate attention and treatment, as a delay in the diagnosis could result in rapid deterioration of the child's condition and death. Bacterial causes should always be considered first. If there is any doubt, the child should be treated with antibiotics without waiting for confirmation of the diagnosis. Common causes of non-blanching (petechial rash) are shown in Table 12.11:

Table 12.11 The differential diagnosis of common causes of petechial rash in children

Causes	Usual findings
• Bacterial Meningococcal septicaemia	High degree of fever, ill-looking, lethargy, headache, peripheral under-perfusion, pallor, mottled skin, prolonged capillary refill time, high CRP, WBC
• Viral CMV, rubella, enteroviruses, HIV, EBV, HHV-6	Low-grade fever, children generally well, absence of signs of shock
• Collagen/vascular SLE, vasculitis	Children are often not ill-looking, fever can be as high as in septicemia, absence of signs of shock. Other organ involvement
• Malignancy Leukemia	Ill-looking, anemia, hepatosplenomegaly, lymphadenopathy. Blood and bone marrow tests are diagnostic
• Thrombocytopenia ITT	Well-looking, usually afebrile (unless associated with an URTI)
• Drugs	Well-looking, low degree of fever, pruritic rash, history of drug intake, eosinophilia, rash disappearing 12–24 h after discontinuation of the drug

12.15
Inflammatory Arthritis (IA)

Polyarthritis (>4 joints within the first 6 months). Main causes are Juvenile idiopathic arthritis (JIA), Rheumatic fever (RF), vasculitis:

* **Juvenile idiopathic arthritis (JIA)** is characterized by arthritis of >1 week duration, presenting <16 years of age and unexplained by known causes. Cases of polyarthritis affect at least five joints either from the onset or within the first 6 months of the onset. There is a broad differential diagnosis for IA (see Chap. 6). ESR (and not CRP) is commonly raised, suggesting that the arthritis is inflammatory but not infectious.
* **Rheumatic fever (RF):** Migratory arthritis, occurring 2–3 weeks following an untreated group A β-hemolytic streptococcal pharyngitis. Fever usually responds dramatically to aspirin (unlike JIA). Diagnosis is established by Jones criteria (see Chap. 6).
* **Polyarthritis due to vasculitis** (e.g., Henoch-Schoenlein Purpura (HSP) or Kawasaki Disease (KD)). HSP manifests with a rash of typical distribution (buttocks, external areas of elbows, and knee joints), abdominal pain, and nephritis. KD is diagnosed by certain criteria (see Chap. 6).

Oligoarthritis (four or fewer joints) and monoarthritis. Main causes are septic arthritis (SA), oligoarhritis of JIA, reactive arthritis, Lyme disease, transient synovitis, neoplastic, and Tb arthritis.

* **Septic arthritis (SA):** This disorder is defined as positive joint fluid culture for bacteria and/or WBC count in the joint fluid of >50,000 cells mm^{-1} (predominately polymorphonuclear cells) with or without positive blood culture (positive in about 50%). Negative gram staining does not exclude the diagnosis. Features in support of this diagnosis are the following:

  – SA is rare in immunocompetent children. Risk factors include hemoglobinopathy, immune compromise
  – It is almost always monoarticular involving predominately large joints
  – Abrupt onset of fever and joint pain
  – Fever is usually high >39.5°C
  – Severe pain and restricted range of joint movement, refusal to walk
  – Joint aspiration is diagnostic (see the definition)
  – Ultrasound or X-ray often show the presence of periosteal reaction
  – MRI may show periosteal abscess
  – Bone scan is positive in the majority of cases

* **Oligoarhritis of JIA:** Diagnostic criteria as in polyarthritis of JIA. In addition, patients commonly have uveitis.
* **Reactive arthritis** (ReA) is an autoimmune arthritis that develops in response to an infection elsewhere in the body, most commonly a viral URT or intestinal infection (Campylobacter, salmonella, Shigella, or Yersinia). ReA is one of the most common causes of arthritis. Characteristic features include the following:

12

- History of infection occurring 1–3 weeks prior to the onset of arthritis
- Arthritis occurring in weight-bearing joints (knee and ankle)
- Commonly associated with the human leukocyte antigen HLA-B27
- Joint aspirate showing an increased WBC but is sterile to culture

Post-streptococcal ReA differs from RF in the absence of heart, CNS, and skin lesions in addition to poor response to aspirin.

- **Lyme disease (LD) arthritis** is characterized by intermittent or chronic monoarthritis or oligoarthritis, particularly affecting the knee. Other clues are as follows:

  - Common arthritis in certain part of the world, for example, USA
  - The patient has not received an antibiotic treatment when LD was acute
  - History of tick bite, erythema migrans

- **Transient Synovitis**

  - Fever is either absent or mild
  - History of a viral infection in the upper respiratory airways
  - One hip is usually affected, children are limping but still walking
  - The child is generally well, symptoms are mild
  - Self-limiting, usually lasting 1–3 weeks
  - Normal WBC, CRP, and ESR
  - WBC count in the joint fluid of <50,000 cells mm^{-1}

- **Neoplastic arthritis** (e.g., leukemia, lymphoma) is uncommon. Diagnostic clues are as follows:

  - Presence of lymphadenopathy, hepatosplenomegaly
  - Presence of anemia, thrombocytopenia, blast cells on the peripheral blood smear
  - Pyrexia is usually not severe (<39.0°C)
  - Bone marrow aspiration is diagnostic

- **TB-arthritis**

  - Lack of response to treatment (antibiotics, NSAIDs, intraocular steroids)
  - Synovial biopsy is diagnostic

12.16
Postoperative Fever

(See also Chap. 6, Sect. 6.4)

Infectious causes include wound infection, peritonitis, intravenous line infection, viral infection, pneumonia Urinary tract infection, infectious diarrhea, bacteremia, osteomyelitis.

Noninfectious causes include dehydration, hematoma, pulmonary atelectasis, transfusion, drug reaction, warm ambient temperature.

The diagnosis of noninfectious causes should only be considered after excluding infectious causes. Although most postoperative fevers are noninfectious, patients are often treated with antibiotics because the differential diagnosis can be difficult. A significant number of cases of infected patients have no fever. Table 12.12 provides key points for each condition.

Table 12.12 Differential diagnosis of fever occurring during the postoperative period

Infectious causes	Noninfectious
Fever usually starts on day 3 or later	Fever day 1–2
Fever height Fever >39°C	Low-grade fever, no chills
Fever pattern may be hectic	Remittent fever
Fever duration 2 day and longer	Duration: 1–2 days
Appearance often ill-looking	Usually well appearing
High CRP, ESR, WBC	Low or mildly increased

12

12.17
Seizures

The main causes of fever in association with seizures are febrile seizures (FS), meningitis, encephalitis, epileptic seizures, or cerebral malaria. See also intracranial infections above [much is a repeat – refer reader to the above section for meningitis. encephalitis, etc]

Condition	Distinguishing clinical features (Diagnostic clues)
Febrile	
FS	This is the most common cause of seizures, age usually 6 months to 5 years Fever is always present at onset, that is, absence of fever excludes FS Usually the child was well prior to onset, child neurologically normal Family history of FS is common Duration of seizure and unconsciousness usually brief. Normal neurological examination before, that is, healthy child, and after the seizure (no neck stiffness or bulging fontanelle, normal LP results)
Meningitis	Child was unwell prior to the onset of seizure, with impaired conscious level, vomiting, headaches, anorexia, lethargy Seizure is a late sign, complex at onset (focal, prolonged and/or multiple) and associated with other neurological features Presence of petechial rash, irritability, bulging fontanelle Diagnosis is established by LP
TB Meningitis	Contact with a case of pulmonary TB More insidious onset, dominated by reduced conscious level Lower degrees of fever, more insidious than with bacterial meningitis Diagnosis is established from CSF findings, a positive PCR for TB DNA, staining and culture of the acid-fast bacilli, positive tuberculin test, and radiological evidence of previous pulmonary infection.
Encephalitis	Usually due to an acute viral encephalitis, most commonly herpes simplex virus (HSV). In milder form, it is also caused by common exanthem (chickenpox, measles, mumps, rubella) or Lyme disease HSE should be suspected clinically in a child with reduced conscious level if one or more of the following four are present [1]: – Focal neurological signs – Fluctuating conscious level for 6 h or more – Contact with herpetic lesions – No other obvious cause The clinical suspicion of HSE is supported by – MRI scan with nonspecific features of HSE – An abnormal EEG with nonspecific features of HSE – A positive CSF result for herpes simplex virus DNA in PCR of CSF

Condition	Distinguishing clinical features (Diagnostic clues)
Intracranial abscess	Should be suspected in a child with a reduced conscious level if – There are focal neurological signs +/− clinical signs of sepsis – There are signs of increased ICP – Diagnosis is confirmed by imaging
Epileptic seizure with fever	Known history of afebrile epileptic seizures or epilepsy Associated with neurodisability Usually low grade-fever provoking the seizure
Cerebral malaria	Living in or traveling to endemic malarious areas Persistence of coma >30 min (often >6 h) after the convulsion Seizure is usually generalized (rarely focal), with high-pitched cry Deep respiration due to acidosis Core-to-skin temperature difference is abnormal, and often >10°C The presence of severe anemia, thrombocytopenia, hemoglobulinuria and parasites on blood smear. Normal CSF
Afebrile	Epileptic seizure, seizure, and loss of consciousness usually longer than in FS Metabolic disorder

Reference

1. The Paediatric Accident and Emergency Research Group. RCPCH Guideline Appraisal & Summary (Decreased Conscious Level), Nov 2005

History of Fever

13

Core Messages

> Fever is perhaps the most ancient hallmark of disease. It dates back as far as civilization itself.

> The oldest civilizations (Egyptian, Mesopotamian, Chinese, Indian, and Greek) demonstrated extensive knowledge of anatomy and physiology, but they tended to view fever as being induced by evil spirits.

> Many ancient physicians, fostered mainly by the Greeks, believed in the beneficial effects of fever (ancient concepts).

> By the eighteenth century, fever was thought to be *a harmful by-product of infection* (the medical renaissance concept). Antipyretics were introduced, and their extensive use has since then been considered beneficial.

> Over the past 40–50 years, intensive research has been carried out to investigate the role of fever. Although still there is disagreement, evidence now indicates that the effects of fever are complex but overall beneficial (current concepts).

13.1
Introduction

Of the many symptoms and signs of diseases, fever has received the most attention throughout medical history. For most of the history, fever was feared by ordinary people as a manifestation of punishment, induced by evil spirits or a marker of death. For medical scholars, however, the biological role of fever in disease was considered as beneficial, particularly so among Greek scholars. This concept underwent a radical transformation in the nineteenth century, and scholars began to regard fever as harmful. The use of antipyretics was considered beneficial. With the introduction of fever therapy in the twentieth

A.S. El-Radhi et al. (Eds.) *Clinical Manual of Fever in Children.*
Doi: 10.1007/978-3-540-78598-9, © Springer-Verlag Berlin Heidelberg 2009

13

Table 13.1 The three evolving concepts of fever

1. Ancient concepts (about 3000 B.C. to A.D. 1800): Fever is beneficial
   Ancient civilization (especially Greek civilization)
   Medicine of the Middle Ages
   Early period of Europeant medicine
2. Medical renaissance concepts (1800–1960): Fever is harmful
   Scholars such as Boerhaave, Bernard, Osler
3. Current concepts: Fever is controversial, predominately beneficial

century, renewed interest in the role of fever began. Currently, there is no consensus as to whether fever is beneficial, neutral, or harmful. This chapter summarizes the knowledge about fever and the changing concepts of its role in diseases from ancient cultures to our present time (Table 13.1).

13.2
Ancient Civilizations

13.2.1
Egyptian Medicine

Egyptian medicine is known to us mainly from medical texts written on papyrus. The most valuable papyri are the Edwin Smith surgical papyrus and the Ebers papyrus, written about 1700 years B.C [1]. These papyri, the oldest known medical texts, contain a description of various infectious diseases such as erysipelas, hepatitis, bilharziasis, ankylostomiasis, gonorrhea, and trachoma. Ancient scholars used splints, bandages, compresses, and other appliances. Specialists existed even at that time as *physician of the belly, physician of the eyes, guardian of the colon,* and *healer of the teeth.* The ancient Egyptians recognized that local inflammation was responsible for fever and that the pulse underwent acceleration during physical exercise and fever.

The Edwin Smith surgical papyrus [2] lists 48 medical cases. Local inflammation was differentiated from general fever, the latter usually meaning high fever: "A diseased wound in his breast inflamed (nsr-y), high fever (smmt-t) comes forth from it." The word *srf* indicated a lesser degree of fever (Fig. 13.1) [3].

Palpation was used to compare high and mild fever. Cold and warm compresses were prescribed for local inflammation, as well as willow leaves, which is the earliest known example of external application of salicylic acid.

13.2.2
Mesopotamian Medicine

Early Sumerian writings in the form of pictograms and later cuneiform (2500–3000 B.C.) indicate that fever as a clinical entity was clearly distinguished from local inflammation [4].

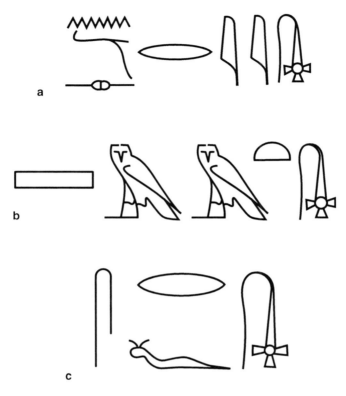

Fig. 13.1 The three words for fever used by the ancient physicians in Egypt were (a) nsr- (b) smm-t and (c) srf. (Redrawn from *Edwin Smith Surgical Papyrus* [3])

The Sumerian pictogram of Ummu (referring to fever) underwent a progressive transformation from about 2500 to 500 B.C. (Fig. 13.2).

   The main source of information about Mesopotamian medicine is a cuneiform writing from about 500 B.C. This writing was found on the 30,000 or so tablets recovered from Nineveh in present-day northern Iraq in 1845 from the ruins of the library of Assurbanipal (668–625 B.C.). Of these, about 1,000 were medical texts, which contain lists of medicine ingredients, diagnoses, and prognoses of various febrile illnesses [5]. Otitis media, for example, was recognized as fire that extends into the interior ear and dulls the hearing [6]. Pneumonia, with its main symptoms of fever, chest pain, cough, and sputum production, was described. Inflammation was related to fever as early as the sixth century B.C. As with many ancient concepts, evil spirits played a major role. Nergal, the god of pestilence, and Ashaka were believed to infest mankind with fever. Priests used exorcism to *expel* the fever.

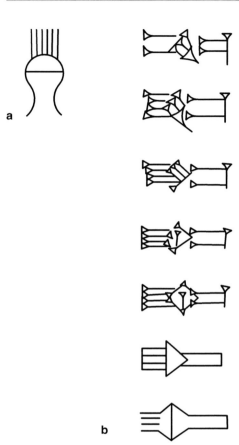

Fig. 13.2 The earliest Sumerian pictogram writing of Ummu (= inflammation or hot thing, meaning fever), written about 2500 BC (a), and the final Akkadian cuneiform writing, about 500 BC (b). (Redrawn by permission of the publishers from *The Healing Hand: Man and Wound in the Ancient World* by Guido Majno, Cambridge, Massachusetts: Harvard University Press © 1975 by the President and Fellows of Harvard College)

13.2.3
Chinese Medicine

The Chinese scholars believed that the soul possessed two antagonistic elements, good and evil, and that health and disease depended upon their balance [7].

The greatest medical Chinese classic is the Canon of Medicine by Nei Ching (Fig. 13.3), written about 3,000 years ago [8]. Although the method of examination was detailed, palpation focused on the pulse only, on which the diagnosis, including that of fever, and the prognosis were based [9]. In typhoid fever, a superficial pulse was considered a good sign, while a thin, thready pulse indicated a bad sign.

Chang-Chung-Ching was known as the Hippocrates of China. In the second century A.D. he wrote an Essay on Typhoid, which is a treatise on various forms of fever. This work, which appeared in 16 volumes, described symptoms of diseases, physical signs, clinical course, methods of treatment and action of drugs.

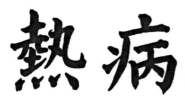

Fig. 13.3 The 'hot disease' mentioned in the *Canon of Medicine* by Nei Ching as a variety of Feverish conditions, including inflammation. Note the flames (bottom left). (Redrawn by permission of the publishers from *The Healing Hand: Man and Wound in the Ancient World* by Guido Majno, Cambridge, Massachusetts: Harvard University Press © 1975 by the President and Fellows of Harvard College)

Treatment of fever by antipyretic drugs and the use of cold applications were also described. Branches of peach trees were used to strike febrile patients to expel the evil spirit and the fever. Watermelon and material from deer horns were prescribed to treat febrile illnesses.

13.2.4
Hindu Medicine

During the earliest period of Indian civilization, medicine was also characterized by belief in magic and demons. Fever was feared since it was begotten by the wrathful fire of the god of destruction, Rudra, hence his name, *destroyer of created beings* [10]. The fire demons, Takman and Yakshma, were also believed to cause various fevers. When the fever was intermittent, the time interval between the peak periods of fever provided the key to prognosis.

The highest development in early Hindu medicine was achieved during the Brahman period (800 B.C. to A.D. 1000) [11]. One of the greatest exponents was Susruta, who wrote the Physiology of Susruta. Like the Greek scholars (it remains debatable which culture influenced the other), he believed that the human body contained three humors: bile, air, and phlegm. Diseases were thought to be due to the disturbance within these humors. Different types of fever were described: some were caused by a disturbance of air and phlegm, others by air and bile. Intermittent, remittent, double quotidian, tertian, and quartan fevers were defined. For treatment of fever, fasting, purging, and drinks from diluted barely gruel were advocated.

13.2.5
Greek Medicine

Greek scholars believed that the body was composed of four humors (or fluids): phlegm, blood, yellow bile, and black bile [12]. Health was maintained when these humors were in equilibrium, while diseases, and most especially fevers, were caused by a disturbance of the four humors. This theory of humoral equilibrium in health, and disequilibrium in disease, which persisted until the middle of the nineteenth century, was the first organized concept of thermoregulation. The present concept also envisages an equilibrium between temperature production and loss.

13

Knowledge about fever was extensive in Greek medicine compared with other ancient cultures. Fevers were divided according to their patterns into continuous (from excess of fire), or intermittent in the form of subtertian and tertian (from excess of water), quotidian (from excess of air), or quartan (from excess of earth). Other classifications described 5-day, 7-day, and 9-day nocturnal and diurnal fevers [13]. Most fevers encountered at that time (for example, continued, quotidian, tertian, and quartan) were also thought to be caused by excess of yellow bile because at that time many infections were associated with both fever and jaundice. Each of these fevers was studied according to the characteristics in its nature and in spacing of the paroxysms. The prognosis for each was determined. The Greek scholars knew that diseases were responsible for producing fever.

The Hippocratic writings characterize many febrile illnesses with such accuracy that diagnosis can be made from the descriptions. These illnesses included the following:

* Malaria is evident, with its paroxysms of fever.
* Mumps with its soft, nonsuppurative swelling and absence of high fever was complicated sometimes by orchitis [14].
* Febrile convulsions, which was noted to occur in children up to the age of 7 years.
* Typhoid fever, a classical example of continuous fever with its ladder-like rise in body temperature during the first week: "The worst, most protracted diseases were the continued fevers, these showed no real remissions; they began mildly but continually increased paroxysm carrying the disease a stage further." Shivering fits and sweat were least frequent and most irregular in these patients. It is remarkable, that these observations were made by palpation only.

There was evidence among scholars that fever was considered beneficial:

* The Hippocratic writings contain evidence that fever was thought to be beneficial to the infected host, "fever was beneficial in ophthalmia," and it cured it [15]. Since Hippocrates believed in the benefit of fever, he placed little emphasis on the treatment of it. When a disease was caused by an excess of one of the four bodily humors, the excess humor was then *cooked* by the fever, "I separated and eventually removed." He considered that nature provided the best medicine, a concept that influenced physicians until the beginning of the twentieth century. The best treatment for fever, if any, was dietary and consisted of starvation, accompanied by cool drinks. Acutely ill patients were usually given barley gruel or barley water, supplemented with hydromel (honey with water) or ioxymel (honey with vinegar). The purpose of the relative starvation and fluid regimen was to reduce the amount of bile and blood in the body.
* Rufus of Ephesus, a surgeon who lived at the beginning of the second century A.D., strongly advocated the beneficial role of fever. He was the first physician to recommend the use of *fever therapy*, such as by malarial fever, to treat epilepsy. He said, "fever is a good remedy for an individual seized with convulsion, and if there were a physician skilful enough to produce a fever it would be useless to seek any other remedy against disease"[16]. About 18 centuries later in 1917, Wagner von Jauregg treated neurosyphilis with malarial fever, for which he received the Nobel Prize 10 years later [17].

* Galen (A.D. 130–200) retained the Hippocratic humoral theory. Fever, according to Galen, could result from either excess of yellow bile, black bile, or phlegm (a condition that he called a cacochymia), or from an excess of blood, a plethora. To restore a healthy balance, Galen advocated bloodletting.

13.2.6
Hebrew Medicine

The roots of Hebrew medicine can be traced to the Bible (compiled between 1500 B.C. and 300 B.C.) and the Talmud (a book of rules and precepts completed between 70 B.C. and the second century A.D.) [18].

Magic, incantation, and mystics appear to be less significant than in other cultures. Certainly, the Biblical record contains no indication that fever was caused by demons or evil spirits. In the Old Testament, fever was part of God's punishment for sins. The Creator of heaven and earth, Yahweh, states "but break my covenant, then be sure that this is what I will do: I will bring upon you sudden terror, wasting disease and recurrent fever" (Leviticus 26: 16; Deuteronomy 28: 22). Fever is also mentioned on several occasions in the New Testament, always without comment on causation. The first time, Jesus saw in Peter's house, "his wife's mother laid and sick of a fever. And he touched her hand and the fever left her" (Matthew 8: 14–16, Mark 1: 29–34, Luke 4: 38–41). Elsewhere, Jesus healed the official's son with his words (John 4: 49–52), and the apostle Paul prayed to God and placed his hands on Publius, who was then healed of fever and a bloody flux, meaning dysentery (Acts 28: 8).

In summary, **the oldest civilizations** (Egyptian, Mesopotamian, Chinese, Indian, and Greek) demonstrated extensive knowledge of fever, but tended to view it as being induced by evil spirits. Hence, exorcism was used in many ancient cultures (to a lesser extent in Greek medicine) in the treatment of fever. Many ancient physicians, however, fostered mainly by the Greeks, believed in the beneficial effects of fever but early Jewish and Christian writers regarded it as a punishment from God.

13.3
Medicine in the Middle Ages

With the beginning of the Middle Ages (ca. 400–1400 A.D.), science and medicine became less important than theology and philosophy [19]. Galen's writings remained a great influence on medicine during the Middle Ages. He had a philosophy embracing body, mind, and soul, which was highly acceptable to the religion of the developing church [20]. The central development of medicine was in anatomy learned mainly from animal dissections but a few were performed on humans. Anatomical studies began at Bologna (ca. 1150 A.D.) and Padua University (ca. 1222 A.D.). Physiology and pathology were still based upon the four humors (blood, phlegm, yellow bile, and black bile). All diseases were characterized as hot, cold, moist, or dry. *Hot diseases* were treated by cooling, *moist diseases* by drying. Bloodletting, was widely practiced in febrile illnesses, as Galen and some of the ancient physicians had done. This was based on the notion

13

of plethora, a theory that attributed disease to part of the body being overfilled with blood. Apart from bloodletting, other methods used in the attempted cure of acute fevers included cooling, emollients, and laxatives.

With the destructive epidemics of the Black Death, which killed as much as one-third (reportedly twenty-five million) of the European population in the fourteenth century (with a peak in 1348), fever became a marker of death. Medicine was not helpful in preventing or treating the illness. The wrath of fever was still attributed to demonic possession, and therefore it required exorcism to expel it in line with evolving theological doctrine. The belief that fever constituted divine punishment also prevailed, particularly among the devout.

13.4
Arabic Medicine in the Middle Ages

*Unlike this "dark period" in Euro*pean medicine, Arabic medicine reached its golden age in the ninth and tenth centuries. The writings of both Hippocrates and Galen were carefully translated from Greek into Syriac and Arabic. Two scholars were outstanding in this period. Abu Ali Husayn ibn Abdulla ibn Sina (A.D. 980–1037), *latinized as Avicenna* [21] was, like Galen, a philosopher and physician. His best work, *Qanun Fit-Tibb*, or *Canon of Medicine* was a vast encyclopedia.

The 2nd great scholar was Abu Bakr Muhammad Zakariya Al-Razi (A.D. 864–923, latinized as Rhazes) was the first scholar to differentiate measles from smallpox with his original treatise on the two diseases [22]. On smallpox he wrote, *"The eruption of the smallpox is preceded by a continued fever, pain in the back, itching in the nose and terror in sleep.* There is redness in both cheeks, a redness of both eyes, a heaviness of the whole body, distress of the whole body, distress and anxiety." Rhazes' best-known medical work, *Kitabul-Hawi Fit-Tibb*, or *Contents of Medicine*, appeared in 25 volumes. The books contain his views on fever and febrile illnesses. He noted that, for example, *"exercise excites fever and fuels it like blowing into fire,"* and that *fever in tuberculosis is mild and blunt.*

*One of Rhaze*s' remarkable observations was his differentiation of fever (elevated central thermoregulatory set point) from heat stroke (normal central thermoregulatory set point): "there is another fever with a higher core temperature than the common fever, where patients are much thirstier and the body feels hot all over" [23]. Rhazes was probably the first scholar to distinguish between the two terms, fever and hyperthermia in the form of heat stroke, often equated even nowadays.

13.5
European Medicine

The concepts of fever in European medicine have gradually evolved over several centuries:

* **Toward the end of the sixteenth century,** medicine achieved an important milestone with the invention of a means to measure body temperature when Galileo (1564–1642)

reinvented the thermoscope. The first thermoscope had been invented by Heron of Alexandria in the second century B.C [24]. Galileo's thermoscope (1592) was an air-filled bulb with an open-ended stem inverted over a container of water. The level of water in the stem varied with ambient temperature but was influenced by the pressure. In 1644, Ferdinand II of Tuscany sealed the neck of the flask thereby eliminating the air pressure variable. Santorio Sanctorius (1561–1636) added thermal graduation to the thermoscope, thereby producing the first thermometer [25]. Temperature was measured by allowing the individual to grasp the bulb of the thermometer. The rate at which the fluid subsequently fell was used as an indicator of body temperature.

* **During the seventeenth century,** fevers were classified as continued (such as typhus), intermittent (such as malaria), or eruptive (such as smallpox). The most prevalent febrile disease in England at that time was malaria, notably the benign tertian form, which was described at that time as the annual spring epidemic of intermittent fevers. Two scholars were outstanding during this period:

  – For **Thomas Sydenham** (1624–1689), the writings of Hippocrates remained the principal source of medical knowledge [26]. He emphasized, however, only one humor, namely blood. In this, he had possibly been influenced by the discovery of the circulation of the blood by William Harvey (1578–1657). The other humors, Sydenham thought, were either contained in, or derived from the blood. Sydenham believed that these spring fevers were attributed to the warmth of the sun acting on humors accumulated in the blood during the winter. He advocated as a treatment a low-calorie diet without meat, with a mild purgative on the day of intermission. He clearly regarded fever as beneficial as witnessed by his remark "fever is a mighty engine which nature brings into the world to remove her enemies."

  – **Hermann Boerhaave** (1668–1738), Professor of Medicine at Leyden, was one of the most well-known physicians of his time. He described the prime symptom of fever as an accelerated pulse and heartbeat, arising from stagnation of the blood at the ends of capillaries and accompanied by an irritation of the heart. He maintained that a rapid pulse was pathognomonic of fever and strongly advocated the measurement of body temperature by means of an alcohol thermometer held in the patient's hand [27].

* **During the eighteenth century,** fever became divided into symptomatic (such as pneumonia or wound infection) and idiopathic or essential. The concept of fever most widely accepted by British physicians was that of William Cullen (1710–1790) [28] of the University of Edinburgh from 1773 to 1790. Cullen divided fevers into a simple inflammatory fever without delirium, and those fevers accompanied by delirium or stupor, which he called "typhus." Although he thought of fever as a general disease that might assume various forms, he believed that the common underlying pathophysiology was a spasm of the arteries.

* **By the mid-1800s,** the ancient humoral theory began to disintegrate, and with it the concept that fever was beneficial. The belief that fever could result from inflammation also evolved further during this century. Francois Broussais (1772–1838) recognized the relationship between the two and suggested that the usual seat of inflammation was the stomach and the intestines.

* **In the nineteenth century,** fever was still regarded as both part of a symptom complex (as it is today) and a disease in its own right [29]. Examples of fever being regarded as a disease were *autumnal fever, jail fever, and hospital fever.* Fever could also be described in terms of the severity of the disease, for example, *malignant fever* or *pestilential fever*, or even in terms of the supposed pathology of the fever, *bilious fever* or *nervous fever.* The multiplicity of names for fever reflects the lack of a breakthrough into an understanding of the causes of febrile illnesses. The breakthrough came with the science of bacteriology, which was able to reveal the etiology of many infectious diseases, such as the identification of the typhoid bacillus in 1880 and the discovery of the tubercle bacillus in 1882. These discoveries relegated fever to a sign of disease. Great scholars of this period include:

  – **Claude Bernhard** (1813–1878), the great French physiologist, recognized that body temperature was regulated in healthy organisms by the balancing of heat production and loss. He demonstrated that animals died quickly when the body temperature exceeded the normal level by 5–6°C, thus suggesting that fever may be harmful and that antipyretics, which were introduced later, may be beneficial [30].
  – **Carl Liebermeister** (1833–1901), a German Physician, elaborated the theory that fever is well controlled by the same mechanisms as in normal body temperature, only at higher set point.
  – **William Osler** declared, "the humanity has three enemies, fever, famine and war, but fever is by far the greatest."
  – **Billroth** (1829–1894) in 1868 attempted to confirm this ancient observation by injecting pus into animals, thereby producing febrile response [31]. His attempt to prove that fever resulted from activity in the host cells themselves failed because the injected material was contaminated with endotoxin, a product of Gram-negative bacteria that induces fever.
  – **Beeson in 1948,** using aseptic techniques to exclude endotoxin, isolated a fever-inducing substance from the host leukocytes, leukocyte pyrogen [32]. This later became known as an endogenous pyrogen identical to interleukin-1.

13.6
History of Fever Therapy

Throughout the history, a variety of diseases have been treated by fever, including the following:

* **Cancer:** The Edwin Smith Surgical papyrus, written about 1700 B.C., contains the use of increased temperatures to treat cancer. In the nineteenth century, Dr. Coley treated cancer patients with bacterial toxins extracted from erysipelas lesions, which caused high fevers. This was based on the observation that some cancers decreased in size or resolved after infection with erysipelas. Malignant tumors were then treated with injection of toxins or erysipelas bacteria. In 1898 Dr. Westermark, a Swedish physician, described local hyperthermia to successfully treat cervical cancers. Research has

shown that malignant cells of certain animal and human tumors are more susceptible to elevated temperatures in the range of 41–44°C than normal tissue.

* **Infectious diseases:** Hippocrates cited hyperthermia in the form of cauterization using a hot iron to treat various ailments. A few centuries later, Refus of Ephesus became the first physician to recommend the use of malarial fever to treat illnesses. Although a variety of diseases have been treated during the past two centuries, it was Wagner von Jauregg in 1917 who gave an enormous impetus to fever as a therapeutic agent by treating neurosyphilis with malarial fever, for which he won the Nobel Prize. Infectious diseases have historically been treated by fever. The best results of fever therapy were observed in gonorrhea and syphilis, including their complications, such as arthritis, keratitis, and orchitis. Approximately 70–80% of the cases treated were arrested using artificial hyperthermia or malarial fever in the range of 40.5–41.0°C or about 50 h administered in several sessions.

* **Other diseases:** Treatment with fever was also practised in patients with rheumatoid arthritis and asthma.

13.7
Present Concepts: Fever May Be Beneficial

Only in the past four decades has there been successful research into the role of fever in disease. One of the most important outcomes of this research has been the discovery of a single mononuclear cell product, interleukin-1 (IL-1), whose effects include induction of fever by its action on the hypothalamic center and activation of T-lymphocytes. The fever induction, which occurs simultaneously with lymphocyte activation, constitutes the clearest and strongest evidence in favor of the beneficial role of fever.

Theoretically, fever could benefit an illness mainly in two ways: It could adversely affect the infecting organisms and/or could enhance the host defenses. The accumulated data now suggest that fever has a protective role in promoting host defense against infection, rather than being a passive by-product (see for details Chap. 9).

References

1. Dawson WR. The Egyptian medical papyri. In: Brothwell D, Sandison AT (Eds.). Diseases in antiquity. Springfield, IL: Thomas CC, 1967, pp. 98–111
2. Breasted J. The Edwin Smith surgical papyrus: The surgical treatise. Chicago: University of Chicago Press, 1930, pp. 37–77
3. Breasted J. Case forty-one. In: Breasted J (Ed.). The Edwin Smith surgical papyrus. Chicago: University of Chicago Press, 1930, pp. 374–91
4. Majno G. The healing hand: Man and wound in the ancient world: The Asu. Cambridge, MA: Harvard University Press, 1975, pp. 374–91
5. Major RH. A history of medicine: Mesopotamia. Springfield, IL: Thomas CC, 1954, pp. 20–32

13

6. Sigerist HE. A history of medicine: Rational elements in Mesopotamia. Oxford: Oxford University Press, 1951, pp. 477–94
7. Major RH. A history of medicine: China. Springfield, IL: Thomas CC, 1954, pp. 83–101
8. Hume EH. The Chinese way in medicine: The universe and Man in Chinese. Baltimore: Johns Hopkins Press, 1940, pp. 5–58
9. Hume EH. Some distinctive contributions of Chinese medicine, 1940, pp. 118–76.
10. Major G. The healing hand. Man and wound in the ancient world: The Vaidya. Cambridge, MA: Harvard University Press, 1975, pp. 261–312
11. Major RH. A history of medicine: India. Springfield, IL: Thomas CC, 1954, pp. 65–81
12. Jones WHS. Philosophy and medicine in ancient Greece. Bull Hist Med 1946; 8(Suppl): 1–15
13. Hippocrates. Epidemic. Book 1 (trans). In: Chadwick J, Mann WN (Eds.). The medical works of Hippocrates. Oxford: Blackwell, 1950, p. 204
14. Hippocrates. Epidemic. Book 1 (trans). In: Chadwick J, Mann WN (Eds.). The medical works of Hippocrates. Oxford: Blackwell, 1950, p. 29.
15. Hippocrates. Coan prognosis. Book 1 (trans). In: Chadwick J, Mann WN (Eds.). The medical works of Hippocrates. Oxford: Blackwell, 1950, p. 351.
16. Major RH. A history of medicine. Precursors of Galen. Springfield, IL: Thomas CC, 1954, pp. 174–88
17. Solomon HC, Kopp I. Fever therapy. N Engl Med 1937; 217: 805–14
18. McGrew RE. Encyclopaedia of medical history: Hebrew medicine. London: Macmillan Press, 1985, p. 129
19. Major RH. A history of medicine: The middle ages. Springfield, IL: Thomas CC, 1954, pp. 223–5
20. Rhodes P. An outline history of medicine: The middle ages. London: Butterworths, 1985, p. 29
21. Sarton G. The history of medicine: Avicenna. Cambridge, MA: Harvard University Press, 1962, pp. 67–77
22. Bollet AJ. The rise and fall of disease. Am Med 1981; 70: 12–18
23. Ar-Razi MZ. Kitabul Hawi Fit-Tibb. Hyderabad, India: Osmania Oriental Publication Bureau, 1963, p. 144
24. Sarton G. Sarton on the history of science. Cambridge, MA: Harvard University Press, 1962
25. Woodhead GS, Varrier-Jones PC. Clinical thermometer. Lancet 1916; 1: 173–80
26. Major RH. A history of medicine: The 17th century; Thomas Sydenham. Springfield, IL: Thomas CC, 1954, p. 524
27. Haller JS. Medical thermometry: A short history. West J Med 1985; 142: 10S–16S
28. Estes JW. Quantitative observations of fever and its treatment before the advent of short clinical thermometers. Med Hist 1991; 35: 189–216
29. Wood WE. Studies on the cause of fever. N Engl J Med 1958; 258: 1023–31
30. Akerren Y. On antipyretic conditions during infancy and childhood. Acta Paediatr 1943; 31: 1–75
31. Major RH. A history of medicine: The predominance of German medicine. Springfield, IL: Thomas CC, 1954, p. 845
32. Beeson PH. Temperature elevating effect of a substance obtained from polymorphonuclear leukocytes. J Clin Invest 1948, 27: 548–53

Fever (Pyrexia)	Fever is defined as a body temperature of 1°C (1.8°F) or more above the mean at the site of temperature recording. For example, the range of body temperature at the axilla is 34.7–37.4°C, with a mean of 36.5°C; 1°C above the mean is 37.5°C, which is fever when the temperature is measured at the axilla.
Aden Fever	See dengue fever.
African Hemorrhage Fever	Refers to Marburg and Ebola virus infections (see Crimean-Congo hemorrhagic fever).
Algid Pernicious Fever	Is a severe malarial attack in which the patient presents with collapse and shock.
American Mountain Fever	See Colorado Tick Fever.
Argentine Haemorrhagic Fever	Is caused by Arboviruses infecting workers who harvest maize and living in rodent-infested shelters.
Autumn Fever	Is a fever similar to Dengue fever occurring at the end of summer in India.
Absorption Fever	Is a fever occurring shortly after birth caused by absorption of uterine discharge through the vaginal wall.
Black Fever	Means kala azar, which is a Hindi name given by the physicians in India to refer to the hyperpigmentation of the skin during the disease.
Blackwater Fever	Is the passage of the dark red urine (hemoglobinuria) due to intravascular hemolysis following infection with falciparum malaria. The condition is occasionally seen in association with hemolysis due to G-6-P-D deficiency. Other features include chills, fever, anemia, jaundice, and hepatosplenomegaly.
Boutonneuse Fever	See Mediterranean Spotted Fever.
Breakbone Fever	See Dengue fever.

N. Klein et al. (Eds.) *Clinical Manual of Fever in Children.*
Doi: 10.1007/978-3-540-78598-9, © Springer-Verlag Berlin Heidelberg 2009

14

Cat-Scratch Fever	(Cat-scratch disease) is a benign infectious disease caused by Gram-negative bacteria (*Bartonella henselae*), which is transmitted to humans by scratch or bite of a cat (or more likely kittens). Symptoms usually appear after 1–2 weeks and consist of tender regional lymphadenopathy and mild fever. The condition usually resolves in 2–5 months. In immunocompromised patients, the condition is life-threatening.
Central Fever	Is the presence of sustained fever resulting from damage of the thermoregulatory centre of the hypothalamus.
Childbed Fever	(Puerperal fever, puerperal septicemia) is a bacterial infection, usually caused by *Streptococcus pyogenes*, of the genital tract occurring in the postneonatal period. The localized infection (puerperal sepsis) can lead to a blood-born spread of infection (puerperal septicemia).
Colorado Tick Fever	(Also Mountain Fever, American Mountain Fever) is a tick-borne, febrile illness caused by Arenavirus, occurring in the Rocky Mountain area of the USA, mostly in May–June months. The virus is transmitted by the wood ticks (*Dermacentor andersoni*). Three to six days after the tick bite there is a sudden onset of fever, myalgia, arthralgia, headaches, weakness, and photophobia.
Congo Hemorrhagic Fever	(See Crimean-Congo Hemorrhagic Fever).
Continuous Fever	(Or Sustained Fever) is characterized by a persistent elevation of body temperature with a maximal fluctuation of 0.4°C during a 24h period. Normal diurnal fluctuation temperature is usually absent or insignificant. Examples of this pattern of fever are typhoid fever and malignant falciparum malaria.
Crimean-Congo Hemorrhagic Fever	(Congo Hemorrhagic Fever, Central Asian Hemorrhagic Fever) is caused by CCHF virus (Nairovirus), which is transmitted by ticks (Ixodid). The disease is characterized by sudden onset of fever, myalgia, headaches, back pain, hemorrhagic tendency, and lymphadenopathy. The disease is primarily a zoonosis, but outbreaks can affect humans causing high mortality.
Dandy Fever	(See Dengue Fever).
Dengue Fever	(Dengue Hemorrhagic Fever) is a disease caused by Arbovirus, which is carried by mosquitoes. The disease is prevalent in Africa. Features include high fever, myalgia, chills, arthralgia, and rash (petechiae). Severe cases are called dengue hemorrhagic fever. Diagnostic criteria by WHO: fever, thrombocytopenia, increased capillary permeability, pleural effusion, or hypoalbuminemia, hypotension, or narrow pulse pressure.

Double Quotidian Fever	(See Quotidian Fever).
Drug Fever	Is a febrile reaction caused by a therapeutic agent, such as antibiotic or cytotoxic drugs.
Dum-Dum Fever	Is a Hindi term given to kala azar disease. Dum-Dum is a town not far away from Calcutta.
Dutton's Relapsing Fever	Referred to as Dutton disease, which is an African tick-borne disease caused by *Borrelia duttonii*, and spread by ticks.
Elephantoid Fever	Is a lymphatic inflammation caused by filariasis. Features include chills, and fever associated with painful swelling of the affected areas (lower legs). The overlying skin may be red.
Enteric Fever	Is a systemic febrile illness with enteric symptoms caused by S. typhi (typhoid fever) and S. paratyphi (paratyphoid fever). The term was used to differentiate typhoid fever from typhus.
Epidemic Hemorrhagic Fever	Is an acute infectious disease characterized by fever, purpura, and vascular collapse, caused by viruses of the genus Hantavirus (see Hemorrhagic Fever with Renal Syndrome).
Eruptive Fever	(See Mediterranean Spotted Fever).
Factitious Fever	Is a creation of fever by manipulation (usually thermometer manipulation). This is occasionally encountered in the differential diagnosis of PUO, occurring in about 2% of mainly adult cases. Sweating and tachycardia are absent.
Familial Hibernian Fever (FHF)	Is the former name for TRAPS (TNF-receptor associated periodic syndrome). FHF resembles the FMF (Familial Mediterranean Fever) and is characterized by recurrent fever with localized myalgia and painful erythema. In contrast to FMF, the FHF has a benign course without amyloid formation.
Familial Mediterranean Fever (FMF)	Is a hereditary (autosomal recessive) disorder characterized by periodic episodes of fever and painful serositis (pleuritis, peritonitis) lasting 24–72 h. The disease is prevalent among the eastern Mediterranean population.
Fever Blisters (cold sores)	Are labial herpetic lesions caused by herpes simplex infection in association with febrile illness.
Fever Phobia	Is exaggerated fear that parents have when their children have fever.
Fever of Unknown Origin FUO	(Or pyrexia of unknown origin PUO). In pediatrics, this term is applied when fever without localizing signs persists for 1 week during which evaluation in the hospital fails to detect the cause. In adults, PUO is the duration of fever of at least 3 weeks, and uncertainty of diagnosis after a 1-week investigation in the hospital is taken as a definition.

Five-Day Fever	(See Trench Fever).
Glandular Fever	(Infectious mononucleosis) is a viral infection caused by Epstein-Barr virus. The illness manifests as a febrile illness, sore throat, and lymphadenopathy. There is often hepatic dysfunction and splenomegaly.
Haverhill Fever	Is the bacillary form of rat-bite fever, caused by *Streptobacillus moniliformis*, and transmitted through contaminated milk and dairy products.
Hay Fever	(Allergic rhinitis) is an acute nasal catarrh consisting of swelling of the nasal mucosa, causing sneezing and itching, associated with conjunctivitis and lacrimation. It is either seasonal (pollen) or perennial (nonseasonal). The illness has actually nothing to do with fever; in the past, patients who suffered from hay fever thought that they had febrile illness until the association to plant pollen became known in 1873.
Hemorrhagic Fever	Is a severe viral infection seen mainly in the tropics, usually transmitted to humans by arthropod bites or contact virus-infected rodents. Common features include fever, hemorrhagic tendency, thrombocytopenia, shock, and neurological disturbance.
Hemorrhagic Fever with Renal Syndrome (HFRS)	Includes several related infections (epidemic hemorrhagic fever, hemorrhagic nephrosonephritis, Songo fever, Korean hemorrhagic fever, hemorrhagic fever, and Nephropathica epidemica) caused by hantavirus and transmitted by rodents. In addition to fever, myalgia, abdominal pain, there is interstitial hemorrhage, renal failure, and shock.
Hepatic Intermittent Fever	(Or Intermittent Hepatic Fever) is an intermittently occurring fever resulting from intermittent impaction of stone in the bile duct, which is causing cholangitis.
Herpetic Fever	(See Fever Blisters).
Hospital Fever	Epidemic typhus (see Jail fever).
Humidifier Fever	Is an illness characterized by fever, cough, and myalgia, caused by inhalation of air contaminated by fungi and blown from humidifiers or air conditioners.
Intermittent Fever	Involves temperature that peaks in the afternoon and returns to normal each day, usually in the morning. This is the second most common type of fever encountered in clinical practice. Examples are malaria, lymphoma, and endocarditis.
Jail Fever	Endemic Typhus is caused by *Rickettsia prowazekii*. Apart from fever, patients develops myalgia, weakness, and headaches.

Katayama Fever	Is an acute manifestation of schistosomiasis (Bilharzia) caused by contact with fresh water that harbors snails infected with *Schistosoma mansoni* or *Schistosoma Japanicum*. Acute manifestations (about 6 weeks after contact) include fever, urticarial rash, and hepatosplenomegaly.
Kenya Fever	(See Boutonnneuse Fever).
Korean Hemorrhagic Fever	Is an infection caused by viruses of the group Hantavirus, and characterized by fever, hemorrhagic tendency, shock, and renal failure (see also Hemorrhagic Fever with Renal Syndrome).
Lassa Fever	Is a viral infection (Arenavirus), with rats being the natural host, seen usually in West Africa. The disease is characterized by fever, myalgia, chest, abdominal and back pain, complicated by hemorrhagic tendency, seizures, and shock. Mortality is high (around 40%).
Malta Fever	(See Undulant Fever = Brucellosis).
Maternal Fever	Denotes fever occurring in term labor, which is often associated with chorioaminionitis.
Mediterranean Spotted Fever	(Boutonneuse Fever) is an acute febrile, zoonotic disease caused by *Rickettsia conorii* and transmitted to humans by the brown dogtick *Rhipicephalus sanguineus*. It is prevalent in southern Europe and central Asia. Features include high fever, myalgia, arthralgia, and a distinct mark: tache noire (black spot) at the site of the tick bite.
Metal Fume Fever	Is an acute allergic reaction caused primarily by inhalation of zinc, magnesium, or copper fumes from welding. A few hours after exposure, workers experience flu-like symptoms with low-grade fever (usually 38–38.5°C), chills, myalgia, and headaches. Symptoms usually last 4–24 h, and recovery occurs within 24–48 h.
Mountain Fever	(See Colorado Tick Fever).
Mud Fever	Is a dermatitis that affects the skin of the heels and back legs of horses, caused by invasion of bacteria (*Dermatophilus congolensis*) when the skin is damaged and exposed to mud and wet conditions.
Nodal Fever	Erythema nodosum is painful and tender erythematous nodules are localized on the shins. Drugs and streptococcal throat infection are most common causes.
Omsk Hemorrhagic Fever	Is caused by Arboviruses, transmitted by moles and muskrats. It occurs in central Russia and Romania. Hemorrhagic tendency by intravascular coagulopathy is typical of the disease.

14

Oroya Fever	(The name refers to an area near La Oroya, Peru) is the potentially fatal form of Bartonellosis, caused the bacteria *Bartonella bacilliformis*, and transmitted by sand flies. The disease occurs mostly in the Andes Mountains of western South America. Manifestations include hemolytic anemia and fever.
Paratyphoid Fever	Is an enteric fever caused by *Salmonella paratyphi* (see Typhoid Fever).
Parrot Fever	(Psittacosis, Ornithosis) is an infectious disease caused by *Chlamydia psittacci* and transmitted to humans by pet birds, including parrots, parakeets, lovebirds, and budgerigars. Humans catch the infection from infected birds by inhaling the organisms from shed features. Symptoms develop 5–12 days after exposure and include fever, myalgia, cough, and in severe cases, pneumonia.
Pel-Ebstein Fever	Described by Pel and Ebstein in 1887, was originally thought to be characteristic of Hodgkin's disease. Only a few patients with Hodgkin's disease develop this pattern, which consists of recurrent episodes of fever lasting 3–10 days, followed by an afebrile period of similar duration. The cause of this type of fever is unknown but may be related to tissue destruction or associated hemolytic anemia.
Periodic Fever	Is characterized by episodes of fever recurring at regular or irregular intervals, and each episode is followed by one to several days, weeks or months, of normal temperature. Examples are seen in malaria.
Pharyngoconjunctival Fever	This disease is associated with type 3 adenovirus infection. It is characterized by fever (usually high and lasts 4–5 days), pharyngitis causing sore throat, rhinitis, conjunctivitis, and posterior cervical lymphadenopathy.
Phlebotomus Fever	(Also called Sandfly Fever) is a febrile viral disease caused by an Arbovirus, which is transmitted by sand flies. It is characterized by influenza-like symptoms, including fever, myalgia, and headaches. The disease occurs mostly in the Balkans and southern Europe.
Pontiac Fever	Is a mild form of legionnaires' disease, caused by bacteria legionella. Symptoms include flu-like illness with fever. In contrast to legionnaires' disease, Pontiac fever does not cause pneumonia. Both forms of legionellosis are caused by breathing mist that comes from a water source (such as air-conditioning cooling towers) contaminated with the bacteria. While legionnaires' disease may cause mortality, Pontiac fever is self-limited.

Pretibial Fever	Is an infection caused by Leptospira bacteria. Characteristic features include an abrupt onset of fever of 39–40°C, abdominal pain, myalgia, and a rash on the pretibial region of the legs.
Prolonged Fever	Describes a single illness in which duration of fever exceeds that expected for this illness, e.g., more than 10 days for a viral URTI.
Protein Fever	Is fever arising from injection of foreign protein such as milk into bloodstream.
Puerperal Fever	(See Childbed Fever).
Pyogenic Fever	Is a invasion of the bloodstream caused by bacteria (mainly staphylococci), which are capable of producing pus.
Q-Fever	(Q for Query Fever) is a zoonotic disease caused by *Coxiella burnettii*. Cattle, sheep, and goats are the primary reservoirs. People working with animal products are at greatest risk of contracting the disease. Common features are fever (39–40.5°C), myalgia, and pneumonia, as well as hepatitis and endocarditis (usually involving the aortic valve).
Quotidian Fever	Caused by P. vivax, denotes febrile paroxysms, which occur daily, while the Double quotidian fever has two spikes within 12 h (12 h cycles. Examples are Kala azar, gonococcal arthritis, juvenile rheumatoid arthritis, and some drug fever (e.g., carbamazepine).
Rat-Bite Fever	Is an infectious disease caused by *Streptobacillus monilliformis* and *Spirillium minus*, which is gram-negative spirochete. In the USA, rat-bite fever is primarily caused by the former bacteria while the latter are the cause of the disease in Asia and Africa. Symptoms occur 2–10 days after a rat bite and include abrupt fever, chills, and myalgia.
Recurrent Fever	Is an illness involving the same organ (e.g., urinary tract) or multiple organ systems in which fever occurs at irregular intervals. An example is Familial Mediterranean fever.
Relapsing Fever	Describes fever alternating with afebrile periods. Examples are tertian or quartan malaria and brucellosis.
Remittent Fever	Is characterized by a fall in temperature each day but not to a normal level. This is the most common type of fever in pediatric practice and is not specific to any disease. Diurnal variation is usually present, particularly if the fever is infectious in origin. Most viral or bacterial diseases present with this pattern.

14

Rheumatic Fever	Is an inflammatory systemic disease of the connective tissue, due to an infection by group A of hemolytic streptococcus. The disease affects joints, heart, central nervous system, skin, and subcutaneous tissue. Fever is a minor criterion for the diagnosis and occurs in about 90% of cases.
Rift Valley Fever	Is a zoonosis, primarily affecting animals, but occasionally humans, caused by a virus, which belongs to the Phlebovirus and transmitted by mosquitoes. Common manifestations include sudden onset of fever, myalgia, headaches, and signs of meningeal irritation. Most cases are mild, resulting in full recovery. In severe cases, there is involvement of the eyes (causing visual impairment), meningoencephalitis, and hemorrhagic tendency, which may cause death.
Rocky Mountain Spotted Fever	Is a serious systemic disease caused by *Rickettsia rickettsii*, transmitted by dog bite. It is mostly prevalent in southeastern areas of the USA (Virginia, Georgia). Patients usually suffer from sudden high fever (39.0–40.5°C), headaches, myalgia, and chills. The associated rash appears as small spots, which begin on the wrists, ankles, palms, and soles. Complications include renal failure, shock, and occasionally death.
Roman Fever	Is a malignant deadly strain of malaria (tertian or falciparum), which affected Rome historically.
Rose Fever	Is the springtime equivalent of hay fever (see Hay Fever).
Ross River Fever	Is epidemic polyarthritis caused by arboviruses and transmitted by mosquito bites. It is most common in Australia.
Sandfly fever	(See Phlebotomus Fever).
Scarlet Fever	Is a bacterial disease caused by a toxin produced by group A hemolytic Streptococci. It usually involves high fever and a characteristic rash, accompanied by tonsillitis.
Sennetsu Fever	Is a rare infection caused by different strains of Ehrlichia bacteria. Common symptoms include sudden high fever, myalgia, and headaches.
Septic Fever	(Or Hectic Fever) occurs when remittent or intermittent fever shows a very large difference between the peak and the nadir. Examples are Kawasaki disease and pyogenic infection.
Sindbis Fever	Is an infection caused by Sindbis virus and characterized by arthralgia, rash, and malaise in addition to fever. It mainly occurs in Africa and Australia. The virus is transmitted by mosquitoe's culex.

Snail Fever	(=Schistosomiasis or Bilharzia) is a parasitic infection caused by an intermediate snails host, which releases parasites known as cercariae.
Songo Fever	(See Hemorrhagic Fever with Renal Syndrome).
South African Tick-Bite Fever	(See Tick-bite Fever).
Splenic Fever (anthrax)	Is a rare and highly lethal infectious disease of humans and animals that is caused by the bacterium *Bacillus anthracis*. Human is infected by ingestion of infected meat, inhalation, or by cutaneous route.
Spotted Fever	(See Rocky Mountain Spotted Fever).
Steroid Fever	Refers to a fever caused by elevated concentration of certain pyrogenic steroids, such as etiocholanolone.
Swamp Fever	Is a viral disease, which affects horses, mules, and donkeys, and is transmitted by horse flies or mosquitoes. The disease is mainly found in the USA.
Thermic fever	Refers to heatstroke.
Three-day fever	Refers to roseola infantum caused by human herpes-6.
Therapeutic Fever	Refers to pyrotherapy or therapy by heat.
Tick-Bite Fever	Is usually a benign disease caused by Rickettsia and is transmitted by tick-bites. Five to seven days after the bite, there is a characteristic black bite mark (eschar or taches noire), associated with severe headaches and lymphadenopathy. It is common in South Africa (caused by *R. conorii*).
Tobia Fever	(See Rocky Mountain Spotted Fever).
Trench Fever	Is caused by Rickettsia quintana, transmitted by body lice, typically attacking the army. Characteristic features are intermittent fever, aches, and pain (particularly in the shins), chills, skin rash, and inflamed eyes. There are often multiple relapses.
Trypanosome Fever	Is the febrile stage of sleeping sickness.
Typhoid Fever	Is an enteric infection caused by *Salmonella typhi*, chiefly involving the lymphoid follicles of the ileum. Characteristic features are fever, which gradually rises during the first week, relative bradycardia, headache, abdominal distension, spelenomegaly, and maculopapular rash.
Undulant Fever	Describes a gradual increase in temperature, followed by a period of high fever for a few days, then a gradual decrease to a normal level. A classical example causing this fever pattern is brucellosis.
Valley Fever	Refers to coccidioidomycosis, which is caused by a soil-borne fungus. The infection mainly occurs in Southern California and is characterized by nonspecific symptoms of fever, chest pain, and cough.

14

West Nile Fever (WNF)	Is caused by the West Nile Virus, which belongs to the genus Flavivirus. Mosquitoes transmit the virus from birds (where it is mostly maintained) to humans. WNF is found in Africa and occasionally reported in some European countries. It is characterized by high fever, influenza-like symptoms, disorientation, tremors, and coma.
Yangtze Valley Fever	Referred to Schistosomiasis Japanicum, which occurs in the Far East.
Yellow Fever	Is a tropical disease caused by a viral infection (Flaviviridae), which is transmitted by infected mosquitoes (*Aedes aegypti*). Mild cases present with flu-like symptoms. Severe forms are life-threatening and present with high fever, myalgia, chills, and headaches leading to shock, bleeding, renal failure, and hepatic failure.

Index